Personalized Immunotherapy for Tumor Diseases and Beyond

Editors

Biaoru Li

Georgia Cancer Center and Department of Pediatrics,
Medical College at GA,
Augusta,
USA

Alan Larson

Rush Cancer Institute,
Rush Presbyterian St. Luke' s Medical Center,
Chicago,
USA

&

Shen Li

Division of Surgical Oncology,
Massachusetts General Hospital Cancer Center and Harvard
Medical School,
Boston, MA, 02114,
USA

Personalized Immunotherapy for Tumor Diseases and Beyond

Editors: Biaoru Li, Alan Larson and Shen Li

ISBN (Online): 978-981-14-8275-5

ISBN (Print): 978-981-14-8273-1

ISBN (Paperback): 978-981-14-8274-8

need for a court order if at any point you breach any terms of this License Agreement. In no event will any delay or failure by Bentham Science Publishers in enforcing your compliance with this License Agreement constitute a waiver of any of its rights.

3. You acknowledge that you have read this License Agreement, and agree to be bound by its terms and conditions. To the extent that any other terms and conditions presented on any website of Bentham Science Publishers conflict with, or are inconsistent with, the terms and conditions set out in this License Agreement, you acknowledge that the terms and conditions set out in this License Agreement shall prevail.

Bentham Science Publishers Pte. Ltd.
80 Robinson Road #02-00
Singapore 068898
Singapore
Email: subscriptions@benthamscience.net

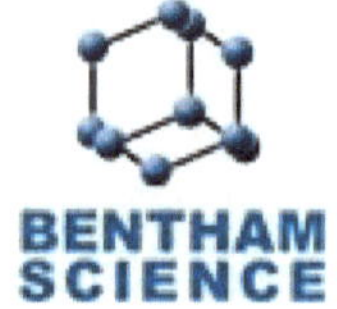

CONTENTS

PREFACE

T-cell adoptive immunotherapy for tumor diseases has been studied for nearly three decades. Steven Rosenberg was a pioneer in the successful use of tumor-infiltrating lymphocytes (TIL) in treating tumor diseases. In 1986, he first discovered that TIL could recognize autologous tumor cells. In 1988, he successfully applied autologous TIL to metastatic melanoma. Since 1989, we have used T-cell adoptive immunotherapy to treat more than 200 cases and published more than 50 papers. T-cell adoptive immunotherapy, along with its newer generation techniques, can be increasingly used to treat various solid tumor diseases such as ovarian, brain, lung, and liver cancers. Before introducing the preface, I will first review T-cell adoptive immunotherapy in three stages to summarize the thirty-year development of T-cell adoptive immunotherapy: (I) the early stages of T-cell adoptive immunotherapy such as TIL adoptive immunotherapy; (II) research and development (R& D) of a new generation of T-cell adoptive immunotherapy; and (III) clinical trials of the next-generation T-cell adoptive immunotherapy.

Early period R& D of T-cell adoptive immunotherapy:

After 1987, Dr. Rosenberg discovered that TILs could be cultured with the aid of the cytokine IL-2 and induced TIL exhibited cytotoxic activity against melanoma cells *in vitro*. TILs isolated from tumor samples were the earliest trials of ACT conducted at the surgical branch of the National Cancer Institute (NCI) in 1988. At the time, objective responses were observed in patients with metastatic melanoma. For the optimal procedure of TIL isolation and proliferation, we carefully studied the NCI protocol and then modified the protocol to establish a new TIL culture and proliferation procedure. Our earliest findings showed that the modified procedures are different from the NCI conventional approaches: (1) enzyme digestion of tumor tissue can result in loss of the signaling of T-cell so that only collagenase IV digestion can keep signaling intactness of T-cell and (2) adding process with a cleaning inhibiting factors and inhibiting cells will increase TIL activity and cytotoxicity to tumors, now the inhibiting factors, inhibiting cells and tissue called as tumor microenvironment (TME) after thirty years. After establishing the modified method, we also routinely employ TIL measurement by the proliferation and cytotoxicity assay since TIL efficacy is variable from a solid tumor. Although TILs effectively used for solid tumor have been debated more than 30 years, a few laboratories have reported that TILs have also been successfully applied to different solid tumors, such as pancreatic cancer, head, and neck cancer, lung cancer, brain cancer and liver cancer under the optimal culture procedures and right therapeutic conditions.

In the early phase of T-cell adoptive immunotherapy, three major breakthroughs were developed to increase TIL efficacy: (I) cytokines induction with IL-2 and IL-12; IL-2 and Anti-CD3 and IL-2 and Anti-CD3/CD28 for their cultures; (II) clinical TIL application combined with chemotherapy or lymphodepletion prior to adoptive cell therapy (ACT); (III) development of TIL location administration. These developments demonstrated the significant benefits in the early TIL clinical application (selected publications from our work as below).

R&D of a new generation of T-cell adoptive immunotherapy: With the maturation of gene transfer technology, three areas developed rapidly:

the affinity of T cells to tumor cells, such as (I) TCR T-cells (T-cell receptor engineered T-cell) and CAR T-cells (chimeric antigen receptor T-cell) related to the reconstructs of the signal structure of TCR molecules; (II) T-cell editing technology; (III) polyclonal TIL combined with a single T-cell genome linking new compounds to improve the efficacy of personalized immunotherapy. TCR T-cells and CAR T-cells on T-cell adoptive immunology have been studied for more than 30 years. Chimeric TCR that achieves T-cell specific affinity was first reported in 1989 by cloning anti-TNP mRNA into TCR V and C chain targeting cells. Since 1989, we had also tried DHBsAb (Duck Hepatitis B virus surface antibody) from duck to clone into human CD3 in TIL to form DHBsAb-CD3 CAR-T cells to treat hepatocellular carcinoma under the guidance of Dr. Shen (Picture **A**), who was my mentor when I was a graduate MD student thirty-five years ago). That time, DHBsAb-CD3 chimeric TIL failed to treat DHBV and HBV HCC cells due to limited knowledge of the early CD3 and TCR structures. Later, Irving and Weiss discovered that CD8 and CD3ζ chains could independently mediate T-cell activation of endogenous TCR; thus, CARs can be reconstructed as an extracellular domain for tumor antigen recognition as well as multiple intracellular signaling domains that mediate T-cell activation. Currently, third-generation chimeric receptors with CD28/4-1BB/CD3ζ can be used to treat chronic lymphocytic leukemia (CLL) with clinical significance. After decoding the TCR signaling protein, we have found that TCRs rely on the patient's human leukocyte antigen (HLA) allele, allowing for class I peptide-MHC binding, and ultimately cancer cell destruction. At present, TCR T-cells are successfully used in solid tumors. Molecular screening techniques of shared or specific tumor antigen/peptides play an essential role in personalized T-cell immunotherapy. We had initiated a phage-display screening system for specific peptides on malignant myeloid cells under the support of Drs. HD. Preisler and G Smiths in 1996 (Picture **B**). After more than 20 years of work, we have set up single-cell techniques, either supporting the specific targeting screening or a new generation T-cell adoptive immunotherapy based on single T-cell genomic profiles. The personalized immunotherapy based on genomics and GWAS from individual T-cell genomic profiles linking to a network and then further linking to the new compounds can be safely and effectively applied to personalized immunotherapy for different patients (selected publications from our work as below).

A   B

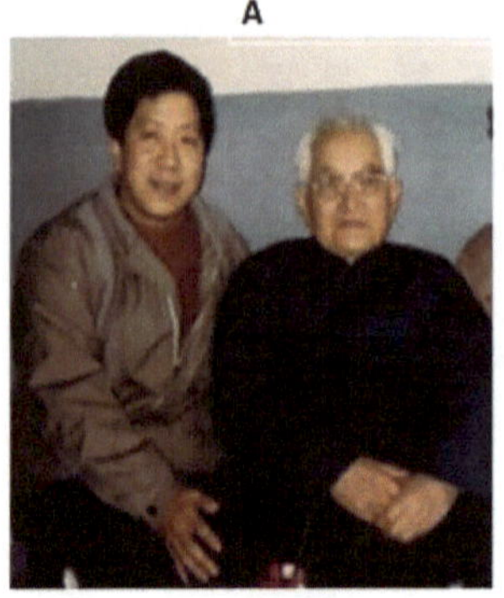

Dr. Shen (1910-2011) first designed CAR T-cell in 1989 (chimeric DHBsAb-CD3 TIL) to treat hepatic cell carcinoma. The picture was made for us to celebrate his 90 years old birthday in 1999.

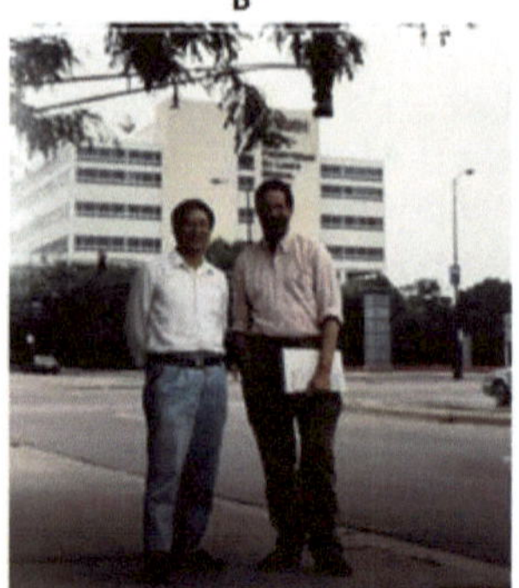

George P Smith and author had worked each other to screen peptides on surface of leukemia cancer stem cell guided by Dr. Preisler by using phage display during 1996-2002. Dr. Smith is awarded 2018-Nobel Laureates in chemistry for his technique.

Clinical trials of the new generation of T-cell adoptive immunotherapy:

Since CAR T-cells have been proven to be effective in treating B-cell hematological malignancies, there are now more than 300 clinical trials on treating hematological malignancies through CAR T-cells. TCR T-cells have been increasingly reported for the treatment of solid tumors. Also, the medical industry is also advancing research on different stages of CAR T-cells and TCR T-cells for various tumor diseases (selected publications as below).

Biaoru Li
Georgia Cancer Center and Department of Pediatrics
Medical College at GA
Augusta
USA

Preamble and Contents

After nearly 30 years of developing T-cell adoptive immunotherapy as summarized above, our book will focus on personalized immunotherapy, a new strategy for cancer treatment in the 21st century. Personalized immunotherapy will involve a set of biochemical, immune, and genomic characterization of the tumors using multi-dimensional analyses in order to lead to an optimal decision on the appropriate immune treatment. Therefore, this book on personalized immunotherapy will first introduce some foundational concepts: MHC research and development, the genomic profiles and genome-wide association study (GWAS) of T-cells and tumor cells from patients, and technologies which provide the basis of personalized immunotherapy. The knowledge has led to the rapid development of personalized immunotherapy in the past decades.

Because recent research in personalized immunotherapy involves targeting therapy, in the book, we will introduce some new immunoassay methods related to personalized immunotherapy. Subsequently, we will present targeting immunotherapy in two chapters: personalized immunotherapies that depend on the tumor immune microenvironment (TIME) (such as PD1 or PDL1-related checkpoint targeted therapy) and immunotherapy dependent on the tumor microenvironment (TME) including IDO (indoleamine 2,3-dioxygenase) inhibitors and ADO (CD39/CD73/adenosine) inhibitors.

The central portion of this book, consisting of eight chapters, is related to personalized T-cell immunotherapy, which includes the basics of personalized T-cell immunotherapy and the essentials of the latest developments in personalized T-cell immunotherapy. The former with three chapters consists of new molecular technologies such as T-cell screening and cloning of tumor neoantigens, a new generation of primary tumor cell culture for T-cell cloning, bioinformatics platform of T-cells and primary tumor cells. The latter or personalized T-cell adoptive immunotherapy with four chapters will present the development and future of adoptive T-cell immunotherapy; the development of T-cell gene therapy and T-cell genome editing; the affinity of transgenic T-cells to tumor cells such as CAR T-cells and TCR T-cells; and systematic modeling of polyclonal specific T-cells. Finally, we will present a biobank for personalized immunotherapy, which we have been studying for more than twenty years.

Personalized immunotherapy is a new immunotherapy model for studying individualized cancer therapy, which involves "providing the right immunotherapy for the right people at the right time." Due to the complexity of individual tumors and immune responses, traditional immunotherapy models have faced challenges. To address this, we have written the book on updated strategies for cancer immunotherapy.

Selected publications for our early period of T-cell adoptive immunotherapy

REFERENCES

[1] Li B. Shanqing Dong, Xiheng Zheng, Yumin Zu, Baoyu Wu and Deyuan Lu. A New Experimental and Clinical Approach of Combining Usage of Highly Active Tumor-infiltrating Lymphocytes and Highly Antitumor Drugs for the Advanced Malignant Tumor. Chinese Medical Journal 1994; 107(11): 803-7.
[PMID: 7867384]

[2] Li B, Shen D. Preliminary Study on the Resting Status of Tumor-infiltrating Lymphocytes. Chinese Microbiology and Immunology 1994; 14(6): 399-402.

[3] Li Biaoru. Tong Shanqing; Hu Baoyu; Zhu Youming; Zhang Xiheng; Wu Jianhe; Lu Deyuan; Lu Jing; Study on the effect of enzymatic digestion on the activity of tumor infiltrating lymphocytes; Journal of Molecular Cell Biology 1994 01

[4] Li B. Tong Shanqing; Zhang Xiheng; Zhu Youming; Hu Baoyu; Lu Deyuan; Lu Jing; Gu Qinlong; Research on TIL proliferation, phenotype and lethality of human malignant solid tumors Modern Immunology199405.

[5] Li Biaoru. Tong Shanqing; Zhu Youming; Hu Baoyu; Zhang Xiheng; Lu Jing; Wu Jianhe; Hu Hongliang; Shen Dinghong; Lu Deyuan; Establishment of a method for separation of tumor infiltrating lymphocytes with high vitality; Journal of Immunology 1994 01

[6] Zhu Y, Zhang X. Biaoru Li; Hu Baoyu; Wu Jianhe; Tong Shanqing; Removal of tumor-doped tumor cells in tumor infiltrating lymphocyte culture; Journal of Shanghai Jiaotong University Medical Science Edition199502.

[7] Jian Tao, Zhang Guochi, Ding Jianqing, Zhang Xiheng. 7. Tao Jian, Zhang Guochi, Ding Jianqing, Zhang Xiheng, **Biaoru Li**, Tong Shanqing, Experimental study of receptor-mediated TNFα gene transfer, Journal of Shanghai Second Medical University, 2000, Vol.20, No.01.

[8] Li Biaoru. Xu Wei, Qian Guanxiang, Zhang Xiheng, Dong Shanqing, Chen Shishu, Methodology of TNF gene transduction of tumor infiltrating lymphocytes, Journal of Shanghai Second Medical University, 1995, Vol. 15 No. 3,

[9] Ding Jianqing, Qian Guanxiang. Xu Wei; Zhu Youming; Hu Liang; Hu Baoyu; Zhang Tengfei; Zhang Xiheng; Xu Rongting; Tong Shanqing; Xu Weizhen; Lu Deyuan; Chen Shishu; A preliminary study of tumor necrosis factor gene transduction of tumor infiltrating lymphocytes Application; Chinese Journal of Cancer Biotherapy 1995 01,

[10] Wang JH, Tong SQ. **Biaoru Li**, Ding JQ, Hu BY, Zhu YM, Lu DY, Hua ZD, Lu J. Immunological Character of TIL in Ovarian Carcinoma. Chin J Cancer Res 2000; 12(2): 99-104.
[http://dx.doi.org/10.1007/BF02983432]

[11] Gu Qinlong. 11. Gu Qinlong, **Biaoru Li**, Electron microscopic observation of human gastric cancer TIL cells *in vitro* killing MKN45 gastric cancer cell lines, Journal of Shanghai Second Medical University, 1995, Vol. 15 No. 4.

[12] Gu Qinlong, Lin Yanqi, Yin Haoran. Zhu Youming, Hu Baoyu; Phenotype and cytotoxic activity of infiltrating lymphocytes in gastrointestinal tumors[J] Journal of Shanghai Second Medical University;1996-03.

[13] Gu Qinlong, Lin Yanqi, Yin Haoran. **Biaoru Li**, Zhu Youming, Hu Baoyu; Preliminary study on cryopreservation of tumor infiltrating lymphocytes. Journal of Immunology, 1995-04

[14] Deng Y, Gu Q. Biaoru Li; Zhang Xiheng; MTT colorimetric assay for LAK and TIL cell activity in cord blood; Journal of Shanghai Jiaotong University Medical Science Edition199502.

[15] Hu Bingcheng, Li Guowen, Wei Cheng, Shen Jiankang, Dong Lin. **Biaoru Li**, Clinical application of infiltrating lymphocytes in malignant brain tumors, Journal of Immunology, 1997-02

[16] Hua Zude, Jing Lu, Li Huifang. Zhu Youming; Tong Qingshan; Clinical study of tumor infiltrating lymphocytes in ovarian cancer. Chinese Journal of Obstetrics and Gynecology 1996 09

[17] Li H, Jing L, Hua Z. Biaoru Li; Tong Shanqing; Lu Deyuan; Study on the killing activity of TIL cells in ovarian cancer Shanghai Medical199505.

[18] Jing Lu. Hua Zude; Zhu Youming; Tong Shanqing; Research on TIL yield and vitality of different materials; Journal of Immunology 1995 03

[19] Jing Lu, Hu Liewei, Hua Zude. **Biaoru Li**, Tong Shanqing; Analysis of the therapeutic effects of different therapeutic approaches for TIL; 1996-02

[20] Jing L, Hua Z, Li H. Biaoru Li, Zhu Youming, Tong Shanqing; In vitro study of ovarian cancer TIL Shanghai Medical Journal199506.J

[21] Jing L, Duan LD, Hua Z. Biaoru Li, Zhu Youming; Tong Shanqing; Preliminary observation of biological characteristics of cord blood lymphocytes, Journal of Shanghai Jiaotong University Medical Science Edition199501.

[22] Tong Shanqing, Wang Jianhua. Ding Jianqing; Hu Baoyu; Zhu Youming; Lu Deyuan; Hua Zude; Lu Jing; Biological characteristics of invasive lymphocytes from ovarian cancer; Chinese Journal of Immunology 2000 03

[23] Cai Xiaomin, Jing Lu, Hua Zude. Tong Shanqing; Clinical Application of TIL from Different Sources; Journal of Immunology 1996 04

[24] Tong S, Wang J. **Biaoru Li**, Ding Jianqing; Hu Baoyu; Zhu Youming; Lu Deyuan; Hua Zude; Lu Jing; Biological characteristics of invasive lymphocytes from ovarian cancer. Chin J Immunol 2000.

List of Contributors

Alan Larson	Department of Virology, Chicago, USA
Amit Datta	Department of Biochemistry, Case Western Reserve University School of Medicine, Cleveland, USA
Biaoru Li	Department of Biochemistry, Case Western Reserve University School of Medicine, Cleveland, USA Department of Pediatrics, Medical College at GA, Augusta, USA
Baoyu Wu	Department of Microbiology, Shanghai Second Medical University, Shanghai, China
Deyuan Lu	Department of Microbiology, Shanghai Second Medical University, Shanghai, China
Emmanuelle Devemy	Rush Cancer Institute, Chicago, USA
George E. Liu	Department of Biochemistry, Case Western Reserve University School of Medicine, Cleveland, USA Beltsville Agricultural Research Center (BARC) – East, Beltsville, USA
GuanXiang Qian	Department of Biochemistry, Shanghai Second Medical University, Shanghai, China
Hong-Liang Hu	Department of Microbiology, Shanghai Second Medical University, Shanghai, China
JianQing Ding	Department of Microbiology, Shanghai Second Medical University, Shanghai, China
Jie Zheng	Department of Microbiology, School of Computer Engineering, Singapore
Li-Hua Jiang	Departments of Immunology and Microbiology, Shanghai Jiao Tong University School of Medicine, Shanghai, China
Meihua Lin	Department of Biochemistry, Case Western Reserve University School of Medicine, Cleveland, USA
Shanqing Tong	Department of Microbiology, Shanghai Second Medical University, Shanghai, China
Shen Li	Division of Surgical Oncology, Boston, USA
Shishu Chen	Department of Microbiology, Shanghai Second Medical University, Shanghai, China
Supriya Perabekam	Rush Cancer Institute, Chicago, USA
Shuzhen Tan	Guangdong Medical University, Zhanjiang, China
Wei-Hua Yan	Medical Research Center, enzhou Medical University, China
Wei Zhang	Department of Biochemistry, Case Western Reserve University School of Medicine, Cleveland, USA
Xihan Zhang	Department of Microbiology, Shanghai Second Medical University, Shanghai, China
Xiao Zhu	Guangdong Medical University, Zhanjiang, China

Youming Zhu   Department of Microbiology, Shanghai Second Medical University, Shanghai, China

Yan Qu   Department of Biochemistry, Case Western Reserve University School of Medicine, Cleveland, USA

INTRODUCTION

After nearly 30 years of developing T-cell adoptive immunotherapy as summarized above, our book will focus on personalized immunotherapy, a new strategy for cancer treatment in the 21st century. Personalized immunotherapy will involve a set of biochemical, immune, and genomic characterization of the tumors using multi-dimensional analyses in order to lead to an optimal decision on the appropriate immune treatment. Therefore, this book on personalized immunotherapy will first introduce some foundational concepts: MHC research and development, the genomic profiles and genome-wide association study (GWAS) of T-cells and tumor cells from patients, and technologies which provide the basis of personalized immunotherapy. The knowledge has led to the rapid development of personalized immunotherapy in the past decades.

Because recent research in personalized immunotherapy involves targeting therapy, in the book, we will introduce some new immunoassay methods related to personalized immunotherapy. Subsequently, we will present targeting immunotherapy in two chapters: personalized immunotherapies that depend on the tumor immune microenvironment (TIME) (such as PD1 or PDL1-related checkpoint targeted therapy) and immunotherapy dependent on the tumor microenvironment (TME) including IDO (indoleamine 2,3-dioxygenase) inhibitors and ADO (CD39/CD73/adenosine) inhibitors.

The central portion of this book, consisting of eight chapters, is related to personalized T-cell immunotherapy, which includes the basics of personalized T-cell immunotherapy and the essentials of the latest developments in personalized T-cell immunotherapy. The former with three chapters consists of new molecular technologies such as T-cell screening and cloning of tumor neoantigens, a new generation of primary tumor cell culture for T-cell cloning, bioinformatics platform of T-cells and primary tumor cells. The latter or personalized T-cell adoptive immunotherapy with four chapters will present the development and future of adoptive T-cell immunotherapy; the development of T-cell gene therapy and T-cell genome editing; the affinity of transgenic T-cells to tumor cells such as CAR T-cells and TCR T-cells; and systematic modeling of polyclonal specific T-cells. Finally, we will present a biobank for personalized immunotherapy, which we have been studying for more than twenty years.

Personalized immunotherapy is a new immunotherapy model for studying individualized cancer therapy, which involves "providing the right immunotherapy for the right people at the right time." Due to the complexity of individual tumors and immune responses, traditional immunotherapy models have faced challenges. To address this, we have written the book on updated strategies for cancer immunotherapy.

CHAPTER 1

MHC and Cancer Immunotherapy

Li-Hua Jiang[1,*] and Wei-Hua Yan[2]

[1] *Departments of Immunology and Microbiology, Shanghai Jiao Tong University School of Medicine, Shanghai, 200025, China*

[2] *Medical Research Center, Taizhou Hospital of Zhejiang Province, Wenzhou Medical University, Linhai, 317000, China*

Abstract: Major Histocompatibility Complex (MHC) is a gene region, which is named human leucocyte antigen (HLA) in humans. The human leukocyte antigen (HLA) system is a highly polymorphic family of genes involved in immunity and responsible for identifying self-cells *versus* no self-cells. Although HLA typing is essential for solid organ and bone marrow transplantation, at present, MHC is going to study on cancer immunotherapy increasingly. In order to introduce MHC related to cancer immunotherapy, the chapter aims at focusing on several MHC issues related to cancer immunotherapy. For example, MHC research and development (R&D) in MHC class I molecular loss related to cancer immunotherapy; tumor immune escape related to nonclassical MHC I; T-cell epitope vaccines; as well as MHC issues in adoptive immune cell therapy and personalized immunotherapy. In each part for MHC related to immune responses for tumor disease, we also introduce clinical uses in a study on MHC issues for T-cell immunotherapy, MHC for T-cell vaccines, and MHC TCR reconstructions for tumor shared/specific antigen related TCR T-cell personalized immunotherapy.

Keywords: Dendritic Cell-Based Cancer Vaccine, Human Leucocyte Antigen (HLA), Major Histocompatibility Complex (MHC), NK Vells, T-Vells, TCR T-Cell Personalized Immunotherapy.

OVERVIEW OF MHC GENES AND MOLECULES

The major histocompatibility complex (MHC) is a common genetic region in vertebrates. It is called human leukocyte antigen (HLA) in humans and histocompatibility-2 (H2) in mice. MHC contains multiple genetic loci, which is highly polymorphic. It was first discovered because it played a decisive role in determining transplant rejection, that is, the degree of histocompatibility between the donor and recipient of organ tissue transplantation [1].

* **Corresponding author Li-Hua Jiang:** Departments of Immunology and Microbiology, Shanghai Jiao Tong University School of Medicine, Shanghai, 200025, China; E-mail:sjtujiang@126.com

It was later uncovered that its main biological role of MHC class I and II molecule-encodes provide antigens that can be recognized by T lymphocytes [2], which are the center of the T cell immune response. Another interesting issue is that MHC class I molecules (including classical and nonclassical Class I molecules) can be used as targets for surface inhibitory receptor recognition by NK, playing an essential role in regulating immune cells' effect for tumor immunotherapy [3].

1. Characteristics of the HLA Gene Complex

The classical HLA gene system is located in the short arm of chromosome 6 (the 6p21 region) and has a length of 3600 kb as Fig. (**1**). It contains 224 gene loci, of which 128 are functional genes with product expression [4].

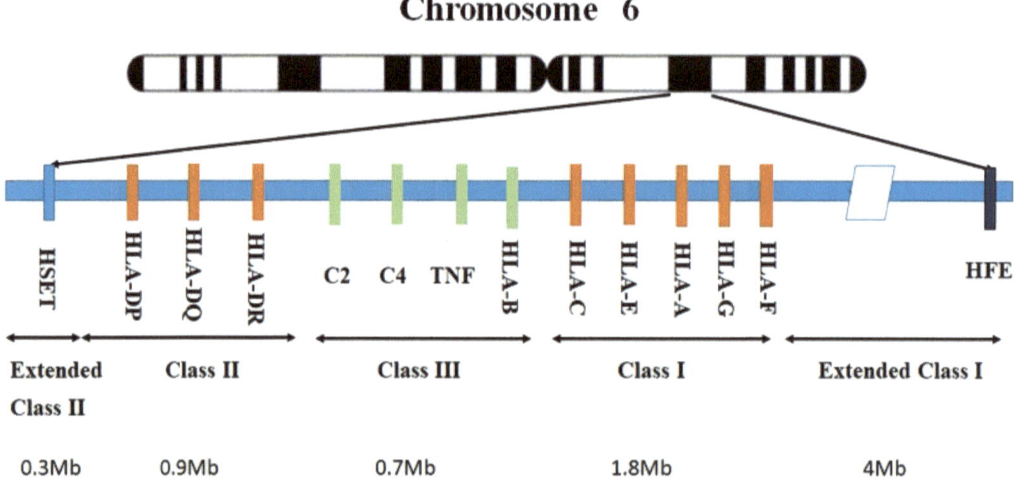

Fig. (1). HLA gene complex.

The most important loci are the classical HLA class I, containing HLA-A, HLA-B and HLA-C genes encoding the classical HLA class I molecules alpha chains; and the classical HLA class II encoding the alpha and beta chains from genes of HLA-DRA, HLA-DRB, HLA-DQA, HLA-DQB, HLA-DPA, HLA-DPB genes. Molecules encoded by HLA-E, HLA-F, HLA-G, and MIC loci, which are located in nonclassical HLA class I loci, play an important role in immune regulation. Other genes are also involved in the body's immunity, such as HLA-DM, HLA-DO, TAP, and PSMB for re-antigen processing and presentation, complement genes, and TNF genes for inflammation.

Most of these genes have polymorphism or be highly polymorphic at each locus with a difference of one base to multiple base pairs, individually, so that clinically HLA polymorphisms have become a major obstacle to allografts, and often also become necessary factors to in immunotherapy of tumors [5].

2. HLA Molecule Structure

The classical HLA class I molecules alpha chain encoded from HLA-A, HLA-B, and HLA-C and β2 micro-globulin (β2M) encoded by the non-HLA gene from chromosome 15 as Fig. (**2**). Classical HLA class II molecules composed of the alpha chain encoded by the A gene of HLA class II and the beta chain encoded by the B gene, encoding from HLA-DR, HLA-DQ, and HLA-DP as Fig. (**2**).

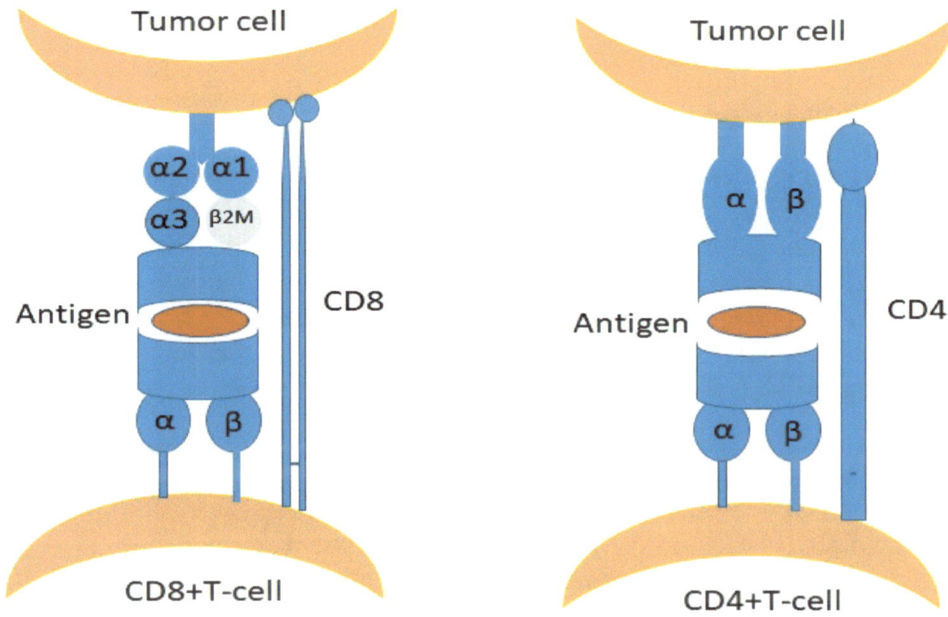

Fig. (2). HLA structure.

The critical difference between Class I molecules and Class II molecules is that the two ends of the peptide-binding groove are closed in Class I molecules so that Class I molecules generally can only accommodate peptides of 9 amino acids. In contrast, Class II molecules are open so that they can accommodate more peptides. For example, the peptide with a length of 16-18 amino acids with nine amino acids are bound in the groove [7]. The Ig-like region is responsible for maintaining the stability of the three-dimensional structure and selectively binds to CD4 or CD8 molecules on the surface of T-cells, thereby limiting the recognition pattern of T-cells. CD8+T-cells recognize antigens presented by MHC class I molecules, while CD4+T-cells recognize the antigen presented by MHC class II molecules.

3. Distribution and Function of HLA Molecules

Classical HLA class-I molecules are distributed on the surface of all nucleated cells, responsible for presenting the antigens produced inside the cells for recognition by CD8+T-cells. In contrast, HLA class II molecules are mainly distributed in antigen-presenting cells (APC), responsible for presenting antigens for recognition by CD4+T-cells.

The presentation of MHC molecules to antigens is a prerequisite for immune recognition of T-cells because the TCR antigen receptor only recognizes the linear epitope (epitope) presented by MHC, affinity short peptide cut off from the protein antigen. Therefore, the recognition of antigens by T-cells is deeply affected by MHC molecules, so-called MHC restriction [8].

MHC class I molecules also have an important function as ligands for some receptors on the surface of NK cells, including KIR2D/KIR3D belonging to the killer cell immunoglobulin-like receptor (KIR) family, killer cell lectin-like receptor (KLR), CD94/NKG2 family, regulating the killing activity of NK cells. The MHC class I molecules play a decisive role in the inhibitory receptors of NK cells because NK cells can recognize and kill tumor cells that lack own MHC class I molecules [3].

4. MHC Allele Detection

The typing of HLA based on the antigenic difference of HLA molecules is to use allotype antisera with complement-dependent micro-lymphocytic methods. Following research and development (R&D) of molecular biology techniques, the molecular typing method has, currently, replaced the serological method. According to the purposes of different laboratories, the technologies currently used are:

1. **PCR-SSO** (Sequence-specific oligonucleotide probes) can use PCR to amplify specific fragments of the HLA gene, fix the PCR amplification product on the hybrid membrane, and then use a series of labeled oligonucleotide oligonucleotide probes for hybridizing various HLA allele-specific DNA sequences, and finally, determine the type of allele according to the hybridization pattern

of each specimen.

2. **PCR-SSP** (Sequence-specific primer assay), based on the DNA sequence differences of various HLA alleles, applies for a series of targeted primers to amplify various allele-specific fragments, and then to determine the HLA allele by electrophoresis based on PCR products.

3. **Real-time PCR**: the basic principle is like PCR-SSP, but it is more convenient and accurate because it does not require electrophoresis operations after PCR. After the first half of the method is the same as PCR-SSO; the PCR products are identified by Sanger sequencing for alleles.

4. **Next-generation sequencing (NGS):** After RNA-seq and DNA-seq are developed since 1995, most scientists working on screening techniques have often used genomic techniques to discover new candidates of neoantigens related to TCR recognizing MHC-peptide. Moreover, engineering T-cells with tumor antigen-specific TCR related to binding MHC can be used to generate TCR T-cells for personalized adoptive T-cell immunotherapy.

MHC CLASS I MOLECULAR LOSS AND CANCER IMMUNOTHERAPY

A variety of biological products have been used for cancer immunotherapy such as BCG, Polysaccharide K (PSK), IL-2, IFN, tumor vaccine, tumor infiltration lymphocytes (TIL). In recent years, novel therapies using antibodies that block immune checkpoint molecules involved in the regulation of T-cell has achieved good results. Unfortunately, only small proportions of patients benefit from these therapies [9]. These immune escaping indicated T-cells in tumor immune surveillance/escape, tumor occurrence and resistance to immunotherapy, for example, loss of tumor antigen, lack of co-stimulatory signals for T cell activation, the resistance of tumor cells to IFN, Resistance of tumor cells to apoptosis, immune negative regulatory cells and immunosuppressive factors in the tumor microenvironment (TME). Considering that the presentation of tumor antigen by MHC I is the premise of T cell immune recognition, the lack or down-regulation of MHC I expression on the tumor cell surface is an important strategy for immune escapes.

1. Loss of Class I HLA Expression in Tumor Tissues

Class I HLA molecules are normally expressed in nearly all nucleated cells, except for trophoblastic placental cells, central nervous system, and an exocrine portion of the pancreas. Hepatocytes and skeletal muscle cells have relatively low expression of Class I HLA proteins. Due to the characteristic of co-dominant expression for Class I HLA alleles, each cell can express six different molecules, including two types of A, B, and C, respectively. All the HLA molecules are thought to be expressed in tumor cells at the early stage of tumorigenesis. However, studies have shown that loss of Class I HLA expression on the tumor cell surface is very common in various types of tumor [10], such as biliary tract carcinoma, bladder carcinoma, breast carcinoma, cervical carcinoma, colorectal carcinoma, endometrial cancer, esophageal carcinoma, gastric carcinoma, glioblastoma, head and neck carcinoma, hepatocellular carcinoma, lymphoma and leukemia, lung carcinoma, melanoma, neuroblastoma, ovarian cancer, pancreas carcinoma, prostate carcinoma, renal cell carcinoma, thyroid carcinoma, and uveal melanoma. The detection rate is estimated to be around 90% in many neoplasms [11].

2. Types of Class I HLA Deletion.

Various types of Class I HLA deletion exist in tumor tissues [11, 12]. Compared with complete deletion, the partial deletion of Class I HLA is found to have higher carcinogenicity. This is because the part of a class I HLA with high efficiency for presenting tumor antigen epitopes is lost, resulting in the failure of T cells to recognize tumor antigen efficiently.

I. **Complete deletion of Class I HLA molecules**. The mechanisms of formation include β2M deletion caused by loss of heterozygosity (LOH) on chromosome 15 and mutation of β2M gene on another chromosome 15, transcriptional down-regulation of antigen presentation machinery (APM), HLA-I or β2M genes, and hypermethylation of Class I HLA genes [11 - 16].

II. **Deletion of haplotypes of HLA.** Deletions occur as a set of HLA genes (type A, B, or C), which may be involved in the loss of an entire or part of chromosome 6 [11].

III. **Down-regulated expression of HLA gene locus** (type A, B, or C). As a result, tumor cells only express the other two gene loci of the four alleles, which can be caused by either decreased transcription level or expression of specific transcription factors. Cytokines secreted by TH1 cells, such as IFN-γ, can reverse the down-regulated expression [11, 12].

IV. **Deletion of HLA alleles.** The deletion occurs at any 1 product from the 3 class I HLA gene loci of the six alleles, which may be caused by somatic mutation of the allele. It is undetectable in most cases since a specific monoclonal antibody against that allele product is required for the detection [11, 12].

V. **Co-occurrence of above-mentioned II, III and IV**. This type of deletion may lead to the expression of 1 allele to the minimum [15 - 17].

VI. **Unresponsive deletion to up-regulation of Class I HLA induced by IFN.** This type may be caused by genetic mutations on molecules related to IFN-γ or IFN-α signal pathway [18, 19].

In summary, loss of Class I HLA expression can be caused through a variety of mechanisms, including abnormalities occurring at any step during synthesis and assembly of Class I HLA molecules. According to whether the deletion can be reversed through interacting with cytokines produced by immunotherapy, the mechanisms are divided into 2 classes [11, 20, 21]: **Irreversible**: including LOH, mutations or deletions on chromosome 6 and 15 (harboring α chain gene and β2M gene, respectively), defect of IFN signal transduction pathway (such as interruption of Jak-STAT pathway); **Reversible**: including down-regulated expression of HLA-A, B or C gene locus, heavy chain gene of Class I, β2M gene, APM genes resulting from abnormal transcription regulation, down-regulation of Class I or APM gene expression caused by hypermethylation, and inhibition upon post-transcriptional modification of Class I MHC mRNAs.

3. Expression of Class I HLA Molecules and Efficiency of Immunotherapy

Several scenarios are raised to predict the immunotherapy efficacy on class-I HLA expression. As for tumors with positive expression of Class I HLA molecules, the immunotherapy efficacy is influenced by other immune escape associated factors, such as tumor antigenicity, apostolicity of tumor cells, and co-stimulatory signals. Appropriate treatment strategies should be put forward towards those impact factors.

I. **Treatment can recover the expression of Class I HLA molecules**. In other words, the deletion belongs to the above-mentioned reversible type. Immunotherapy can lead to local release of cytokines produced from TH1 T-cells in the tumor microenvironment, such as IFN-α and IFN-γ, which reversely upregulate Class I HLA molecule expression on tumor cells and the tumor antigens presented by the class-I HLA molecules can re-activate specific T cells to recognize and kill tumor cells. Studies have shown a positive correlation between expression recovery of Class I HLA molecules and immunotherapy efficacy on tumors [11, 20, 21].

II. **Treatment cannot recover the expression of Class I HLA molecules since the deletion belongs to the above-mentioned irreversible type.** Immunotherapy is generally ineffective on tumors with such type of deletion, and the effort in the future is to find a way of increasing the expression of Class I HLA molecules. For instance, blocking antibodies for immune checkpoint usually have no effect on patients with mutated β2M and LOH on chromosome 15, which can cause inefficient antigen presentation [11, 22, 23].

III. **Expression of Class I HLA molecules is restorable**, while the treatment itself has no impact on its expression. In order to have a better clinical effect in such a situation, other methods are required to enhance the expression of Class I HLA molecules. Therefore, it is imperative to identify the types of Class I HLA deletion for the prediction of therapeutic efficiency.

4. The Relation Between Selective Pressure of Immunocyte and Changes of Class-I HLA Expression Pattern in Tumor Cells

Tumor cells are evolved from normal cells containing a positive expression of Class I HLA molecules. Loss of class-I HLA molecules occurs during the progressive development of neoplasms. Studies have shown that deletion is a gradual process with different cellular clones and various expression levels of class-I HLA molecules. AT the 12th International Conference on HLA, Garrido *et al.* proposed that tumor tissue could be classified into three types based on the expression of class-I HLA molecules, including positive, heterozygosity, and negative types. It is commonly believed that these three types of tumors reflect the transformation process of class-I HLA molecule expression from positive to negative. Tumor cells display positive expression at the early stage of tumor formation, and then heterozygous state with the gradual appearance of negative clones. Pure negative state indicates a late stage of tumorigenesis. Tumor cell clones with positive expression of class-I HLA molecules can be recognized and destroyed by activated anti-tumor T-cells. However, tumor cell clones of negative expression gradually form through a mechanism such as mutation and escape from recognition and elimination. As a result, only clones with negative expression of class-I HLA molecules finally remain in tumor tissues under such selective pressure [11, 24, 25].

Many kinds of researches have demonstrated a positive correlation between expression of class-I HLA molecules and the infiltration of immune cells, such as T-cells and M1 cells in tumor tissues. During the development of tumorigenesis, tumor cells gradually lose class-I HLA molecules accompany structure change of tumor tissue. In a positive and heterozygous state, there are lymphocytes and macrophages infiltrated in the tumor tissue due to the ability of class-I HLA molecule expressed cells to activate T-cells. However, in a negative expression state, the tumor tissues have deficient infiltration of immune cells, and tumor cells with class-I HLA molecules locate at tumor surrounding stroma region, forming an obvious boundary from negatively expressed tumor cells in the center of the lesion. Meanwhile, many fibroblasts emerge in peritumoral tissues, which mix with various immune cells to form a granulomatous structure of tumor tissue surrounded by non-neoplastic tissues. Such kind of granulomatous structure can be observed in many tumors, which continue to progress due to the inactive state of surrounding immune cells [15, 25, 26].

Although studies are still limited, comparison of class-I HLA molecule expression between metastatic and primary tumor tissues can inspire additional perspectives: 1) metastases with either expressed or not expressed class-I HLA molecules can derive from both primary tumor with positive and negative expression of class-I HLA molecules; 2) the type of deletion in metastatic and primary tumors can be same or different; 3) metastases can have a complete positive expression of class-I HLA molecules even if the primary lesion is negative. These interesting phenomena suggest that selective pressure posed by T-cells and NK cells plays an important role in the expression state of class-I HLA molecules in metastases and primary tumors [11, 27, 28].

There is also a relationship between the expression level of class-I HLA molecules in metastases and the immune status of the body. In the immunosuppressive state, metastasis can be induced, and then an expression of class-I HLA molecules can be restored as well. Studies in mouse models revealed that among multiple tumor cell clones, H-2 positive clones have higher immunogenicity and metastatic ability in comparison to H-2 negative clones. More significantly, sarcoma cell clones with reversible deletion of class-I HLA molecules after induction of IFN could enter a state of so-called immune quiescence in mice with normal immune function. However, metastases with positive expressed class-I HLA molecules were formed after T-cell deficiency was induced in mice. Immune quiescence refers to a static condition that tumor cells are neither progressive nor destroyed by the immune system. The status of equilibrium between tumor cells and the body's immune system can be maintained for a long period of time without any clinical symptoms unless the body immunity is decreased [11, 29 - 31].

EXPRESSION LEVELS OF NONCLASSICAL MHC CLASS I AND TUMOR IMMUNE ESCAPE

1. The HLA Class I Antigen Expression and Cancer

The HLA class I antigens play essential roles in immune response, for example, HLA can present peptide to T-cells and serve for ligands for a panel of receptors expressed on immune cells. Based on the tissue expression pattern, genetic polymorphism, and molecular function, HLA class I antigens can be grouped as the classical (HLA Ia for HLA-A, -B, and -C) and nonclassical antigens (HLA Ib for HLA-E, -F and -G). Unlike highly polymorphic and ubiquitously expressed HLA Ia antigens on nucleated cells, HLA Ib molecules have features such as limited tissue localization, low genetic diversity, limited peptide repertoire, and distinct functional profiles [32]. In the context of malignancies, alternation of HLA Ia antigen expression abnormalities can escape from host anti-tumor immune responses while induction of HLA Ib antigen expression on cancer cells can be involved in HLA Ib antigens to bind immunoinhibitory receptors such as immunoglobulin-like transcripts (ILT)2, ILT4 and NK receptor group 2 (NKG2) [33].

2. Roles of HLA Ib Antigens in Immune Modulation

The nonclassical HLA I antigens HLA-E, HLA-F, and HLA-G, were identified during the late 1980s. Contrary to the high polymorphic of HLA Ia antigens, only 43, 44, and 69 alleles with 11, 6, and 19 different proteins for HLA-E, HLA-F, and HLA-G, respectively (http://hla.alleles.org/nomenclature/stats.html). During the past three decades, the biological function and related clinical significance of HLA-E and HLA-G have been widely investigated in various physiological and pathological conditions [33].

HLA-E binds to the inhibitory receptors CD94/NKG2A and the activating receptor CD94/NKG2C. However, HLA-E preferentially binds to the inhibitory receptor CD94/NKG2A with much higher avidity than that of the activating receptor CD94/NKG2C. Consequently, HLA-E interacts with CD94/NKG2A can inhibit the activation and proliferation of NK cells and impair survival of the CD8+ tumor-infiltrating T lymphocytes in the tumor microenvironment [34].

HLA-G is the most intensively investigated molecule among the HLA Ib family, and seven HLA-G isoforms (HLA-G1~ HLA-G7) generated by its primary transcripts alternative splicing have been identified. Isoforms HLA-G1~HLA-G4 are membrane-bound while HLA-G5~HLA-G7 is soluble. Different HLA-G isoforms are distinguished by the number of extracellular immunoglobulin-like domains and by the transmembrane residues they have or not. HLA-G1 is encoded by the full-length HLA-G mRNA, and with three extracellular immunoglobulin-like domains (α1, α2, and α3), other isoforms may lack the α2, α3 domain or both, respectively. HLA-G can render comprehensive immune suppressive function by binding to receptors such as ILT2 and ILT4. ILT2 can be expressed on B-cell, T cells, NK cells, DCs, myeloid-derived suppressor cells (MDSCs), and monocytes, while ILT4 is expressed on DCs and monocytes, neutrophils and MDSCs. HLA-G/ILT2/4 inhibitory signal pathway can impair immune cell proliferation, differentiation, cytotoxicity, cytokine secretion, and chemotaxis. Moreover, HLA-G/ILT2/4 interaction can induce regulatory cells and promote the generation of MDSCs or polarization of M1 type macrophage to the M2 type. ILT2/4 recognizes HLA-G in its extra cellar $\alpha3$ domain. However, the binding specificity of ILT2 and ILT4 is different according to the structure of the HLA-G molecule, that ILT4 recognizes both HLA-G associated with β_2M and free HLA-G heavy chains, whereas ILT2 only recognizes HLA-G associated with β_2M [35]. Given immune-suppressive functions resulted from the HLA-E and HLA-G and the interaction of their receptors in cancer immunology, HLA-G/ILT2/4 and HLA-E/NKG2A signaling pathway have been proposed as new immune checkpoints as the well established cytotoxic T lymphocyte-associated protein 4 (CTLA-4)/B7 and programmed cell death protein-1 (PD-1)/PD-L1. Antibodies target to these immune checkpoints can restore or re-activate T-cell and NK cell anti-tumor responses. Several approaches based on the HLA-G/ILT2/4 and HLA-E/NKG2A signaling pathway are currently under development for cancer immunotherapy [36, 37].

HLA-F is the least investigated molecule among HLA Ib antigens until recent data addressed that HLA-F can interact with either activating or inhibitory receptors on immune cells, depending on the conformation of HLA-F molecule. ILT2 and ILT4 can bind HLA-F/β_2m/peptide complex through a docking strategy that precludes HLA-F open conformer recognition. However, KIRs (3DL1, 3DL2, 3DS1, and 2DS4) can bind HLA-F open conformer, where KIR3DS1 is of the highest binding affinity for HLA-F open conformer [38, 39]. These important findings Therefore, it is imperative to identifyprovide new evidence that HLA-F functions as an important immune regulatory molecule in human physiological and pathological conditions have been emerging. Though relative information of HLA-F/KIRs in cancer immunology is limited, the biological significance of HLA-F/KIR3DS1 in the viral infectious diseases has been highlighted in recent studies. For example, HLA-F open conformer /KIR3DS1 interaction can activate NK cell function in the control of viruses such as HIV and HCV replication [39, 40]. However, the inhibitory pathway between HLA-F/β_2m/peptide complex/ILTs and HLA-F open conformer/KIR3DL1 remains to be investigated.

3. Clinical Relevance of HLA Ib Expression in Cancers

Cancer cells harness different strategies to escape surveillance from host both adaptive and innate anti-tumor immune responses. Abnormal expression and impaired function of HLA antigens on tumor cells frequently occurred in cancer immune evasion. In most cases, accompany with HLA Ia antigens down-regulated high-regulation of HLA-E, -F and -G have been detected in a wide variety of cancers associated with the progression and unfavorable clinical outcome of tumor diseases [41].

HLA-E expression has been found in many types of cancers, such as breast cancer, cervical cancer, colorectal cancer, gastric cancer, glioblastoma, hepatocellular carcinoma, lung cancer, melanoma, renal cancer, thyroid cancer, and vulvar squamous cell carcinoma. Among these studies, increased HLA-E expression in cancer lesions has been observed to be related to the cancer cell metastasis, recruitment of regulatory immune cells, or associated with a worse prognosis in various cancer patients [33]. HLA-F expression has been observed in breast cancer, bladder cancer, oesophageal squamous cell cancer, gastric cancer, hepatocellular carcinoma, nasopharyngeal cancer, neuroblastoma, and lung cancer. Among these studies, HLA-F expression in gastric adenocarcinoma has observed to be significantly correlated with the depth of invasion, nodal involvement, lymphatic and venous invasions, and with a worse prognosis [42]. In patients with HLA-F positive had a worse survival than those with HLA-F negative. In another study, upregulated HLA-F expression (lesion *vs.* normal tissue) was found to have significantly worse survival than those with HLA-F unchanged and downregulated in patients with oesophageal squamous cell carcinoma [43].

HLA-G expression in cancers was firstly reported in 1998. Later, HLA-G expression has been analyzed and evaluated worldwide in thousands of malignant samples with various types of cancers such as breast cancer, colorectal cancer (CRC), cervical cancer, endometrial cancer, oesophageal squamous cell carcinoma (ESCC), Ewing sarcoma, gastric cancer, glioblastoma, HCC, lung cancer, lymphoma, nasopharyngeal carcinoma, oral squamous cell carcinoma, ovarian cancer, pancreatic adenocarcinoma, thyroid cancer, and vulvar squamous cell carcinoma. Aberrant HLA-G expression in cancers has been found to be associated with advanced tumor stage, metastasis, and worse prognosis [35].

4. Prospective of HLA-E and HLA-G Targeted Cancer Immunotherapy

Cancer therapy has made significant improvements due to the development of new approaches to increase anti-tumor immune responses. Tumor immunotherapies currently are mainly focused on the antibodies (Ab) to block immune checkpoints such as CTLA-4 and PD-1 to restore or re-activate T-cell anti-tumor immune responses, or the generation of T cells expressing chimeric antigen receptor (CARs) specific for tumor antigens. However, but only nearly 20% of patients received the benefit from the targeted cancer immunotherapy. Therefore, combination therapy for targeting immune checkpoint pathways could significantly increase therapeutic response [44]. Indeed, besides the well-acknowledged CTLA-4/B7 and PD-1/PD-L1 signaling pathway, other potential immune checkpoints such as HLA-G/ILT2/4 and HLA-E/NKG2A signaling pathway blockade are currently under development or clinical trial for cancer immunotherapy [33].

Protein expression blockers (PEBLs) by constructs containing a single-chain variable fragment derived from an anti-NKG2A antibody can block NKG2A expression on NK cells. Kamiya *et al.* reported that NKG2A null NK cells had higher cytotoxicity against HLA-E+ tumor cells [45]. Furthermore, André *et al.* [46] recently reported that HLA-E-specific inhibitory receptor NKG2A is an important checkpoint on NK and CD8+ T cells. NKG2A blocked with Monalizumab can restore the anti-tumor function of NKG2A+ NK and T-cells. Moreover, combination with the anti-PD-L1 blocking mAb (Durvalumab) has a synergistic effect in NKG2A+ and PD-1+ NK cells against HLA-E+ and PD-L1+ target cells, which can further improve the control of tumor growth and mice from death.

Cancer immune therapy based on the HLA-G/ILT2/4 immune checkpoint pathway has been proposed *in vivo* studies. In previous preclinical investigations, restoring the functions of NK cell or T-cell against target cancer cells has been observed with blocking tumor cell-expressed HLA-G or immune cell surface ILT2/4 with specific mAbs [35]. Moreover, the generation of T cells to express chimeric antigen receptors (CAR) specific for HLA-G are currently under development for cancer immunotherapy.

However, a few critical aspects should be taken into consideration before application in a clinical trial. First, the inter-tumor and intratumor heterogeneity of HLA-E/G expression vary dramatically, as indicated in numerous previous studies. Second, at least seven HLA-G isoforms have been identified so that HLA-G and ILT2/4 binding depends on the molecular structure of the different molecular structures of HLA-G isoforms make the HLA-G /ILT2/4 signaling pathway even more complex.

MHC FOR T-CELL EPITOPE AND ACTIVE IMMUNE VACCINES

As mentioned earlier, due to the differences in the amino acid sequence of different MHC molecules, the three-dimensional structure of the peptide-binding groove may also be different, the bag-like structure that directly and closely binds to the different peptides, resulting in its ability to bind. The types of peptides are also different, but this selective recognition is not as specific as the recognition between antigens and antibodies. It only requires that certain positions of the peptide must be specific amino acids, resulting in meeting the characteristics of the consensus motif [47].

Therefore, when designing a T-cell epitope vaccine, it must be accurately designed according to the HLA type of each patient. This is particularly important in neoantigen vaccines based on the detection of neonatal mutations in tumor cells. Many new mutations caused by amino acid sequence changes can be detected in tumor cells. Synthetic peptides containing T-cell epitopes at higher concentrations can be used as vaccines to stimulate them more effectively. However, only some of those neonatal tumor mutations are suitable for designing vaccines, that is, a common motif that conforms to the HLA category owned by patients, and the others are ineffective. Based on the HLA-peptide structure as described above, at present, because constructs of specific vaccines require MHC-peptides matching, dendritic cell-based cancer vaccines by specific peptides forming peptide-MHC complex have been increasingly and easily used to produce active immunotherapy by vaccines [48].

MHC FOR ADOPTIVE IMMUNE CELL THERAPY

Due to the health status, immune status of tumor patients and convenience of cell preparation, it is often necessary to consider the use of allogeneic immune cells, such as CIK cells, CAR-T cells, CAR-NK cells, *etc.*, but these strategies must be carefully considered the issue of HLA matching between donors and recipients because there are several factors can affect the effectiveness of treatment.

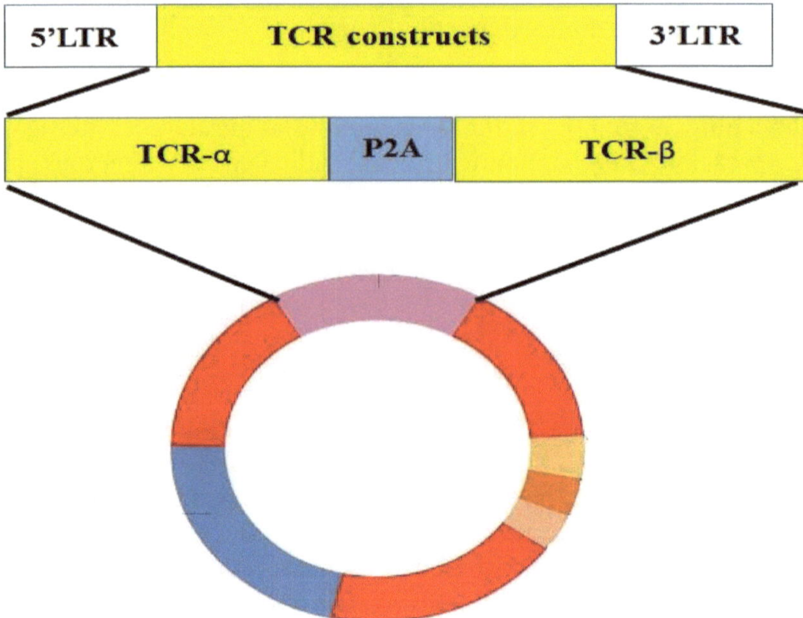

Fig. (3). HLA based-TCR constructs for TCR T-cells.

For example, if an immune cell recognizes tumor antigens, resulting in killing tumor cells, the MHC restriction needs to be in priority considered. That is, the epitopes presented by different MHC are different from an individual patient. Therefore, tumor antigen presented by the different MHC molecules cannot produce the effect of immunotherapy for patient tumor cells. However, considering the high frequency of some HLA alleles, for example, half of the individuals in the general population carry the HLA-A2 series alleles, so that adoptive treatment of T-lymphocytes among some individuals with the same HLA gene is still feasible, but the T-lymphocytes requires careful analysis of the HLA type and the common motifs that it can present antigens [48].

Based on HLA-peptide restriction as described above, at present, TCR recognizing peptides bound to major histocompatibility complex (MHC) molecules have increasingly reported [49]. In order to avoid MHC screening techniques for T-cell therapy as described above, if we achieve TIL to have been conferring MHC recognition, a construct of TCR as Fig. (**3**) is made up of two protein chains (TCR-α and TCR-β) with a P2A self-cleaving peptides, after overlapping extension PCR to achieves TCR complex from TIL, selective TCR domain can recognize and bind to a tumor-specific peptide target presented in the context of HLA class I receptor so that the TCR can be directly used to packaging viral vectors for TCR T-cell personalized immunotherapy [50].

CONCLUSION

MHC is essential to a target of tumor-specific T-cells such as TIL and TCR T-cells for adoptive T-cell immunotherapy and target of tumor vaccines for active immunotherapy. Because tumor cells often accumulate hundreds of mutations with several immunogenic neoantigens under MHC restriction, four strategies are going to be used to immunotherapy: (1) DC-based tumor vaccines by specific peptides forming peptide-MHC complex *in vivo*; (2) TCR based T-cell immunotherapy for adoptive T-cell immunotherapy; (III) NK based immunotherapy and (IV) checkpoint inhibitory therapy-related MHC function. These new strategies, which will be discussed in chapter 12, are increasingly supporting clinical oncologists to apply for a new generation of immunotherapy for patients.

CONSENT FOR PUBLICATION

Not applicable.

CONFLICT OF INTEREST

The authors confirm that the content of this chapter has no conflict of interest.

ACKNOWLEDGEMENTS

In order to support writing quality, two editors (Nancy Debry is editor in our America Society of Pediatrics) have been invited to modify some grammar in the writings.

The mention of trade names or commercial products in this article is solely to provide specific information and does not imply recommendation.

Competing interest statements

REFERENCES

[1]   Snell GD. Some recollections of Peter Gorer and his work on this fiftieth anniversary of his discovery of H-2. Immunogenetics 1986; 24(6): 339-40.
[http://dx.doi.org/10.1007/BF00377948] [PMID: 3539776]

[2]   Zinkernagel RM, Doherty PC. The discovery of MHC restriction. Immunol Today 1997; 18(1): 14-7.
[http://dx.doi.org/10.1016/S0167-5699(97)80008-4] [PMID: 9018968]

[3]   Ljunggren HG, Kärre K. In search of the 'missing self': MHC molecules and NK cell recognition. Immunol Today 1990; 11(7): 237-44.
[http://dx.doi.org/10.1016/0167-5699(90)90097-S] [PMID: 2201309]

[4]   The MHC sequencing consortium. Complete sequence and gene map of a human major histocompatibility complex. Nature 1999; 401(6756): 921-3.
[http://dx.doi.org/10.1038/44853] [PMID: 10553908]

[5]   Mosaad YM. Clinical role of human leukocyte antigen in health and disease. Scand J Immunol 2015; 82(4): 283-306.
[http://dx.doi.org/10.1111/sji.12329] [PMID: 26099424]

[6]   Klein J, Sato A. The HLA system. First of two parts. N Engl J Med 2000; 343(10): 702-9. Review.2

[7]   Sharma G, Holt RA. T-cell epitope discovery technologies. Hum Immunol 2014; 75(6): 514-9.
[http://dx.doi.org/10.1016/j.humimm.2014.03.003] [PMID: 24755351]

[8]   Castro CD, Luoma AM, Adams EJ. Coevolution of T-cell receptors with MHC and non-MHC ligands. Immunol Rev 2015; 267(1): 30-55.
[http://dx.doi.org/10.1111/imr.12327] [PMID: 26284470]

[9]   Sharma P, Allison JP. The future of immune checkpoint therapy. Science 2015; 348(6230): 56-61.
[http://dx.doi.org/10.1126/science.aaa8172] [PMID: 25838373]

[10]   Garrido F, Aptsiauri N. Cancer immune escape: MHC expression in primary tumours *versus* metastases. Immunology 2019; 158(4): 255-66.
[http://dx.doi.org/10.1111/imm.13114] [PMID: 31509607]

[11]   Garrido F. MHC/HLA Class I Loss in Cancer Cells. Adv Exp Med Biol 2019; 1151: 15-78.
[http://dx.doi.org/10.1007/978-3-030-17864-2_2] [PMID: 31140106]

[12]   Garcia-Lora A, Algarra I, Garrido F. MHC class I antigens, immune surveillance, and tumor immune escape. J Cell Physiol 2003; 195(3): 346-55.
[http://dx.doi.org/10.1002/jcp.10290] [PMID: 12704644]

[13]   del Campo AB, Kyte JA, Carretero J, *et al.* Immune escape of cancer cells with beta2-microglobulin loss over the course of metastatic melanoma. Int J Cancer 2014; 134(1): 102-13.
[http://dx.doi.org/10.1002/ijc.28338] [PMID: 23784959]

[14]   Carretero FJ, Del Campo AB, Flores-Martín JF, *et al.* Frequent HLA class I alterations in human prostate cancer: molecular mechanisms and clinical relevance. Cancer Immunol Immunother 2016; 65(1): 47-59.
[http://dx.doi.org/10.1007/s00262-015-1774-5] [PMID: 26611618]

[15]   Perea F, Bernal M, Sánchez-Palencia A, *et al.* The absence of HLA class I expression in non-small cell lung cancer correlates with the tumor tissue structure and the pattern of T cell infiltration. Int J Cancer 2017; 140(4): 888-99.
[http://dx.doi.org/10.1002/ijc.30489] [PMID: 27785783]

[16]   Serrano A, Tanzarella S, Lionello I, *et al.* Rexpression of HLA class I antigens and restoration of antigen-specific CTL response in melanoma cells following 5-aza-2'-deoxycytidine treatment. Int J Cancer 2001; 94(2): 243-51.
[http://dx.doi.org/10.1002/ijc.1452] [PMID: 11668505]

[17]   Koopman LA, Corver WE, van der Slik AR, Giphart MJ, Fleuren GJ. Multiple genetic alterations cause frequent and heterogeneous human histocompatibility leukocyte antigen class I loss in cervical cancer. J Exp Med 2000; 191(6): 961-76.
[http://dx.doi.org/10.1084/jem.191.6.961] [PMID: 10727458]

[18]   Seliger B, Ruiz-Cabello F, Garrido F. IFN inducibility of major histocompatibility antigens in tumors. Adv Cancer Res 2008; 101: 249-76.
[http://dx.doi.org/10.1016/S0065-230X(08)00407-7] [PMID: 19055946]

[19]   Sucker A, Zhao F, Pieper N, *et al.* Acquired IFNγ resistance impairs anti-tumor immunity and gives rise to T-cell-resistant melanoma lesions. Nat Commun 2017; 8: 15440.
[http://dx.doi.org/10.1038/ncomms15440] [PMID: 28561041]

[20]   Aptsiauri N, Garcia-Lora A, Garrido F. "Hard" and "Soft" loss of MHC class I expression in cancer cells.Tumour immunology & immunotherapy. Oxford University Press 2014; pp. 63-78.
[http://dx.doi.org/10.1093/med/9780199676866.003.0005]

[21]   Garrido F, Cabrera T, Aptsiauri N. "Hard" and "soft" lesions underlying the HLA class I alterations in cancer cells: implications for immunotherapy. Int J Cancer 2010; 127(2): 249-56.
[http://dx.doi.org/10.1002/ijc.25270] [PMID: 20178101]

[22]   Zaretsky JM, Garcia-Diaz A, Shin DS, *et al.* Mutations associated with acquired resistance to PD-1 blockade in melanoma. N Engl J Med 2016; 375(9): 819-29.
[http://dx.doi.org/10.1056/NEJMoa1604958] [PMID: 27433843]

[23]   Sade-Feldman M, Jiao YJ, Chen JH, *et al.* Resistance to checkpoint blockade therapy through inactivation of antigen presentation. Nat Commun 2017; 8(1): 1136.
[http://dx.doi.org/10.1038/s41467-017-01062-w] [PMID: 29070816]

[24]   Garrido F, Ruiz-Cabello F, Cabrera T, *et al.* Implications for immunosurveillance of altered HLA class I phenotypes in human tumours. Immunol Today 1997; 18(2): 89-95.
[http://dx.doi.org/10.1016/S0167-5699(96)10075-X] [PMID: 9057360]

[25]   Aptsiauri N, Ruiz-Cabello F, Garrido F. The transition from HLA-I positive to HLA-I negative primary tumors: the road to escape from T-cell responses. Curr Opin Immunol 2018; 51: 123-32.
[http://dx.doi.org/10.1016/j.coi.2018.03.006] [PMID: 29567511]

[26]   Garrido F, Perea F, Bernal M, Sánchez-Palencia A, Aptsiauri N, Ruiz-Cabello F. The escape of cancer from T cell-mediated immune surveillance: HLA class I loss and tumor tissue architecture. Vaccines (Basel) 2017; 5(1): 7.
[http://dx.doi.org/10.3390/vaccines5010007] [PMID: 28264447]

[27]   Carretero R, Romero JM, Ruiz-Cabello F, *et al.* Analysis of HLA class I expression in progressing and regressing metastatic melanoma lesions after immunotherapy. Immunogenetics 2008; 60(8): 439-47.
[http://dx.doi.org/10.1007/s00251-008-0303-5] [PMID: 18545995]

[28]   Kloor M, Michel S, von Knebel Doeberitz M. Immune evasion of microsatellite unstable colorectal

cancers. Int J Cancer 2010; 127(5): 1001-10.
[http://dx.doi.org/10.1002/ijc.25283] [PMID: 20198617]

[29]   Cozar JM, Aptsiauri N, Tallada M, Garrido F, Ruiz-Cabello F. Late pulmonary metastases of renal cell carcinoma immediately after post-transplantation immunosuppressive treatment: a case report. J Med Case Reports 2008; 2: 111.
[http://dx.doi.org/10.1186/1752-1947-2-111] [PMID: 18423038]

[30]   Garcia-Lora A, Algarra I, Gaforio JJ, Ruiz-Cabello F, Garrido F. Immunoselection by T lymphocytes generates repeated MHC class I-deficient metastatic tumor variants. Int J Cancer 2001; 91(1): 109-19.
[http://dx.doi.org/10.1002/1097-0215(20010101)91:1<109::AID-IJC1017>3.0.CO;2-E]   [PMID: 11149409]

[31]   Aguirre-Ghiso JA. Models, mechanisms and clinical evidence for cancer dormancy. Nat Rev Cancer 2007; 7(11): 834-46.
[http://dx.doi.org/10.1038/nrc2256] [PMID: 17957189]

[32]   Adams EJ, Luoma AM. The adaptable major histocompatibility complex (MHC) fold: structure and function of nonclassical and MHC class I-like molecules. Annu Rev Immunol 2013; 31: 529-61.
[http://dx.doi.org/10.1146/annurev-immunol-032712-095912] [PMID: 23298204]

[33]   Würfel FM, Winterhalter C, Trenkwalder P, *et al.*   European Patent in Immunoncology: From Immunological Principles of Implantation to Cancer Treatment. Int J Mol Sci Apr 12 2019; 20(8) E1830.

[34]   Wieten L, Mahaweni NM, Voorter CE, Bos GM, Tilanus MG. Clinical and immunological significance of HLA-E in stem cell transplantation and cancer. Tissue Antigens 2014; 84(6): 523-35.
[http://dx.doi.org/10.1111/tan.12478] [PMID: 25413103]

[35]   Lin A, Yan WH. Heterogeneity of HLA-G Expression in Cancers: Facing the Challenges. Front Immunol 2018; 9: 2164.
[http://dx.doi.org/10.3389/fimmu.2018.02164] [PMID: 30319626]

[36]   van Hall T, André P, Horowitz A, *et al.* Monalizumab: inhibiting the novel immune checkpoint NKG2A. J Immunother Cancer 2019; 7(1): 263.
[http://dx.doi.org/10.1186/s40425-019-0761-3] [PMID: 31623687]

[37]   Friedrich M, Jasinski-Bergner S, Lazaridou MF, *et al.* Tumor-induced escape mechanisms and their association with resistance to checkpoint inhibitor therapy. Cancer Immunol Immunother 2019; 68(10): 1689-700.
[http://dx.doi.org/10.1007/s00262-019-02373-1] [PMID: 31375885]

[38]   Dulberger CL, McMurtrey CP, Hölzemer A, *et al.* Human Leukocyte Antigen F Presents Peptides and Regulates Immunity through Interactions with NK Cell Receptors. Immunity 2017; 46(6): 1018-1029.e7.
[http://dx.doi.org/10.1016/j.immuni.2017.06.002] [PMID: 28636952]

[39]   Garcia-Beltran WF, Hölzemer A, Martrus G, *et al.* Open conformers of HLA-F are high-affinity ligands of the activating NK-cell receptor KIR3DS1. Nat Immunol 2016; 17(9): 1067-74.
[http://dx.doi.org/10.1038/ni.3513] [PMID: 27455421]

[40]   Lunemann S, Schöbel A, Kah J, *et al.* Interactions Between KIR3DS1 and HLA-F Activate Natural Killer Cells to Control HCV Replication in Cell Culture. Gastroenterology 2018; 155(5): 1366-1371.e3.
[http://dx.doi.org/10.1053/j.gastro.2018.07.019] [PMID: 30031767]

[41]   Kochan G, Escors D, Breckpot K, Guerrero-Setas D. Role of non-classical MHC class I molecules in cancer immunosuppression. OncoImmunology 2013; 2(11): e26491.
[http://dx.doi.org/10.4161/onci.26491] [PMID: 24482746]

[42]   Ishigami S, Arigami T, Setoyama T, *et al.* Clinical-pathological implication of human leukocyte antigen-F-positive gastric adenocarcinoma. J Surg Res 2013; 184(2): 802-6.

[http://dx.doi.org/10.1016/j.jss.2013.04.003] [PMID: 23706560]

[43]   Zhang X, Lin A, Zhang JG, *et al.* Alteration of HLA-F and HLA I antigen expression in the tumor is associated with survival in patients with esophageal squamous cell carcinoma. Int J Cancer 2013; 132(1): 82-9.
[http://dx.doi.org/10.1002/ijc.27621] [PMID: 22544725]

[44]   Khalil DN, Smith EL, Brentjens RJ, Wolchok JD. The future of cancer treatment: immunomodulation, CARs and combination immunotherapy. Nat Rev Clin Oncol 2016; 13(5): 273-90.
[http://dx.doi.org/10.1038/nrclinonc.2016.25] [PMID: 26977780]

[45]   Kamiya T, Seow SV, Wong D, Robinson M, Campana D. Blocking expression of inhibitory receptor NKG2A overcomes tumor resistance to NK cells. J Clin Invest 2019; 129(5): 2094-106.
[http://dx.doi.org/10.1172/JCI123955] [PMID: 30860984]

[46]   André P, Denis C, Soulas C, *et al.* Anti-NKG2A mAb Is a Checkpoint Inhibitor that Promotes Anti-tumor Immunity by Unleashing Both T and NK Cells. Cell 2018; 175(7): 1731-1743.e13.
[http://dx.doi.org/10.1016/j.cell.2018.10.014] [PMID: 30503213]

[47]   Lundegaard C, Lund O, Buus S, Nielsen M. Major histocompatibility complex class I binding predictions as a tool in epitope discovery. Immunology 2010; 130(3): 309-18.
[http://dx.doi.org/10.1111/j.1365-2567.2010.03300.x] [PMID: 20518827]

[48]   Kawakami Y, Eliyahu S, Sakaguchi K, *et al.* Identification of the immunodominant peptides of the MART-1 human melanoma antigen recognized by the majority of HLA-A2-restricted tumor infiltrating lymphocytes. J Exp Med 1994; 180(1): 347-52.
[http://dx.doi.org/10.1084/jem.180.1.347] [PMID: 7516411]

[49]   McCormack E, Adams KJ, Hassan NJ, *et al.* Bi-specific TCR-anti CD3 redirected T-cell targeting of NY-ESO-1- and LAGE-1-positive tumors. Cancer Immunol Immunother 2013; 62(4): 773-85.
[http://dx.doi.org/10.1007/s00262-012-1384-4] [PMID: 23263452]

[50]   Vita R, Mahajan S, Overton JA, *et al.* The immune epitope database (IEDB): 2018 update. Nucleic Acids Res 2019; 47(D1): D339-43.
[http://dx.doi.org/10.1093/nar/gky1006] [PMID: 30357391]

CHAPTER 2

Immune Cells Signaling-Pathway and Genomic Profiles for Personalized Immunotherapy

Wei Zhang[1], Yan Qu[1], Meihua Lin[1], Amit Datta[1], George E. Liu[1,2] and Biaoru Li[1,3,*]

[1] *Department of Biochemistry, Case Western Reserve University School of Medicine, Cleveland, OH, USA*

[2] *USDA, ARS, ANRI, Bovine Functional Genomics Laboratory, Beltsville Agricultural Research Center (BARC) – East, Beltsville, MD, USA*

[3] *Georgia Cancer Center and Department of Pediatrics, Medical College at GA, Augusta, GA 30912, USA*

Abstract: Lymphocytes play important roles in body defense for a few diseases, such as tumor diseases, autoimmune diseases, allergic inflammation. The genomic profiles with their analyses for body defense of lymphocytes have been applied to identify and verify disease-associated and disease-specific biomarkers. The genomic profiles of lymphocytes also can provide more information to understand their functions and roles in the development of tumor diseases, although genomic profiles from lymphocytes are still not completed for different tumor diseases. The chapter first reviews subtypes/functions and signaling/pathways of different lymphocytes and then introduce genomic profiles with their networks on these types of lymphocytes to highlight the genomic profiles of lymphocytes in tumor diseases. The genomic profiles are going to produce clinical potentials of precision medicine such as tumor prediction, tumor prevention, and prognostic estimation and personalized therapy of lymphocytes so that, here, we will more focus on the study of genomic expression and network of personalized immunotherapy because the profiles of gene expression with their network in lymphocytes start a new chance to develop personalized immunotherapy soon.

Keywords: B-cells, Genomic Expression Profiles, NK Cells, Network, Pathway, Personalized Immunotherapy, Precision Medicine, Single-Cell RNA-seq, T-Cells.

INTRODUCTION

Genomic profiles with their networks of lymphocytes are subject to studying of different responses to tumor diseases. Also, the profiles have been applied to

* Corresponding author Biaoru Li: Georgia Cancer Center and Department of Pediatrics, Medical College at GA, Augusta, GA 30912, USA; Tel: 440-317-1443; E-mail: bli@augusta.edu

identify biomarkers for therapeutic strategies of tumor diseases. The chapter first reviews types/function, signaling/pathway of lymphocytes, finally allowing genomic profiles with their network analyses of these lymphocytes to apply for immunotherapy of different patients with different tumor diseases.

Lymphocytes include T-cells (CD4 for cell-mediated regulation and CD8 for cell-mediated cytotoxicity), B-cells (for humoral antibody-driven) and natural killer cells (NK cells critical for innate cell-mediated cytotoxicity) as well as other T-cells (NKT-cells and γδ T-cells) found in peripheral blood, lymph and some tissues [1 - 3]. The functions of T-cells and B-cells are initiated by recognizing specifically foreign antigen (Ag) during a process called Ag presentation by Ag presentation cells (APC) such as by macrophage [4]. NK cells are involved in innate immunity to kill infected cells and tumor cells, although NK cells have some adaptive immunity activated by cytokines and then release cytotoxic molecules to kill the altered cells [5]. Usually, flow-cytometry can use specific markers to define the percentage of lymphocytes from blood, lymph, and tissues as Fig. (**1**) and Table **1**.

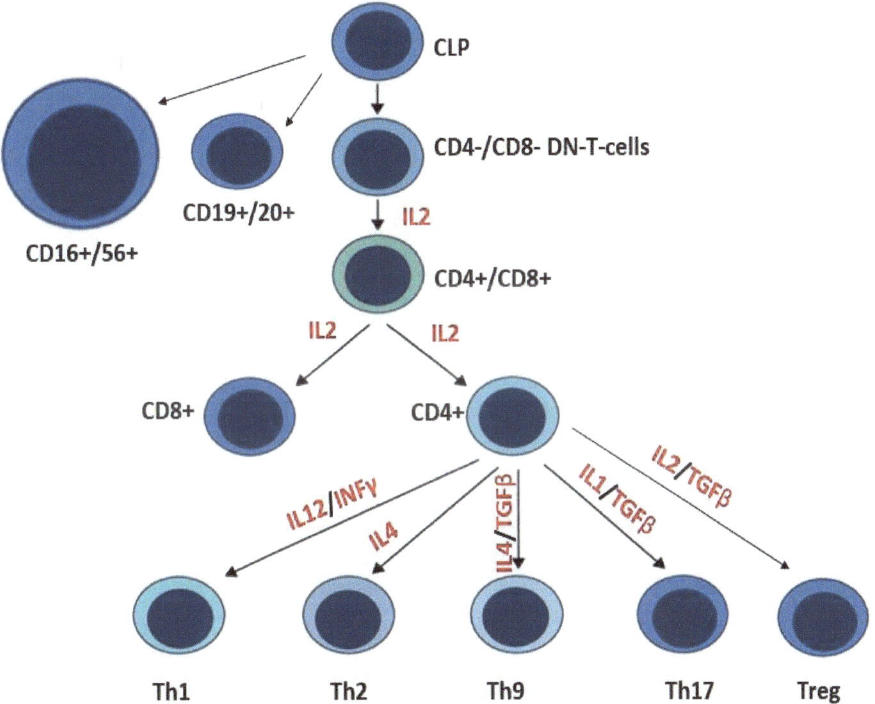

Fig. (1). Differentiation of Common Lymphocyte progenitor (CLP). The development of lymphopoiesis of B-cells, T-cells and NK cells identified by their biomarkers with induction of cytokines (red).

Table 1. Percentage of lymphocytes.

Class	Phenotypic Markers	Function	Percent (range)
T helper cells	TCRαβ , CD3/CD4	Release cytokines to regulate other immune cells	46% (28–59%)
T cytotoxic cells	TCRαβ, CD3/CD8	Lysis of virally infected, tumor cells and allografts	19% (13–32%)
NK cells	CD16/CD56	Lysis of virally infected cells and tumor cells	7% (2–13%)
γδ T cells	TCR γδ/CD3	Immunoregulation and cytotoxicity	5% (2–8%)
B cells	CD19/CD20	Production of antibodies	23% (18–47%)

CD3+CD4+T-cells of CD3+T-cells can be further divided by their surface biomarkers, gene expression, and functions after induced by cytokines *in vitro* and stimulated by diseases *in vivo* [6, 7]. Once activated *in vitro* and *in vivo*, they secrete different cytokines regulating the different immune responses. In detail, the CD4+T-cells induced by different cytokines and stimulated by different diseases for several subtypes are demonstrated in Fig. (**1**) and functioned as Table **2**.

Table 2. The function of CD4+ Helper T-cells.

Cell Type	Cytokines Produced	Key Transcription Factor	Role in Immune Defense
Th1	IFNγ, IL2	T-bet	Produce defense against intracellular bacteria, viruses, and cancer.
Th2	IL4, IL5, IL6, IL10, IL13	GATA-3	Aid the differentiation and antibody production by B cells
Th9	IL9	IRF4, PU.1	Defense against helminths
Th17	IL17	RORγ	Defense against gut pathogens and at mucosal barriers
Treg	IL10, TGFâ	*Foxp3*	Help B cells produce antibody

T-CELL MEMBRANE SIGNALING

Immune cells initiate an immune response based on T-cell membrane signaling proteins as Fig. (**2A**) [8]. As demonstrated in the Fig. (**2B**), cytotoxic CD8+ T-cells can kill tumor cells and virus-infected cells based on the expression of CD8+ molecule on the cell surface [9]. The CD8+ T-cells first recognize their targets by binding to short peptides associated with MHC class I molecule, present on the surface of tumor cells to kill those cells [10]. After activated, CD8+ T-cells also produce IL-2 and IFN-γ to further influence macrophages and NK cells [11]. Helper CD4+ T-cells as Fig. (**2B**) defined CD4 molecules on their surfaces, assist other lymphocytes (such as B-cells, CD8+ T-cell, and macrophages) [12]. The CD4+ T-cells become activated when they presented by peptides associated with the MHC class II molecule expressed on the surface of APC [13]. Moreover, once T-cells are activated, T-cells differentiate into effector T-cells and memory cells expressing CD45RO, CCR7, and CD62L [14]. In CD4+ T-cell subfamily, regulatory T-cells as shown in Fig. (**1**), called CD4$^+$ Treg cells, maintain immune tolerance, and suppress immune reaction [15]. Some of CD4+ Treg cells have higher expression of FOXP3 gene as Table **2** [16]. Several other types of T-cells, such as Tr1 cells and Th3 cells, without FOXP3 gene expression, also have suppressive activity by producing suppressive molecules [17]. T-cell activation also demonstrates a high expression of some biomarkers such as CD25, CD69, CD71, HLA-DR, and CTLA-4 [18]. As concluded in Fig. (**2A**) and Fig. (**2B**), T-cell's activations are a very complex

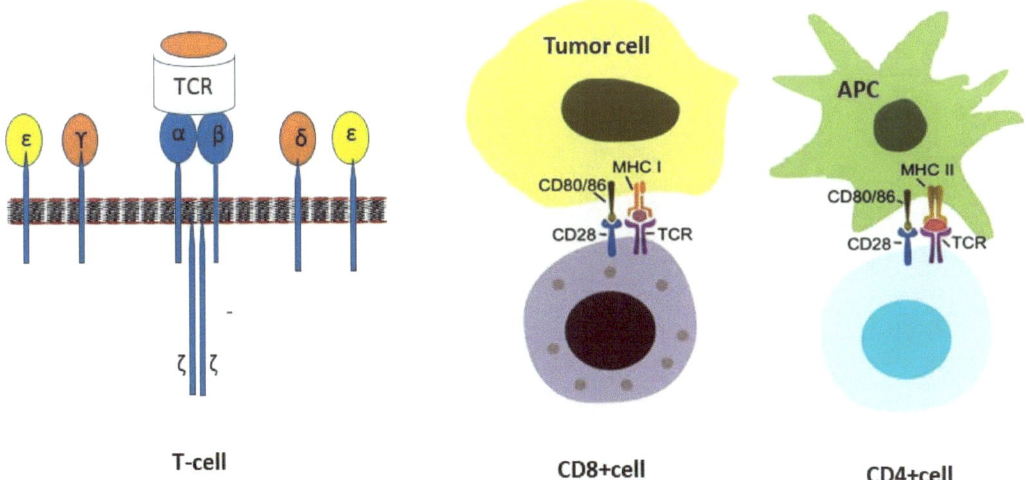

Fig. (2). T-cells and CD8+cell and CD4+cell Membrane Signaling Protein. Fig. (**2A**) describes T-cells membrane signaling molecules, and Fig. (**2B**) shows the difference CD8 and CD4.

process in CD+4 and CD+8 cells. Activation of CD4+ T-cells occurs through the simultaneous engagement of the T-cell receptor (TCR) and CD28 on the T-cell for stimulatory molecule by MHC class II-Ag and co-stimulatory molecule by B7 (CD80/86) on the APC [19], while activation of CD8+T-cells occurs with the simultaneous engagement of the T-cell receptor (TCR) and CD28 on the T cell for stimulatory molecule by MHC class I-Ag and a co-stimulatory molecule by B7 (CD80/86) on the surface of tumor cells [20]. According to recent researches of lymphocytes killing tumor cells, several new T-cell receptors are discovered, including inhibitory receptors and activating receptors. Inhibitory receptors include CTLA4 (cytotoxic T-lymphocyte antigen-4), PD-1 (Programmed cell death protein 1), and TIM-3 (T cell immunoglobulin and mucin-domain containing-3) as Fig. (**3**). They can actively induce T cell exhaustion at the site of a tumor so that these kinds of inhibitory receptors can be used to block to study killing tumor cells [21 - 24]. Now more and more data show that T-cell exhaustion plays a vital role in tumor relapses so that in recent years, there are a few experiments and clinical trials with immune checkpoint blockers in targeting therapy of tumor diseases [25, 26]. Some of them have confirmed good responses for treatment, allowing them to apply for patients [27]. Furthermore, SIT (SHP2-interacting transmembrane adaptor protein) is also an identified transmembrane adaptor protein, which interacts with the SHP2 (SH2-containing protein tyrosine phosphatase-2) *via* an ITIM (immunoreceptor tyrosine-based inhibition motif) so that the complex also acts as a critical negative regulator of TCR-mediated signaling [28].

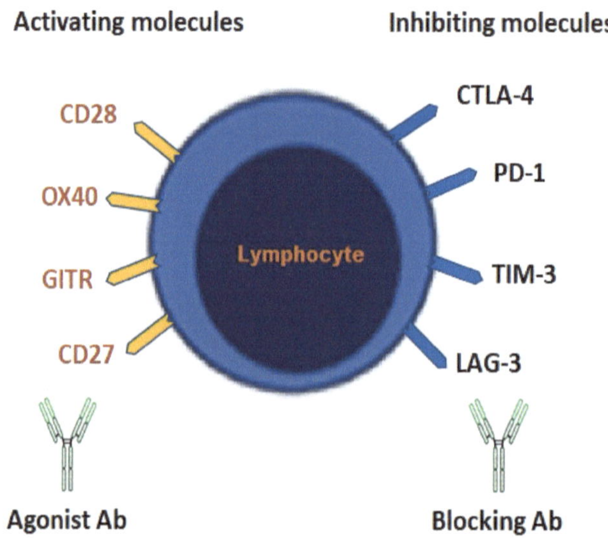

Fig. (3). T-cells Targeting Signaling. T-cell is activated by TCR-CD28 and CD4/8 membrane signaling protein so that the network involves cytokine production and CD4/8 related functions. Inhibitory molecules such as CTLA-4, PD-1, TIM-3, and LAG-3 can be blocked to decrease T-cell exhaustion to kill tumor cells, and activating molecules such as CD28 can be used to stimulate T-cell function for kill tumor cells.

T-CELLS PATHWAY AND NETWORKS

After T-cell is activated by both TCR-CD28 and CD4/8 membrane signaling proteins, several pathways (or network) of the T-cell process so that the T-cells release cytokines and produce CD4/8 related functions. T-cell signaling proteins downstream with co-stimulatory molecules form a combined network with at least seven pathways as Fig. (**4**) (both networks of CD4+cells and CD8+cells are a few differences so that they are discussed, respectively, in the chapter of personalized therapy).

1. **PI3K Pathway**: The most crucial pathway in T-cells is the PI3K pathway, which is co-activated by CD28. If the absence of CD28, T-cell receptor signaling results in an anergic status [29];

2. **p38 MAPK Pathway**: CD4+ molecules binding lymphocyte-specific kinases (lck) recruit ZAP-70 to activate p38 MAPK pathway which is the core of protein kinases for different protein kinases of lymphocytes [30];

3. **RAS-MEK-ERK Pathway**: ZAP-70 activates LAT for RAS-MEK-ERK pathway, by which terminal transcriptional factors bind FOS response element allowing activation and production of the IL-2 gene [31];

4. **JNK Pathway**: Their terminal transcriptional factors bind Jun response element allowing complete CD4+/C8+ functions [32];

5. **NF-kB Pathway**: The most complex pathway in T cells is the NF-kB pathway. As Fig. (**4**), phosphorylated LAT recruits SLP-76 to the membrane to create the active diacylglycerol (DAG), and PKC acts on PIP2, phosphorylating it to produce phosphatidylinositol-3,4,5-trisphosphate (PIP3). DAG binds and activates some PKCs. PLCγ initiates the NF-kB pathway. In other fields, DAG also activates PKCθ, which then phosphorylates CARMA1. TAK1 phosphorylates IKK-β introduces some molecules into the nucleus and binds the NF-κB response element. This product coupled with NFAT signaling allows complete activation of the IL-2 gene [33]; **JNK pathway.** Their terminal transcriptional factors bind Jun response element allowing complete CD4+/C8+ functions [32]; **NF-kB pathway.** The most complex pathway in T cells is the NF-kB pathway. As Fig. (**4**), phosphorylated LAT recruits SLP-76 to the membrane to create the active diacylglycerol (DAG), and PKC acts on PIP2, phosphorylating it to produce phosphatidylinositol-3,4,5-trisphosphate (PIP3). DAG binds and activates some PKCs. PLCγ initiates the NF-kB pathway. In other fields, DAG also activates PKCθ, which then phosphorylates CARMA1. TAK1 phosphorylates IKK-β introduces some molecules into the nucleus and binds the NF-κB response element. This product coupled with NFAT signaling allows complete activation of the IL-2 gene [33];

6. **Calcium Channel Pathway**: The second important factor in T cells is PKCθ, which can increase calcium release, critical for activating the transcription factors NF-κB. IP3 is also released from the membrane by PLC-γ and diffuses

rapidly to activate calcium channel receptors on the ER to induce the release of calcium into the cytosol. The cytosolic calcium binds calmodulin, which then activates calcineurin, in turn, activates NFAT, which trans-locates to the nucleus. NFAT activates the transcriptions of a set of genes, for instance, IL-2, a cytokine that promotes the long-term proliferation of activated T cells [34];

7. **Alternative Pathways**: Once the activation of TCR recognition of antigen, some alternative membrane signaling pathways for activation and inhibition have been described as Fig. (**3**), for example, CTLA4, PD-1, and TIM-3, which actively induce T cell exhaustion.

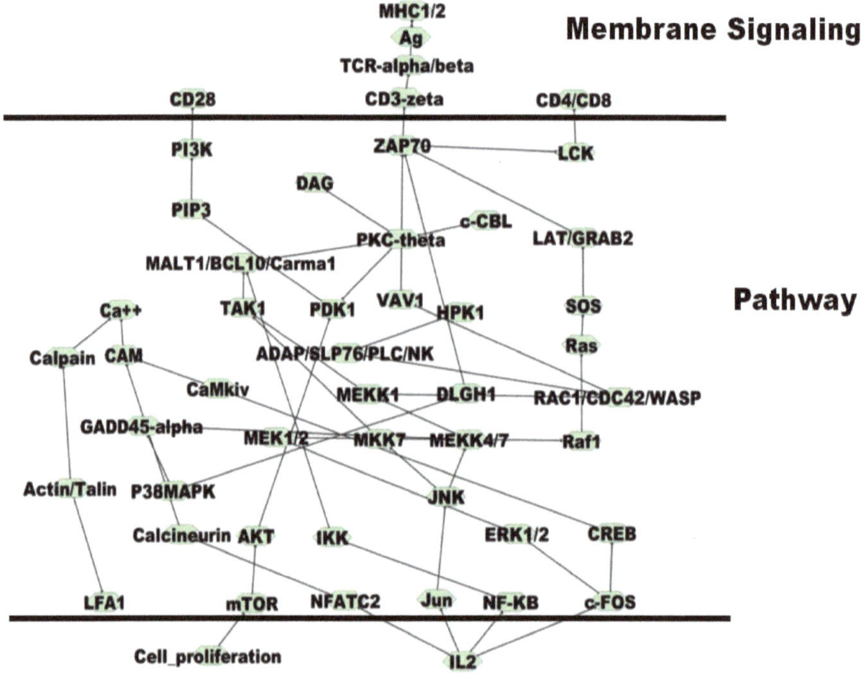

Fig. (4). T-cells Network.

GENOMIC EXPRESSION PROFILE OF T-CELLS

1. Genomic Expression Profiles of TIL

Rosenberg and his colleagues have demonstrated that TILs immunotherapy is more than 100-fold to kill tumor cells to compare T-cells from peripheral blood in the 1980s [35]. We have been studying TIL immunotherapy for more than two decades because we discovered that TILs are in the quiescent status when those located at tumor sites [36]. To study TIL quiescent status for immunotherapy and personalized immunotherapy, quiescent gene expression and genomic expression profiles of CD3+T-cells and CD3+CD8+ T-cells from TIL have been primarily studied by our laboratory so that following questions were addressed: (1) quiescence of the TIL CD8 cells is, mainly, an actively maintained state rather a default state in the absence of the stimulating signals; (2) signaling pathways involved in the quiescent status [37 - 39]. In the genomics era, a study on TIL genomic profile begins to be involved in prediction, prevention, prognostic estimation of tumor diseases, and personalized immunotherapy of TILs for tumor diseases. For example, some scientists studied TIL genomics profiles from breast cancer with a response to neoadjuvant chemotherapy under grouping TIL pre-treated and post-treatment. They purified TIL subtypes (CD3, CD4, CD8, CD20, CD68, Foxp3) and analyzed genomics of tumor-infiltrating immune cells (CD3, CD4, CD8, CD20, CD68, Foxp3) from pre-treatment and post-treatment. They identified tumor-infiltrating immune cell profiles to predict the pathological complete response (pCR) to neoadjuvant chemotherapy. A higher chemotherapy effect and good prognosis on lymphocytic infiltration were an inversion of CD4/CD8 ratio associated with better prognosis while high CD3 and CD68 infiltration were a worse disease-free survival. Finally, they uncovered immune cell subpopulation profiles with the mechanisms which largely support understanding immune cells responses to chemotherapy, and therefore, their results assist a new plan for new immune-targeted therapies [40]. In the field of tumor prevention of TIL profiles, another group of clinical scientists studied coeliac disease and Crohn's disease, which develop into small bowel carcinoma. Their results indicated that better outcome was related to high TIL from analysis of MSI (microsatellite instability). This result might help patients to find targeted anti-cancer prevention with coeliac disease and Crohn's disease [41].

Opposite to TIL genomic profiles for prediction, prevention, prognostic estimation of tumor diseases as described above, our long-term aims of TIL projects focus on TIL quiescent status related to immunotherapy and personalized immunotherapy. During 2000-2009, we studied genomic profiles with their analysis of quiescent CD3+cells and CD3+CD8+T-cells of TILs by single-cell mRNA differential display (DD) [42]. Our results demonstrated that multiple genes (Tob, TGF-b, Sno-A, Ski, LKLF, Myc, ERF, and the REST/NRSF complex) expressed in the actively maintained quiescent state of CD8 T-cells as compared to the natural state of T-cells. In 2013, we further reported single CD8+T-cell RNA-seq (obtained from TIL) to support results from the DD. The genomic profile and quantitative real-time PCR demonstrate that TILs are in quiescent status as Table **3**. Single-cell RNA-seq harvested 19.6 million sequencing reads, 11.6 million aligned reads, the mapped genes, mapped transcripts, and mapped exons were 18,356, 25,717, and 113,089, respectively. We also found that 14,062 genes (54.6%) with more than 3 RPKM [43].

Table 3. CD8+Cell results of single-cell differential display and RNA-seq.

| Genes | Single-Cell DD | Single-Cell qPCR | | Single-Cell RNA-Seq |
| | Positive screening | Fold change | SE | RPKM/beta-actin |
		(TIL CD8 cell)	(TIL CD8 cell)	
Beta-actin	Yes	1	0	1.4
Tob	Yes	2.72	0.012	2.2
Ski	Yes	1.91	0.076	3.2
Sno-A	Yes	1.32	0.021	2.1
TGF-beta	Yes	7.23	0.0127	3.76
LKLF	Yes	0.87	0.0854	1.4
ERF	Yes	3.95	0.065	2.43
REST/NRSF	Yes	1.24	0.076	1.32
c-Myc	Yes	0.89	0.0932	1.11

2. Genomic Expression Profiles from Peripheral Blood Immune Cells

Blood is a complex tissue consisting of T-cells, B-cells, NK cells, monocytes, and granulocytes. The relative proportion of each of these cell types largely changes among individuals and in response to stimuli. In whole blood, neutrophils usually are the most abundant cell type, normally varying range 30%–70%. Monocytes can change from 2% to 10%. The relative proportion of T-lymphocytes and B-lymphocytes can range 61%–85% and 7%–23% in lymphocyte obtained from PBMCs, respectively [44]. The ratio of CD4+T-cells to CD8+T-cells can vary from <1.0 to 2.0 [45]. Circulating immune cells comprise rich information about the health status and disease status of an individual. In order to explore and develop these potentials, gene expression profiling of peripheral blood cells has been increasingly reported.

In 2006, some scientists used cDNA microarray to study purified B-cells, CD4+T-cells, CD8+T-cells, granulocytes, and lymphocytes to explore their gene expression pattern. After supervised clustering analysis, they identified gene expression signatures for B-cells (427 genes), T-cells (222 genes), CD8+ T-cells (23 genes), granulocytes (411 genes), and lymphocytes (67 genes) [46].

At a similar period, other scientists used Affymetrix Human Genome U133 arrays to study genomic profile switch from the development and mature of lymphocytes, including those from the thymus, cord blood, and adult. After purified subpopulations of human thymocytes and circulating T-cells, their results have uncovered profiles for human thymopoiesis so that the profile can monitor the development and production of T-cells (especially for CD4+T-cells) [47].

Soon, these genomic expression profiles of peripheral blood cells can support personalized immunotherapy. For example, if we understand genomic profiles, we can study the genomic profile to produce a network related to the immune cells of an individual patient, so that we can use those to induce or inhibit genes for personalized immunotherapy. Genomic profiles of the lymphocyte of PBMC also can assist genetically engineering T-cells. For instance, T-cells are transduced by particular substances, such as TNF-α, TGF-β, IL2, IL12, and IFN-γ if this kind of gene is discovered by a lower expression in the genomics file of an individual patient. Moreover, the genomic profiles can support current new techniques such as genetically engineering higher affinity substances between tumor cells and T-cell such as modified TCR (T-cell receptor) and chimeric antigen receptors T-cell (CAR-T cells) if the genomics profile tells us a lower TCR process-related network.

GENOMIC EXPRESSION PROFILE OF B-CELL

1. Genomic Expression Profiles of B-Lymphocyte

B-lymphocytes (also called B-cell), approximately 15% of lymphocytes in healthy adults [48], function primarily in humoral (antibody-mediated) immunity. Now B-cells have been discovered not only producers of antibodies but also cellular immune function as antigen-presenting cells (APC) [49]. The APC potential of B-cell is increasingly studied to antitumor effects on animals and humans. Because CD40-activated B-cells functionally induce specific T-cell responses as APC, CD40-activated B-cell immunotherapy has begun to apply for antitumor adoptive immunotherapy at levels of translational medicine and clinical trial *in vivo* and *ex vivo* [50].

Relied on researches of B-cell function and those of their application, immunological scientists have applied for genomic files by significance analysis of microarrays (SAM) algorithm to study B-cell profiles such as comparing profiles between B-cells and T-cells. Their results demonstrated that expression was a significant difference between B-cells and T-cells. They uncovered 427 genes as B-cell signature (specific expression pattern in B-cells). The genomic expression pattern includes B-cell surface markers (CD20, CD24, CD38, CD72, CD74, CD79A/B, CD83, CD86), B-cell associated genes including B-cell co-receptor molecules (CD19, CD21, CD22, FCGR2B), immunoglobulins expression molecules (IG gamma, kappa, lambda; light and heavy), MHC class II receptors (HLA-DM/O/P/Q/R), signal transduction molecules (SYK, LYN, BTK, BLNK, BLK) and transcriptional regulators (EBF, PAX5/BSAP, OBF1/POU2AF1, SPIB, PU.1/SPI1, IRF4, IRF8, CEBPB). The B-cell signature is analyzed by enriched

GO annotations to classical B-cell functions include MHC Class II receptor activity, antigen presentation, antigen binding, and antigen processing. The 427 genes with their network can integrate membrane signaling proteins with the eventual production of Ab. Although the genomic results of B-cells have uncovered for IgG production rather than APC function by CD40-activated B cells, hopefully, the genomics profile can be further studied for CD40-activated B cells [46, 51].

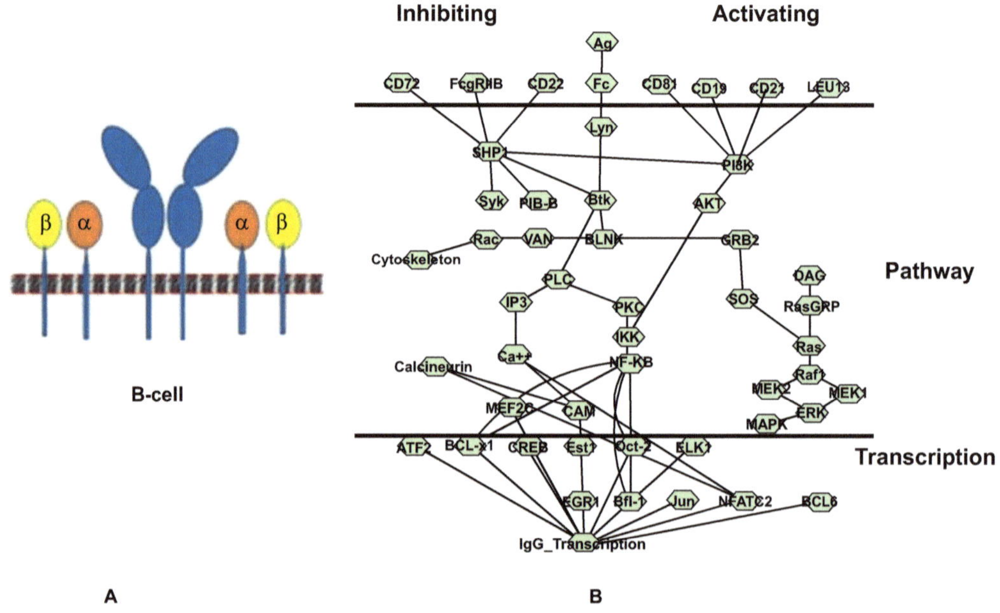

Fig. (5). B-5. B-cell membrane signaling and network. (Fig. **5A**). B-cell is activated by Ag-Fc membrane signaling protein and Fig. (**5B**). B-cell network involves IgG production and APC related functions.

2. Network of B-lymphocyte

After B-cell is activated by B-cell receptor on membrane signaling proteins as Fig. (**5A**), a network of B-cell can cascade so that the B-cells produce Ab as Fig. (**5B**). The B-cell signaling proteins downstream can be involved in a combined network with at least five pathways:

1. **Ag-Fc-Lyn pathway**. The most crucial pathway in B-cells is Ag-Fc-Lyn pathway, which is co-activated by CD19, CD21, and CD81 as well as others to increase immunoglobin production. Moreover, the pathway can be co-inhibited by CD22 and CD71 and so on to block immunoglobin production [52];

2. **p38 MAPK pathway**. p38 MAPK pathway is the core of protein kinases for

different protein kinases in B-lymphocytes [30];

3. **RAS-MEK-ERK pathway**. RAS-MEK-ERK pathway are activating terminal transcriptional factors bind response element allowing activation and production of the immunoglobin gene [31];

4. **NF-kB pathway**. The most complex pathway in B cells is the NF-kB pathway. As Fig. (**5B**), phosphorylates IKK-β introduce some molecules into the nucleus and bind the NF-κB response element for activation and production of the immunoglobin gene [33];

5. **Calcium channel pathway.** Calcium pathway in B-cells can increase calcium release, critical for activating the transcription factors NF-κB and IP3. The cytosolic calcium binds calmodulin, which then activates calcineurin to activate NFAT, which relocates to the nucleus for the production of the immunoglobin gene [34].

These genomic expression profiles of B-cells with their network are increasingly reporting for immunoglobin production. Now B-cells have been discovered to produce APC function by CD40-activated B-cells so that these genomic expression profiles of B-cells can be further studied for the cell therapy potential of CD40-activated B cells shortly.

GENOMIC EXPRESSION PROFILE AND NETWORK OF NK-CELL

1. NK-Lymphocyte

NK cells provide cell-mediated immune responses to virus-infected cells and tumor cells, most functions of NK cells, similar to those of CD8 cells. However, NK cells can recognize tumor cells in the absence of antibodies and MHC, allowing for a much faster immune reaction. The NK cells are large granular lymphocytes (LGL) with CD16/CD56 surface markers in humans [53]. Their signaling proteins on cell membranes consist of activating receptors and inhibitory receptors, killing the cells absent self MHC and Ab. As demonstrated in Fig. (**6A**), NK cells, usually, contain activating receptors (NKG2D; NCR, a natural cytotoxicity receptor; CD16, or FcΥRIII) and inhibitory receptors (KIR, Killer-cell immunoglobulin-like receptors; LIR, an immunoglobulin-like receptor; CD94/NKG2) [54]. Once tumor cells lose MHC molecules, which can bind inhibitory receptor on the surface of NK cells, NK cells can kill them by activating receptors with mechanisms regarding granule-mediated immune response (perforin and granzymes), Ab-mediated immune response (FcΥRIII, CD16) and cytokine-mediated immune response (IFNγ and TNFα).

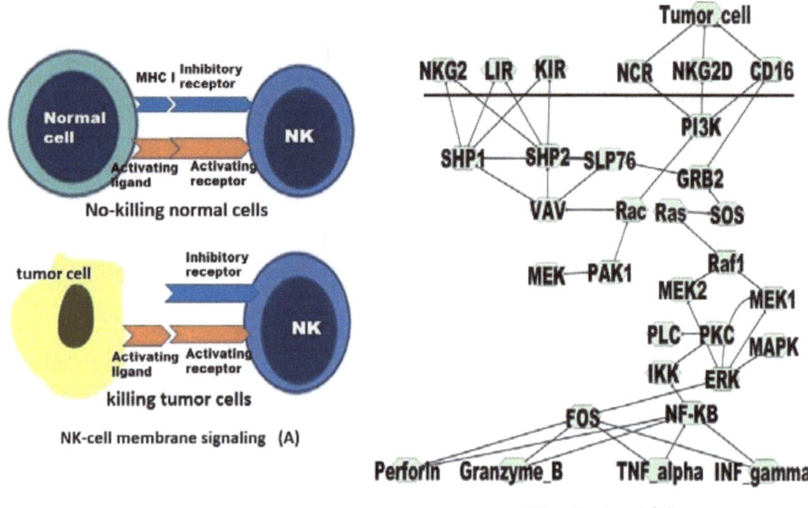

Fig. (6). NK-cells membrane signaling and network. Fig. (**6A**). NK-cell membrane signaling protein and thus NK-cell is activated by tumor cells. On the surface of NK cells, inhibitory molecules such as NKG2, KIR, and LIR binding normal cell MHCI to block NK to kill healthy cells while tumor cells without MHC molecules blocking so that NK cells are activated to kill the tumor cell. Fig. (**6B**). Activating molecules such as NKG2D, CD16, and NCR to kill tumor cells by NK-cell network by TNF-alpha, INF-gamma, perforin, and granzymes-B.

2. Genomic Expression Profiles of NK-Lymphocyte

Because NK cells play critical roles in host defense against tumors and infectious pathogens in innate immunity, genomic profiles of NK cells can provide us extensive information, including NK cell therapy. To better study NK cell function and development, a group of scientists deeply study genomic expression profiles of NK cells with their subpopulations in resting/stimulated states, differentiation stages, and disease situations. Their results of microarray analysis demonstrated that NK-cells had comprehensive cellular responses (induced under IL-2, IL-8, IL-12, IL-21, and IFN-α) to activated NK cells (for example, proliferation, cytotoxicity, and cytokine/chemokine production). Their results further show upregulated gene profiles including activating receptors (KLRC1, KLRC3), granule molecules (death receptor ligands FasL, TNFSF10, granzyme A/B, and CTLA1) to cytotoxicity, cytokine receptors (IL2RG, IL18RAB, IL27RA), chemokine receptors (CX3CR1, CCR5, CCR7), members of secretory pathways (DEGS1, FKBP11, SLC3A2), and the TF T-bet. Their analyses showed that IL-2-activated CD16+ NK cells overexpress several genes (OX40 ligand, CD86, Tim3, and galectins) and genes associated with cell-cycle progression and proliferation (cyclins, CDKs) and downregulate quiescence associated genes (FOXO3A, CDKN1B) [55].

3. Network of NK-Lymphocyte

After NK-cell is activated by N-cell receptor on membrane signaling proteins as demonstrated at Fig. (**6B**), a network of NK-cell cascades so that the NK-cells produce cytotoxicity function. The NK-cell signaling proteins could be involved in a combined network with at least four pathways:

1. **PI3K pathway**. The most critical pathway in NK-cells is the PI3K pathway, which is activated by CD16, NKG2D, and NCR. If the absence of MHC molecules which bind NKG2, KIR, and LIR, PI3K pathway of NK cells signaling results in NK cells killing tumor cells by the granule-mediated immune response (perforin and granzymes) and cytokine-mediated immune response (IFNγ and TNFα) [29];

2. **p38 MAPK pathway**. Activated p38 MAPK pathway which is to help protein kinases of lymphocytes [30];

3. **RAS-MEK-ERK pathway**. RAS-MEK-ERK pathway co-activate FOS response element allowing activation and production of the granule-mediated immune response [31];

4. **NF-kB pathway**. NF-kB pathway allows complete activation of the cytokine-mediated immune response (IFNγ and TNFα) [33].

GENOMIC EXPRESSION PROFILE OF NKT-CELL

1. NKT-Lymphocyte

NKT cells are a subset of T cells that co-express an $\alpha\beta$ T-cell receptor, and those are also partially similar to the function of NK cells, such as natural killer function. Although NKT cells have been discovered five subtypes, the most popular NKT cells are NKT type-1 (one of Vα24$^+$NKT), a far more limited NKT cells in diversity so-called as invariant NKT (iNKT). NKT type-1 and other NKT cells have $\alpha\beta$TCR to recognize lipids and glycolipids presented by CD1d molecules from Ag presentation cells as Fig. (**7A**) [56], which are different from those of CD8+T-cells by MHC class-1 to recognize tumor cells or class-2 (CD4+T-cell) to recognize APC. Now, most of the laboratories used Vα24$^+$NKT cells as the NKT cell marker to count NKT cells by flow cytometry (0.05% to 0.2% in healthy human).

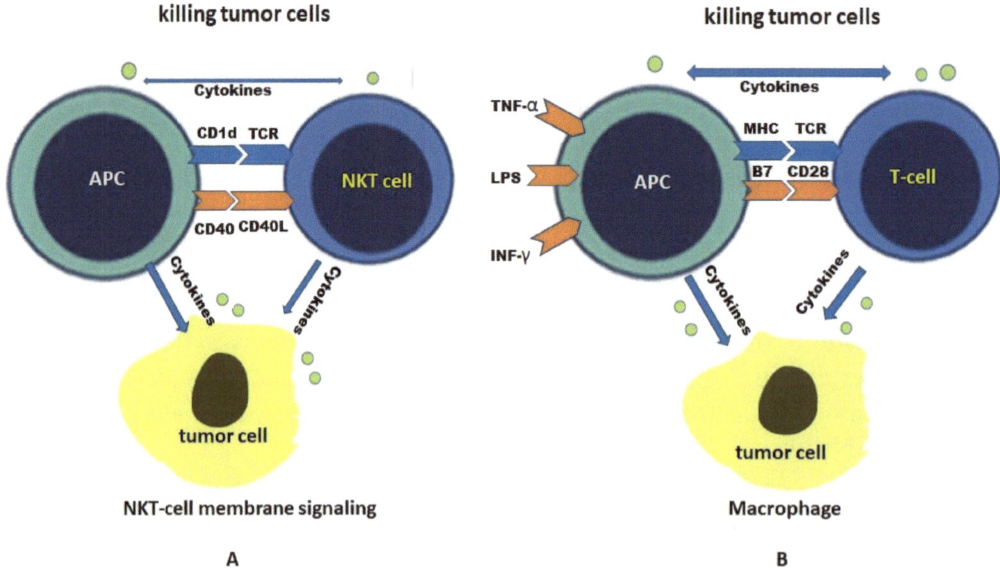

Fig. (7). NKT-cells and macrophage membrane signaling. Fig. (**7A**). NKT-cell membrane signaling protein. Thus NKT-cell is activated by tumor cells. On the surface of NKT cells, TCR molecules binding APC CD1d to activate NTK cell to kill tumor cells by cytokines while Fig. (**7B**) macrophage is activated by TNF-α, INF-γ, and LPS molecules to activate T-cells to kill tumor cell by macrophage molecules such as TNF-α and INF-γ.

2. Genomic Expression Profiles and Network of NKT-Lymphocyte

Although NKT-cells are poorly understood for NKT subtype, function and genomic profiles, 18 mice genomics files of NKT cells have been registered in GEO database (Gene Expression Omnibus in NCBI) including NKT cell development and microRNA control, NKT related arthritis, lymphoma as well as a genomic comparison between T-cell and NKT-cells. Because NKT-cell is a unique T-cell subset with the ability to regulate the immune system in response to a broad range of diseases, to study NKT-cell to control different diseases under the current knowledge of NKT-cell, some scientists begin to study, in details, control-point [57] for NTK related diseases rather than network related to genomic profiles:

1. Some scientists used a deleting-dicer technique, which generates functional miRNAs to study the iNKT cell-specific miRNA profile. The genomics results confirmed a post-transcription controlled by microRNA by comparing microRNA expression among T-cells and NKT-cells. For example, iNKT and Treg cells expressing miR-21 in iNKT and Treg cells while miR-30c, miR-106a, miR-106b, miR-150, and Let-7 family are down-regulated in both iNKT and Treg cells [58];

2. Because NKT-cell is a developmentally and functionally distinct lineage of T cells restricted by CD1d–lipid antigen complexes, CD1d-lipid microarray is used to study their response to different LPSs;

3. Because T-cell receptor (TCR) and CD1d specifically bind glycolipid antigen, mammalian glycolipid agonist ligand for NKT cells were studied their NKT-cell selection;

4. Although the NKT-cell TCRα is invariant, a more diverse TCRβ can support NKT-cell selection, the results demonstrated TCRβ contributes to the affinity of interaction with distinct glycolipid ligands to endow the NKT-cell lineage with some flexibility in the types of the antigen recognized;

5. Because two crucial control points in NKT-cell development, control-point 1 represents NKT-cell selection only in the thymus and control point-2 both in thymus and periphery, some scientists confirmed that functional transition from an immature NK1.1− (CD161− in humans) phenotype to the mature NK1.1+ stage;

6. Although the developmental relationships between subsets of functionally distinct mature NKT cells are not well understood, some subsets including CD4+, CD4−CD8−, and CD8 NKT cells and others are going to study control-point by other cells and factors that regulate these additional differentiation steps;

7. Because a broad range of secreted and intracellular signaling factors have been identified that are selectively important for NKT-cell development, some cytokines from NKT-cell have been discovered, such as IL-15, CSF, NF-κB family members (SLAM and FYN).

GENOMIC EXPRESSION PROFILE OF MACROPHAGE

1. Macrophage

Macrophages are an extremely diverse cell population, even in homeostasis. They infiltrate and reside in all of our organs and the local microenvironment. These different compartments play a critical role in establishing and maintaining this diversity of macrophages. Macrophage has two subtypes, M1 responses to inflammatory signals (IFNγ and LPS) while M2 responses to IL4 and IL13 so that M2 (anti-inflammatory role) could be required by tumor growth called as a tumor-associated macrophage (TAM) which has been demonstrated to secrete pro-tumoral signals [59, 60]. However, the macrophages are receptors activated by IFN-γ, TNF-α, and LPS as Fig. (**7B**) [61]. After they are activated, macrophage's MHC class II with Ag peptides bind to TCR of CD4+T-cells to process T-cell receptor signaling pathways.

2. Genomic Expression Profiles and Network of Macrophages

Macrophage phenotypes vary primarily based on their location, developmental origin, local microenvironment, and genetic and epigenetic situation, and thus now at least 23 genomics profiles are registered in GEO including those from different inhibitors or inducers such as IL-27 and IL-17A, those of differentiation from monocyte to macrophage and those of different responses to different diseases [62].

The network of macrophage is so complicated that scientists focus on a basic process known as polarization (activation in tissue-resident and circulating monocyte-derived macrophages with their other changes) [63]. M1 is polarized to the inflammatory pathway processed by IFN-γ and LPS characterized by their transcriptional, morphological, and secretory profiles. Gene expression changes of M1 include the upregulation of Nos2 and the secretion of pro-inflammatory signals, such as IL6 and IL12 [64] while alternatively activated macrophages (known as AAMs) or M2 macrophages are polarized by anti-inflammatory signals, such as IL4 and IL13 and upregulate genes (Arg1, Mrc1, and Cd163). Scientists further discovered that M2 macrophages process Notch (and not to Stat6) signaling with their IL4 and IL13 to be induced into M2 macrophages [65, 66]. Although M2 macrophages favor tumor growth, the repolarization of M2 of phenotypes into M1 macrophages has successfully produced anti-tumoral responses.

CONCLUSION

Immune cells play pivot roles in immune responses to tumor cells and control of the immune regulations, including response to tumor disease and regulation against tumor-specific or tumor-associated cells. The emergence of genomics with bioinformatic analysis allows defining gene expression in lymphocytes to realize their networks from different types of immune cells, even though a few genomic files are not transparent. The genomic expression profiles by microarray and RNA-seq techniques can explore functional interactions between genomics and tumor disease-specific biomarkers by integrating with clinical bioinformatics analysis. The present chapter reviews the signaling membrane proteins on lymphocytes to highlight the genomic profiles of lymphocyte's response to tumor diseases; and then, we introduce the potential significance of network-related personalized immunotherapy from the current genomic profiles of lymphocytes and discuss the value of the currently available genomics data to perform personalized immunotherapy.

On other hands, in the previous and below-mentioned chapter, DNA lever change such as SNPs or DRC (an innate DNA repair capacity) is introduced to control multi-stage carcinogenesis so that a suboptimal DRC or SNPs in peripheral lymphocytes is reported as a cancer susceptibility marker and functional response to DNA damage sensing, cell-cycle checkpoint as well as DNA repair [67 - 69]. Because the level of gene/protein expressions in lymphocytes indirectly demonstrates DNA change (such as DRC levels or SNPs), the phenotypes of genomics can support the level of DNA damage or repair in affected or unaffected lymphocytes.

Moreover, immune cells such as CD8$^+$ T cells are considered as the major players in immune responses against cancer with cytotoxic activity by releasing various cytokines and granules. If we understand the genomic profiles-related network of the immune cells, we can discover network change from genomics expression of patients, finally defining resting genes to activated CD8+T-cells, a key to perform personalized immunotherapy [70].

As described above, personalized immunotherapy relies on a change of genetics information and genomics profiles of T-cells and tumor cells of an individual patient. Eventually, the genomic/genetic database with their network linking drug banks are established, medical doctors can readily use patient genetic/genomic file to decide types of immune cells (such as TIL, NK, CAR-T-cells or others) and decide the type of inducers or inhibitors (based on genomics data) to treat or target *ex vivo* cultured immune cells to opt for undergoing personalized immunotherapy of individual patient with tumor disease.

CONSENT FOR PUBLICATION

The authors declare no financial interests.

CONFLICT OF INTEREST

The authors confirm that the content of this chapter has no conflict of interest.

ACKNOWLEDGEMENTS

We had set up single-cell methods to analyze genomic profiles, including CD3+, CD3+CD8+ from liver cancer during 1999-2007 when we worked in Case Western Reserve University. WZ and YQ both were Ph.D. students during the period, ML and AD were research assistant. BL set up a single cell genomic technique to analyze the immune cells, and GL set up bioinformatics analysis. The research was previously supported by National Cancer Institute IRG-91-0-2-09, USA (to BL).

Mention of trade names or commercial products in this article is solely to provide specific information and does not imply recommendation.

REFERENCES

[1]   Trabolsi A, Arumov A, Schatz JHT. T Cell-Activating Bispecific Antibodies in Cancer Therapy. J Immunol 2019; 203(3): 585-92.
[http://dx.doi.org/10.4049/jimmunol.1900496] [PMID: 31332079]

[2]   Lee JY, Han AR, Lee DR. T Lymphocyte Development and Activation in Humanized Mouse Model. Dev Reprod 2019; 23(2): 79-92.
[http://dx.doi.org/10.12717/DR.2019.23.2.079] [PMID: 31321348]

[3]   Vitale M, Cantoni C, Della Chiesa M, *et al.* An Historical Overview: The Discovery of How NK Cells Can Kill Enemies, Recruit Defense Troops, and More. Front Immunol 2019; 10: 1415.
[http://dx.doi.org/10.3389/fimmu.2019.01415] [PMID: 31316503]

[4]   Torralba D, Martín-Cófreces NB, Sanchez-Madrid F. Mechanisms of polarized cell-cell communication of T lymphocytes. Immunol Lett 2019; 209: 11-20.
[http://dx.doi.org/10.1016/j.imlet.2019.03.009] [PMID: 30954509]

[5]   Varani M, Auletta S, Signore A, Galli F. State of the Art of Natural Killer Cell Imaging: A Systematic Review. Cancers (Basel) 2019; 11(7): E967.
[http://dx.doi.org/10.3390/cancers11070967] [PMID: 31324064]

[6]   Fike AJ, Kumova OK, Carey AJ. Dissecting the defects in the neonatal CD8$^+$ T-cell response. J Leukoc Biol 2019; 106(5): 1051-61.
[http://dx.doi.org/10.1002/JLB.5RU0319-105R] [PMID: 31260598]

[7]   Park SL, Gebhardt T, Mackay LK. Tissue-Resident Memory T Cells in Cancer Immunosurveillance. Trends Immunol 2019; 4906(19): 5-30125.

[8]   Leclerc M, Mezquita L, Guillebot De Nerville G, *et al.* Recent advances in lung cancer immunotherapy: Input of t-cell epitopes associated with impaired peptide processing. Front Immunol 2019; 10: 1505.
[http://dx.doi.org/10.3389/fimmu.2019.01505] [PMID: 31333652]

[9]   Khavari P. Cytotoxic cellular mediators of the immune response to neoplasia: a review. Yale J Biol Med 1987; 60(5): 409-19.
[PMID: 3321723]

[10]   Quaranta V, Schmid MC. Macrophage-Mediated Subversion of Anti-Tumour Immunity. Cells 2019; 8(7): E747.
[http://dx.doi.org/10.3390/cells8070747] [PMID: 31331034]

[11]   Lin Y, Xu J, Lan H. Tumor-associated macrophages in tumor metastasis: biological roles and clinical therapeutic applications. J Hematol Oncol 2019; 12(1): 76.
[http://dx.doi.org/10.1186/s13045-019-0760-3] [PMID: 31300030]

[12]   Neamatallah T. Mitogen-Activated Protein Kinase Pathway: A Critical Regulator in Tumor-associated Macrophage Polarization. J Microsc Ultrastruct 2019; 7(2): 53-6.
[http://dx.doi.org/10.4103/JMAU.JMAU_68_18] [PMID: 31293885]

[13]   Mahlbacher GE, Reihmer KC, Frieboes HB. Mathematical modeling of tumor-immune cell interactions. J Theor Biol 2019; 469: 47-60.
[http://dx.doi.org/10.1016/j.jtbi.2019.03.002] [PMID: 30836073]

[14]   de Mey S, Jiang H, Wang H, *et al.* Potential of memory T cells in bridging preoperative chemoradiation and immunotherapy in rectal cancer. Radiother Oncol 2018; 127(3): 361-9.
[http://dx.doi.org/10.1016/j.radonc.2018.04.003] [PMID: 29871814]

[15]   Rezalotfi A, Ahmadian E, Aazami H, Solgi G, Ebrahimi M. Gastric Cancer Stem Cells Effect on

Th17/Treg Balance; A Bench to Beside Perspective. Front Oncol 2019; 9: 226.
[http://dx.doi.org/10.3389/fonc.2019.00226] [PMID: 31024835]

[16]   Copsel S, Wolf D, Komanduri KV, Levy RB. The promise of CD4⁻FoxP3⁺ regulatory T-cell manipulation *in vivo*: applications for allogeneic hematopoietic stem cell transplantation. Haematologica 2019; 104(7): 1309-21.
[http://dx.doi.org/10.3324/haematol.2018.198838] [PMID: 31221786]

[17]   Raverdeau M, Christofi M, Malara A, *et al.* Retinoic acid-induced autoantigen-specific type 1 regulatory T cells suppress autoimmunity. EMBO Rep 2019; 20(5): e47121.
[http://dx.doi.org/10.15252/embr.201847121] [PMID: 30894405]

[18]   Chen X, Du Y, Lin X, Qian Y, Zhou T, Huang Z. CD4+CD25+ regulatory T cells in tumor immunity. Int Immunopharmacol 2016; 34: 244-9.
[http://dx.doi.org/10.1016/j.intimp.2016.03.009] [PMID: 26994448]

[19]   Huff WX, Kwon JH, Henriquez M, Fetcko K, Dey M. The Evolving Role of CD8⁺CD28⁻ Immunosenescent T Cells in Cancer Immunology. Int J Mol Sci 2019; 20(11): E2810.
[http://dx.doi.org/10.3390/ijms20112810] [PMID: 31181772]

[20]   Bano A, Pera A, Almoukayed A, *et al.* CD28 null CD4 T-cell expansions in autoimmune disease suggest a link with cytomegalovirus infection F1000Res 8 pii: F1000 Faculty Rev-327 2019.

[21]   Wu X, Gu Z, Chen Y, *et al.* Application of PD-1 Blockade in Cancer Immunotherapy. Comput Struct Biotechnol J 2019; 17: 661-74.
[http://dx.doi.org/10.1016/j.csbj.2019.03.006] [PMID: 31205619]

[22]   Heath BR, Michmerhuizen NL, Donnelly CR, *et al.* Head and Neck Cancer Immunotherapy beyond the Checkpoint Blockade. J Dent Res 2019; 98(10): 1073-80.
[http://dx.doi.org/10.1177/0022034519864112] [PMID: 31340724]

[23]   Wartewig T, Ruland J. PD-1 Tumor Suppressor Signaling in T Cell Lymphomas. Trends Immunol 2019; 40(5): 403-14.
[http://dx.doi.org/10.1016/j.it.2019.03.005] [PMID: 30979616]

[24]   Kurachi M. CD8⁺ T cell exhaustion. Semin Immunopathol 2019; 41(3): 327-37.
[http://dx.doi.org/10.1007/s00281-019-00744-5] [PMID: 30989321]

[25]   Brunner-Weinzierl MC, Rudd CE. CTLA-4 and PD-1 Control of T-Cell Motility and Migration: Implications for Tumor Immunotherapy. Front Immunol 2018; 9: 2737.
[http://dx.doi.org/10.3389/fimmu.2018.02737] [PMID: 30542345]

[26]   D'Arrigo P, Tufano M, Rea A, Vigorito V, *et al.* Manipulation of the immune system for cancer defeat: a focus on the T cell inhibitory checkpoint molecules. Curr Med Chem 2018.
[http://dx.doi.org/10.2174/0929867325666181106114421] [PMID: 30398102]

[27]   Numakura K, Horikawa Y, Kamada S, *et al.* Efficacy of anti-PD-1 antibody nivolumab in Japanese patients with metastatic renal cell carcinoma: A retrospective multicenter analysis. Mol Clin Oncol 2019; 11(3): 320-4.
[http://dx.doi.org/10.3892/mco.2019.1887] [PMID: 31341623]

[28]   Liu WS, Jin WY, Zhou L, *et al.* Structure based design of selective SHP2 inhibitors by De novo design, synthesis and biological evaluation. J Comput Aided Mol Des 2019; 33(8): 759-74.
[http://dx.doi.org/10.1007/s10822-019-00213-z] [PMID: 31300938]

[29]   Pompura SL, Dominguez-Villar M. The PI3K/AKT signaling pathway in regulatory T-cell development, stability, and function. J Leukoc Biol 2018.
[http://dx.doi.org/10.1002/JLB.2MIR0817-349R] [PMID: 29357116]

[30]   Farber DL. Biochemical signaling pathways for memory T cell recall. Semin Immunol 2009; 21(2): 84-91.
[http://dx.doi.org/10.1016/j.smim.2009.02.003] [PMID: 19298946]

[31]   Jun JE, Rubio I, Roose JP. Regulation of ras exchange factors and cellular localization of ras activation by lipid messengers in T cells. Front Immunol 2013; 4: 239.
[http://dx.doi.org/10.3389/fimmu.2013.00239] [PMID: 24027568]

[32]   Alshamsan A. Paradoxical signaling pathways in developing thymocytes. J Pharm Pharm Sci 2011; 14(3): 378-86.
[http://dx.doi.org/10.18433/J3CG6G] [PMID: 22202221]

[33]   Fulford TS, Ellis D, Gerondakis S. Understanding the Roles of the NF-κB Pathway in Regulatory T Cell Development, Differentiation and Function. Prog Mol Biol Transl Sci 2015; 136: 57-67.
[http://dx.doi.org/10.1016/bs.pmbts.2015.08.002] [PMID: 26615092]

[34]   Srikanth S, Woo JS, Sun Z, Gwack Y. Immunological Disorders: Regulation of Ca^{2+} Signaling in T Lymphocytes. Adv Exp Med Biol 2017; 993: 397-424.
[http://dx.doi.org/10.1007/978-3-319-57732-6_21] [PMID: 28900926]

[35]   Topalian SL, Muul LM, Solomon D, Rosenberg SA. Expansion of human tumor infiltrating lymphocytes for use in immunotherapy trials. J Immunol Methods 1987; 102(1): 127-41.
[http://dx.doi.org/10.1016/S0022-1759(87)80018-2] [PMID: 3305708]

[36]   Li B, Shen DH. Preliminary Study on the Resting Status of Tumor-infiltrating Lymphocytes. Chinese Microbiology and Immunology 1994; 14(6): 399-402.

[37]   Li BR, Tong SQ, Hu BY, *et al.* [Study on the influence of enzymatic digestion upon tumor-infiltrating lymphocytes]. Shi Yan Sheng Wu Xue Bao 1994; 27(1): 103-7.
[PMID: 8042406]

[38]   Li B, Tong SQ, Zhang XH, Zhu YM, *et al.* Research on TIL proliferation, phenotype and lethality of human malignant solid tumors. Modern Immunology 1994; p. 05.

[39]   Li B, Perabekam S, Liu G, Yin M, Song S, Larson A. Experimental and bioinformatics comparison of gene expression between T cells from TIL of liver cancer and T cells from UniGene. J Gastroenterol 2002; 37(4): 275-82.
[http://dx.doi.org/10.1007/s005350200035] [PMID: 11993511]

[40]   Kochi M, Iwamoto T, Niikura N, *et al.* Tumour-infiltrating lymphocytes (TILs)-related genomic signature predicts chemotherapy response in breast cancer. Breast Cancer Res Treat 2018; 167(1): 39-47.
[http://dx.doi.org/10.1007/s10549-017-4502-3] [PMID: 28905250]

[41]   Vanoli A, Di Sabatino A, Martino M, *et al.* Small bowel carcinomas in celiac or Crohn's disease: distinctive histophenotypic, molecular and histogenetic patterns. Mod Pathol 2017; 30(10): 1453-66.
[http://dx.doi.org/10.1038/modpathol.2017.40] [PMID: 28664941]

[42]   Zhang W, Ding J, Qu Y, *et al.* Genomic expression analysis by single-cell mRNA differential display of quiescent CD8 T cells from tumour-infiltrating lymphocytes obtained from *in vivo* liver tumours. Immunology 2009; 127(1): 83-90.
[http://dx.doi.org/10.1111/j.1365-2567.2008.02926.x] [PMID: 18778280]

[43]   Xu Y, Hu H, Zheng J, Li B. Feasibility of whole RNA sequencing from single-cell mRNA amplification. Genet Res Int 2013; 2013: 724124.
[http://dx.doi.org/10.1155/2013/724124] [PMID: 24455282]

[44]   Li M, Deng Q, Zhang L, He S, Rong J, Zheng F. The pretreatment lymphocyte to monocyte ratio predicts clinical outcome for patients with urological cancers: A meta-analysis. Pathol Res Pract 2019; 215(1): 5-11.
[http://dx.doi.org/10.1016/j.prp.2018.10.026] [PMID: 30401580]

[45]   Hernberg M. Lymphocyte subsets as prognostic markers for cancer patients receiving immunomodulative therapy. Med Oncol 1999; 16(3): 145-53.
[http://dx.doi.org/10.1007/BF02906126] [PMID: 10523794]

[46]   Palmer C, Diehn M, Alizadeh AA, Brown PO. Cell-type specific gene expression profiles of leukocytes in human peripheral blood. BMC Genomics 2006; 7: 115.
[http://dx.doi.org/10.1186/1471-2164-7-115] [PMID: 16704732]

[47]   Lee MS, Hanspers K, Barker CS, Korn AP, McCune JM. Gene expression profiles during human CD4+ T cell differentiation. Int Immunol 2004; 16(8): 1109-24.
[http://dx.doi.org/10.1093/intimm/dxh112] [PMID: 15210650]

[48]   Mowery YM, Lanasa MC. Clinical aspects of monoclonal B-cell lymphocytosis. Cancer Contr 2012; 19(1): 8-17.
[http://dx.doi.org/10.1177/107327481201900102] [PMID: 22143058]

[49]   Cai X, Zhang L, Wei W. Regulatory B cells in inflammatory diseases and tumor. Int Immunopharmacol 2019; 67: 281-6.
[http://dx.doi.org/10.1016/j.intimp.2018.12.007] [PMID: 30572252]

[50]   Rossetti RAM, Lorenzi NPC, Yokochi K, *et al.* B lymphocytes can be activated to act as antigen presenting cells to promote anti-tumor responses. PLoS One 2018; 13(7): e0199034.
[http://dx.doi.org/10.1371/journal.pone.0199034] [PMID: 29975708]

[51]   Braylan RC, Orfao A, Borowitz MJ, Davis BH. Optimal number of reagents required to evaluate hematolymphoid neoplasias: results of an international consensus meeting. Cytometry 2001; 46(1): 23-7.
[http://dx.doi.org/10.1002/1097-0320(20010215)46:1<23::AID-CYTO1033>3.0.CO;2-Z]   [PMID: 11241503]

[52]   Dörner T, Lipsky PE. Signalling pathways in B cells: implications for autoimmunity. Curr Top Microbiol Immunol 2006; 305: 213-40.
[http://dx.doi.org/10.1007/3-540-29714-6_11] [PMID: 16724808]

[53]   Lima M. Extranodal NK/T cell lymphoma and aggressive NK cell leukaemia: evidence for their origin on CD56+bright CD16-/+dim NK cells. Pathology 2015; 47(6): 503-14.
[http://dx.doi.org/10.1097/PAT.0000000000000275] [PMID: 26166665]

[54]   Sivori S, Vacca P, Del Zotto G, Munari E, Mingari MC, Moretta L. Human NK cells: surface receptors, inhibitory checkpoints, and translational applications. Cell Mol Immunol 2019; 16(5): 430-41.
[http://dx.doi.org/10.1038/s41423-019-0206-4] [PMID: 30778167]

[55]   Wang F, Tian Z, Wei H. Genomic expression profiling of NK cells in health and disease. Eur J Immunol 2015; 45(3): 661-78.
[http://dx.doi.org/10.1002/eji.201444998] [PMID: 25476835]

[56]   Shissler SC, Webb TJ. The ins and outs of type I iNKT cell development. Mol Immunol 2019; 105: 116-30.
[http://dx.doi.org/10.1016/j.molimm.2018.09.023] [PMID: 30502719]

[57]   Podbielska M, O'Keeffe J, Hogan EL. Autoimmunity in multiple sclerosis: role of sphingolipids, invariant NKT cells and other immune elements in control of inflammation and neurodegeneration. J Neurol Sci 2018; 385: 198-214.
[http://dx.doi.org/10.1016/j.jns.2017.12.022] [PMID: 29406905]

[58]   Fedeli M, Napolitano A, Wong MP, *et al.* Dicer-dependent microRNA pathway controls invariant NKT cell development. J Immunol 2009; 183(4): 2506-12.
[http://dx.doi.org/10.4049/jimmunol.0901361] [PMID: 19625646]

[59]   França GM, Carmo AFD, Costa Neto H, Andrade ALDL, Lima KC, Galvão HC. Macrophages subpopulations in chronic periapical lesions according to clinical and morphological aspects. Braz Oral Res 2019; 33: e047.
[http://dx.doi.org/10.1590/1807-3107bor-2019.vol33.0047] [PMID: 31141038]

[60]   Jeong H, Hwang I, Kang SH, Shin HC, Kwon SY. Tumor-Associated Macrophages as Potential

Prognostic Biomarkers of Invasive Breast Cancer. J Breast Cancer 2019; 22(1): 38-51.
[http://dx.doi.org/10.4048/jbc.2019.22.e5] [PMID: 30941232]

[61]   Wang J, Pendurthi UR, Rao LVM. 2019.

[62]   Rolvering C, Zimmer AD, Kozar I, *et al.* Crosstalk between different family members: IL27 recapitulates IFNγ responses in HCC cells, but is inhibited by IL6-type cytokines. Biochim Biophys Acta Mol Cell Res 2017; 1864(3): 516-26.
[http://dx.doi.org/10.1016/j.bbamcr.2016.12.006] [PMID: 27939431]

[63]   Zhu Y, Dai J, Yao X, *et al.* [IL-16 aggravates dextran sulfate sodium (DSS)-induced mouse inflammatory bowel disease by promoting M1 polarization of macrophages]. Xibao Yu Fenzi Mianyixue Zazhi 2018; 34(8): 695-701.
[PMID: 30384867]

[64]   Wei W, Li ZP, Bian ZX, Han QB. *Astragalus* Polysaccharide RAP Induces Macrophage Phenotype Polarization to M1 *via* the Notch Signaling Pathway. Molecules 2019; 24(10): E2016.
[http://dx.doi.org/10.3390/molecules24102016] [PMID: 31137782]

[65]   Sakamoto T, Obara N, Nishikii H, *et al.* Notch Signaling in Nestin-Expressing Cells in the Bone Marrow Maintains Erythropoiesis *via* Macrophage Integrity. Stem Cells 2019; 37(7): 924-36.
[http://dx.doi.org/10.1002/stem.3011] [PMID: 30932281]

[66]   Jiandong L, Yang Y, Peng J, *et al.* Trichosanthes kirilowii lectin ameliorates streptozocin-induced kidney injury *via* modulation of the balance between M1/M2 phenotype macrophage. Biomed Pharmacother 2019; 109: 93-102.
[http://dx.doi.org/10.1016/j.biopha.2018.10.060] [PMID: 30396096]

[67]   Nagel ZD, Chaim IA, Samson LD. Inter-individual variation in DNA repair capacity: a need for multi-pathway functional assays to promote translational DNA repair research. DNA Repair (Amst) 2014; 19: 199-213.
[http://dx.doi.org/10.1016/j.dnarep.2014.03.009] [PMID: 24780560]

[68]   Matta J, Morales L, Ortiz C, *et al.* Estrogen Receptor Expression Is Associated with DNA Repair Capacity in Breast Cancer. PLoS One 2016; 11(3): e0152422.
[http://dx.doi.org/10.1371/journal.pone.0152422] [PMID: 27032101]

[69]   Guo Y, Yu H, Samuels DC, Yue W, Ness S, Zhao YY. Single-nucleotide variants in human RNA: RNA editing and beyond. Brief Funct Genomics 2019; 18(1): 30-9.
[http://dx.doi.org/10.1093/bfgp/ely032] [PMID: 30312373]

[70]   Li B, Hu HL, Ding JQ, Yan D, Yang LM. Functional cell-proliferation and differentiation by system modeling for cell therapy. International Journal of Latest Research in Science and Technology 2015; 4(2): 180-7.

CHAPTER 3

Immunoassay of Personalized Immunotherapy

Li-Hua Jiang[1] and **Biaoru Li**[1,2,*]

[1] *Departments of Immunology and Microbiology, Shanghai Second Medical University, Shanghai*

[2] *Georgia Cancer Center and Department of Pediatrics, Medical College at GA, Augusta, GA 30912, USA*

Abstract: The immune response is a dynamic reaction of a body, allowing to fight against tumor cells. However, an unbalanced host immune response is highlighted in tumor disease. Abnormal responses lead to autoimmune diseases, whereas low responses favor opportunistic infections and host with tumor cells. The conflicting situations make it difficult to arrange an appropriate immunoassay for immunotherapy. Before human genomics decode in 2004, testing the immune response with this profile of patients remains a challenge. This is due to individual variability so that it impedes immunoassay for personalized immunotherapy. After the fifteen years' effort, immunoassays are committed to personalized immunotherapy of tumor diseases for precise prediction/prevention, immune targeting therapy, and personalized immunotherapy. Now, identifying new targets at the protein level, SNP at the DNA level, and mRNA expression at the RNA level may guide a new generation of immunoassay. The techniques to test the immune responses to tumor diseases are currently being studied, but they still have many influence factors such as technical standardization and technique selection, and interpretation, and therefore, the chapter gives a comprehensive insight into the immunoassay for personalized immunotherapy.

Keywords: Cytotoxic T-cell assay (CTL), ELISA (Enzyme-linked immunosorbent assay), Immunoassay, Single Nucleic Polymorphism (SNP), Targets.

INTRODUCTION

The immune system plays an essential function in protecting human beings from external factors such as biological factors (bacteria and virus infection), chemical and physically stimulating, as well as internal factors such as abnormal cells from mutant genes and epigenetics changes, helping the maintenance of the functional balance of cells and tissues. A quiescent response, inborn or acquired, may lead to host easy to suffer from tumor diseases [1].

* **Corresponding author Biaoru Li:** Georgia Cancer Center and Department of Pediatrics, Medical College at GA, Augusta, GA 30912, USA; Tel: 440-317-1443; E-mail: bli@augusta.edu

Defined as host quiescent response to tumor cells in tumor disease, the immune system cannot produce enough immune cells, immune factors, and functional responses or cannot affect specific kill tumor cells by macrophage, T-cell, B-cells with their target factors [2]. Current assaying fundamental of anti-tumor responses are involved in the complex process including assay of immune cells, immune factors, and immune functions, which contributes evaluation of the immune system of patients with tumor diseases, allowing them to monitor the immune change, so that this may help medical doctors to select an optimal immune medication of personalized care.

However, monitoring the immune system is individual and complex interactions between its components [3]. Even if counting cells, measuring soluble or cell surface biomarkers are to assess the immune system, these routine assays cannot demonstrate complex interactions without host system biology. After human genomics decode, evaluating the immune response with this profile is the possibility from the genomic level for an individual patient [4]. Following fifteen years' effort after the human genome decode, immunoassays are undertaken to personalized immunotherapy of tumor diseases, such as precise prediction/prevention, immune checkpoint blocking (ICB) therapy, and personalized active/adoptive immunotherapy. Now, identifying new immune targets at the protein level, SNP at the DNA level, and mRNA expression at the RNA level of immune dysfunction with tumor diseases are going to guide targeted immune therapies [5].

In the chapter, we introduce three sections for immunoassays of cancer immunotherapy: (1) assays record a response *in vivo/ex vivo/in vitro* or response to a given stimulation; (2) assay immune targets (ICB) related immunotherapy with genomics support; (3) technical standardization, biomarkers selection, and systematic interpretation. In the conclusion part, we present an immunoassay selection of personalized immunotherapy for an individual patient.

BASIC RECORD OF IMMUNE FUNCTION AND RESPONSE

A few of immunoassay strategies are currently being recorded in clinical immunotherapy for tumor diseases. These assays include (I) *in vivo* delayed-type hypersensitivity (DTH); (II) *in vitro* measuring T-cell number/T-cell function by ELISA and flow cytometry analysis of cytokine expression and CTL function; (III) *in vitro* measuring specific T-cells with their responses by assay tetramer and complementarity determining region (CDR); (IV) PCR-based detection of T-cell receptors, genes, and cytokine productions; (V) Ab assay for tumor-associated antigens or other antigens.

Delayed-Type Hypersensitivity *In Vivo*

DTH test, a traditional method using antigen in the form of soluble protein alone or as antigen loaded onto antigen-presenting cells, is injected intradermally, measuring the diameter of erythema after 48–72 hours [6]. CD4+T-cells that recognize the antigen presented on local antigen-presenting cells induce the response by releasing cytokines, increasing vascular permeability, and recruiting monocytes to the site. DTH assay can support the immune analysis of cancer vaccines [7]. The ability to isolate, expand, and assess the phenotype or function of antigen-specific T-cells from skin biopsies of DTH sites may serve as an additional strategy to evaluate antigen-specific immune responses [8].

Measures of Immune Function *Ex Vivo*

Functional assays of T-cells include the T-cell number and functional cytokine production measured by ELISA and FACS, T-cell proliferation, and CD8+T-cell cytotoxicity (CTL).

1. Detection of T-cell Number with Intracellular Cytokines by Flow Cytometry

After T-cells are harvested and stimulated, fluorochrome-conjugated anti-CD4, and anti-CD8 antibodies to allow to gate T-cells and anti-CD69 to monitor the activation of T cells by FACS [9]. Different patterns of cytokine secretion in the T-cells could be used to study memory/effector T-cells with different immune functions. For example, IL-2, IFN-γ, and TNF-α secreted by helper-1 and IL-4, IL-5, IL-6, IL-10, and IL-13 secreted by T helper-2 so that the measurement can monitor immune cells with their functional responses from peripheral blood, lymph nodes and tumor tissues [10].

2. Detection of Secreted Cytokines by ELISA Assays

Cytokine secretion by T-cells response to antigen can be detected by measuring either cytokine production directly from blood or T-cells from PBMC are incubated with antigen measured by an ELISA [11]. Although current techniques can run 15 cytokines in a single sample, it is rarely used to evaluate the cytokine profile of different T-cells in the site of tumor tissues. However, an ELISPOT assay represents one single cell secreting the cytokine of interest, so that antigen-specific T-cell is determined by the number of spots (cytokine-secreting cells) or evaluated by the number of cells placed into the well with reliable detection known-quantities of antigen-specific T-cells with cytokine secretion [12]. At present, computerized methods provide an ELISPOT assay high throughput screening with antigen-specific T-cell responses by using a large-scale analysis.

3. Lymphoproliferation Assay

In our early TIL researches and clinical application, we had used the lymphoproliferation assay to study the TIL function [13]. TILs are mixed with tumor cells, after 72–120 h, [^{3}H] thymidine was added, and DNA synthesis (as a measure of proliferation) was quantified by using a gamma counter to measure the amount of radiolabeled thymidine incorporated into the DNA. The proliferation assay has been used frequently in clinical trials to compare T-cell responses before and after immunization *in vivo* or before and after T-cell culture and inducing *in vitro* [14].

4. CTL and Quantifying CTL

In our TIL researches with the clinical application, we often used TIL CTL assay to screen and determine TIL efficacy [15]. The direct cytotoxicity assays measure the ability of CD8+ CTLs to lyse autogenous tumor or tumor cell-line so that the result is thought to be an important indicator for *ex vivo* anti-tumor activity. We had previously used ^{51}Cr release to measure CTL, whereas, currently, MTT assay protocol with the available kit has routinely used the CTL micro-cytotoxicity [16]. Additionally, limiting dilution analysis (LDA), a quantitative assay for CTL, is more correlated with T-cell numbers from functional activity. LDA analyses involve the serial dilution of T-cells in a very large number of wells, followed by an *in vitro* stimulation phase and target lysis phase [17]. Poisson distribution analysis determines the results of wells at a T-cell dilution.

Measures of Antigen-Specific Immune Responses *In Vitro/Ex Vivo*

1. Peptide MHC Tetramers

TCR staining has been used for T-cell antigen-specific immune response determined by flow cytometric or PCR-based techniques. During flow cytometric analysis, a scientist can gate CD8+T-cells and assay expression of antigen-specific TCRs. The usefulness of tetramers is derived from studies of viral epitope-specific CTLs so that T-cells specific for CMV and EBV demonstrated that CD8+ T-cells were specific for peptides representing these antigens [18]. Recently, it has become possible to visualize antigen-specific T-cells under flow cytometry by using fluorescently labeled multimeric MHC peptide complexes that bind specifically to antigen-specific T-cells. Some reports have found a positive MHC tetramer related to CTL cytotoxicity in immune assays, and thus, the intensity of staining of CD8+T-cells with peptide MHC tetramers appears to correlate with T-cell affinity to antigen [19]. Several recent studies also demonstrated the utility of flow cytometric analysis using peptide MHC tetramers to quantitate CD8+T-cells specific for tumor antigens or control antigens used frequently in immunotherapy protocols. These selected T cells were cloned for the analysis, and were further shown to respond to the specific antigen, including cytokine-producing [20]. Moreover, the peptide/MHC tetramers for quantitating antigen-specific T-cells can demonstrate the CD45 memory phenotype [21]. In general, tetramers FACS is important to assess antigen-specific T-cells, memory T-cells, and cytokine expression T-cells as well.

2. TCR Complementarity Determining Region

Antigen-specific T-cells can be detected by PCR techniques for detecting a restricted TCR repertoire by sequencing the complementarity determining the region (CDR) [22]. One of CDR, CDR3, encodes the highly polymorphic portion of the TCR, mainly responsible for recognizing peptide-MHC complexes. Some studies in melanoma patients and renal cell carcinoma patients have confirmed a restricted TCR gene for immune responses [23]. At present, a fluorescence-based method for CDR3 length analysis can support the determination of polyclonal, oligoclonal, and monoclonal T-cells [24].

Measurement of Cytokine mRNA

Quantitative real-time PCR is a highly accurate method for measuring the levels of genes of interest in sample RNA. We have routinely applied the technique to the analysis of cytokine mRNA from fresh or cryopreserved specimens of patients as our reports [25]. We have also used the quantitative real-time PCR to study quiescent T-cells of TIL and their activity for more than 20 years. Recently, some scientists used the technique to detect antigen-specific T-cell responses from melanoma patients after clinical trials of melanoma peptide-based vaccines. Their results showed that quantitative real-time PCR could be used to detect antigen-specific T-cell responses in peripheral blood samples [26].

Based on the description above, immunoassays can evaluate immune responses against tumor cells. In addition, the selection of immunoassay relies on the requirement and selection of immunotherapy. For example, T-cell adoptive immunotherapy is subject to using T-cell proliferation assay and CTL assay, while active immunotherapy or TCR T-cell immunotherapy can use MHC-peptide tetramer and ELISPOT assay. Moreover, according to reported data obtained from MHC-peptide tetramer staining and those obtained from ELISPOT assays and LDA, flow cytometric analysis of tetramer is more sensitive than those of LDA for CTL precursors and ELISPOT.

Measurement of Tumor Antibodies

Although the tumor antigens are undetectable in sera at the early stage of tumorigenesis, the nature of an antibody amplification response to antigens makes tumor-associated autoantibodies as promising early diagnosis in cancer. For example, lung cancers can trigger host immune responses and elicit antibodies against tumor antigens. This response occurs because of some proteins by mutated P53, misfolded overexpressed NY-ESO, and aberrantly glycosylated MUC-1. The antibodies against tumor antigens have two advantages. The first is to detect not only at initial diagnosis but also up to 5 years when cancer is diagnosed. Secondly, the Abs have long half-lives in serum with that enhancement after tumor development [27].

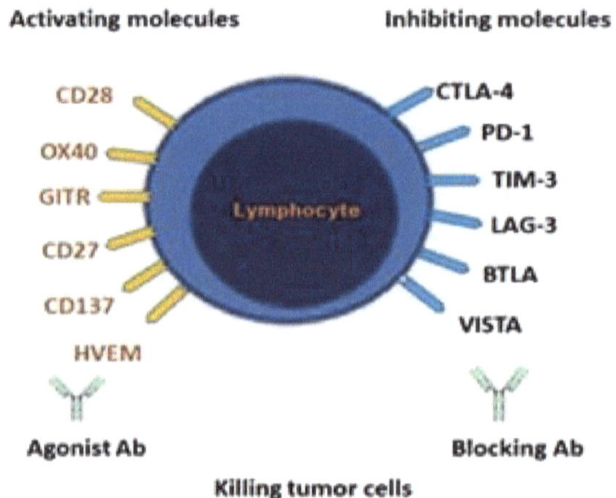

Fig. (1). T-cells Targeting Signaling.

MEASUREMENT OF IMMUNE TARGETS FOR IMMUNOTHERAPY

Inhibitory molecules such as CTLA-4, PD-1, TIM-3, and LAG-3 can be blocked to decrease T-cell exhaustion to kill tumor cells, and activating molecules such as CD28 can be used to stimulate T-cell function for kill tumor cells.

According to recent researches on targeting immunotherapy, several new targets of T-cell receptors are discovered, including inhibitory receptors and activating receptors. Inhibitory receptors such as CTLA4 (cytotoxic T-lymphocyte antigen-4), PD-1 (Programmed cell death protein 1), and TIM-3 (T cell immunoglobulin and mucin-domain containing-3) as Fig. (**1**) can actively induce T-cell exhaustion at the site of tumor [28], so that these antibodies of inhibitory receptors, called immune checkpoint blocking antibody (ICB), can be used to block to T-cell exhaustion, resulting in killing tumor cells. Now more and more data show that T-cell exhaustion plays a very important role in tumor relapses, and therefore, more ICBs are discovered for targeting therapy of tumor diseases as Table **1**. Some of them have been approved by the FDA for good clinical responses, allowing them to apply for patients [29]. Moreover, activating receptors such as CD28, CD27, CD137 are going to be studied by agonists to killing tumor cells [30]. In order to make good responses for clinical patients, a few immunoassay strategies of the new target therapy are currently being reported for tumor diseases in clinical immunotherapy.

Table 1. Different targets with molecular immunotherapy.

Targets	Agents
PD-1	Pembrolizumab, nivolumab, pidilizumab, MEDI0680, REGN2810, AMP-224, AMP-514
PD-L1	Durvalumab, atezolizumab, avelumab
PD-L2	rHIgM12B7
CTLA-4	ipilimumab,Tremelimumab,
LAG3	IMP321
OX40	MEDI6469, MEDI6383, MEDI0562, MOXR0916
GITR	TRX518
CD137	Urelumab
CD40	CP-870
CD27	Varlilumab

These assays include (I) measuring inhibitory receptors and activating receptors by immunohistochemistry (IHC) staining; (II) measuring mRNA or SNP of inhibitory receptors/activating receptors by quantitative RT-PCR and by SNP detection at DNA/RNA level; (III) measuring inhibitory receptors/activating receptors by ELISA or FACS at the protein level.

Measuring Inhibitory and Activating Receptors by IHC Staining

Several immunohistochemistry (IHC) kits with their protocols have been developed to assess inhibitory receptors, including PD-1, PD-L1, CTLA-4, which can measure expression levels in patients, who are candidates for targeting inhibitor of immunotherapy. Now, PD-L1 IHC 28-8 pharmDx kit has been approved as a diagnostic kit with Dako Autostainer Link 48 platform support [31]. After the study, the kits for melanoma, squamous cell carcinoma of the head and neck, urothelial carcinoma, nivolumab therapy have supported the target of inhibitory receptors [32]. At present, several platforms have been used the diagnosis, such as Dako Autostainer Link-48, Dako Omnis, Leica Bond-III, and

Ventana BenchMark ULTRA. For example, PD-L1 IHC 28-8 pharmDx kit on Dako Autostainer Link-48 was used to evaluate PD-L1 expression levels [33].

Although a few of IHC platforms are going to be studied on targets of inhibitory receptors/activating receptors, a good IHC platform requires measurement of (I) multiple and quantitative targets in one slide such as CTLA-4, PD-1, TIM-3 and LAG-3 for inhibitory receptors and activating receptors such as CD28, CD27, CD137; (II) sensitivity and specificity with the reports; (III) auto-reading system with computerized methods for a large-scale analysis; (IV) computerized methods providing clinical responses by high throughput targeting drugs. In order to address the questions, some scientists have studied the density and quantified the distribution of positive cells so that they can determine the associations with anti-PD-1 response reported a 56% objective response rate in patients with advanced Merkel cell carcinoma (MCC) receiving pembrolizumab [34]. Their results show that quantitative assessments of PD-1+cell and PD-L1+cell densities, as well as the geographic interactions, can correlate with clinical response.

Measurement of mRNA and SNPs in Inhibitory and Activating Receptor

Quantitative real-time PCR is a highly accurate method for measuring the levels of genes of receptors in sample RNA. We have routinely applied the technique to the analysis of cytokine mRNA from fresh or cryopreserved specimens from patients as reports [35]. The quantitative real-time PCR is going to be increasingly used to detect inhibitory and activating receptors from T-cells and tumor cells of peripheral blood samples and tumor tissues.

Moreover, genotyping SNP selection will open one new field detecting the inhibitory and activating receptor. SNP detection by TaqMan genotypes assay is going to be increasingly used to detect SNPs of inhibitory and activating receptors from T-cells and tumor cells from peripheral blood samples and tumor tissues. Several pieces of evidence have confirmed SNP in PD-1/PDL-1 related to immunotherapy response for immunotherapy. For example, a result suggested that rs2282055 and rs4143815 may be a biomarker for the efficacy of nivolumab [36].

Measuring Inhibitory Receptors by ELISA or FACS at the Cell Level

1. Detection of Inhibitory Receptors by Flow Cytometry

After T-cells are harvested and/or stimulated, fluorochrome-conjugated anti-CD4 and anti-CD8 antibodies allow to gate T-cells and anti-receptor targets to monitor receptors of T cells by FACS. Different patterns of inhibitory receptors in the T-cells could be used to study receptors assay of immunotherapy so that the measurement can monitor inhibitory receptors in peripheral blood, lymph nodes, or tumor tissues [37].

2. Detection of Inhibitory Receptors by ELISA Assays

Inhibitory and activating receptors of T-cells and tumor cells can be detected by measuring either T-cells from PBMC or TIL and primary tumor cells. Although current techniques can run several receptors in a single sample, it cannot be used to evaluate all profiles of different T-cells and tumor cells in the site of tumor tissues. An ELISPOT assay represents one single cell receptors so that T-cell is determined by the number of spots (cytokine-secreting cells) or evaluated by the number of cells placed into the well with reliable detection known quantities of T-cells and tumor cells with receptors [38]. At present, computerized methods provide high throughput screening receptors from T-cell and tumor cells with a large-scale analysis.

The three assays can determine inhibitory and activating receptors from T-cell and tumor cells. According to reported data obtained from IHC at the tissue level, quantitative real-time PCR combined with SNPs at the molecule level, and FACS staining/ELISA assays at the cell level, quantitative real-time PCR/SNPs and flow cytometric analysis is more sensitive than ELISA, while receptor data from IHC staining are very specific.

TECHNICAL CONSIDERATION AND STANDARDIZATION

Before selecting immunological assays to monitor anti-tumor immune responses, it is important to consider the performance characteristics of detecting immune responses, immune response-related with tumor diseases, and assaying-results predicting clinical outcome.

Desirable performance characteristics detecting T-cell responses include (I) adequate sensitivity and specificity; (II) measurement of reliability and reproducibility; (III) simple and rapid to perform; (IV) small quantities of specimens. As described above, tetramer analysis is highly sensitive, quick to perform while ELISA and ELISPOT plates can be prepared in bulk by using automated pipettes, plate washers, and plate readers so that large numbers can be set up efficiently. The PCR-based techniques for detecting TCR gene or cytokine mRNA transcription require the smallest quantity of specimens. The cutoff should be accepted as indicative of an effective level of immunological response with their standardization for immunological assays. Tumor cell (tumor cell line or primary tumor cells) may be measured by CTLs CD8+T-cells, so that modified cytotoxicity assays to measure target cell apoptosis for active immunotherapy by tumor vaccine, T-cell adoptive immunotherapy, and molecular targeting therapy. It is possible that currently available assays can measure a function with direct relevance to immunotherapy, demonstrating the importance in the correlation of immune response with clinical outcome.

CONCLUSION

Current immunoassay, as described above, has four clinical applications: immune prediction/prevention, molecular targeting immunotherapy, active immunotherapy, and adoptive T-cell immunotherapy.

Prediction and Prevention: Ability is to conduct a precise analysis of risk for tumor disease and then the effective prediction of immune balance in the body. Although the traditional concept of immunotherapy is involved in T-cell infused into the body to play immunotherapy, current immunoassay has prediction function as same as precision medicine. For example, the patient was discovered genetic profiles with an SNP, which is sensitive to imatinib to treat so that medical doctors can use the imatinib to administer the patient [39].

Molecular Targeting Therapy: A panel of CTLA-4, PD-1, TIM-3, and LAG-3 for inhibitory receptors and CD28, CD27, CD137 for activating receptors are going to study molecular targeting immunotherapy of tumor diseases. For example, as we mentioned above, techniques of multiple staining IHC, ELISA, and quantitative real-time PCR seem to have possibilities as a tool for molecular targeting therapy [40].

Active immunotherapy: In the near future, it will be possible to evaluate the response of the tumor vaccine if we set up a clinical index for immunoassay [41]. The immunoassay finally leads physicians to enable to estimate the right treatment on tumor vaccine for patients with tumor diseases. Several reports have indicated that TCR MHC-peptide tetramer and ELISPOT assay can measure DC cells tumor vaccines.

Adoptive T-cell immunotherapy: If T-cell proliferation assay and CD8+T-cell CTL assay are combined with data from different SNPs and genomic expression from tumor cells and T-cells, the combined results have importantly impacted on adoptive immunotherapy, such as measurement efficacy of T-cell treatment. We have reported T-cell proliferation assay and CD8+T-cell CTL assay more than 100 cases to support T-cell personalized immunotherapy [42]. Recently next generation sequences are more affordable so that the precision diagnosis can significantly increase the effect of the treatment.

CONSENT FOR PUBLICATION

The authors declare no financial interests.

CONFLICT OF INTEREST

The authors declare no financial interests.

ACKNOWLEDGEMENTS

In the early period, BL with his colleagues set up the first TIL CTL assay by 51Cr release as described in the chapter (1985-1993). BL further study more than 25 years, including setting up single-cell methods to analyze genomic profiles with quantitative real-time PCR for cytokine and receptor measurement. Now LHJ is going to develop the new techniques for immunotherapy.

The mention of trade names or commercial products in this article is solely to provide specific information and does not imply recommendation.

REFERENCES

[1]   Russo V, Protti MP. Tumor-derived factors affecting immune cells. Cytokine Growth Factor Rev 2017; 36: 79-87.
       [http://dx.doi.org/10.1016/j.cytogfr.2017.06.005] [PMID: 28606733]

[2]   Markowitz J, Wesolowski R, Papenfuss T, Brooks TR, Carson WE III. Myeloid-derived suppressor cells in breast cancer. Breast Cancer Res Treat 2013; 140(1): 13-21.
       [http://dx.doi.org/10.1007/s10549-013-2618-7] [PMID: 23828498]

[3]   Guo WF, Zhang SW, Zeng T, Li Y, Gao J, Chen L. A novel network control model for identifying personalized driver genes in cancer. PLOS Comput Biol 2019; 15(11)e1007520
       [http://dx.doi.org/10.1371/journal.pcbi.1007520] [PMID: 31765387]

[4]   Lanzós A, Elliott K. EACR Cancer Genomics 2019 conference: from tumour evolution to personalised immunotherapy. FEBS J 2019; 286(21): 4209-14.
       [http://dx.doi.org/10.1111/febs.15063] [PMID: 31556220]

[5]   Albin N, Mc Leer A, Sakhri L. [Precision medicine: A major step forward in specific situations, a myth in refractory cancers?]. Bull Cancer 2018; 105(4): 375-96.
       [http://dx.doi.org/10.1016/j.bulcan.2018.01.009] [PMID: 29501208]

[6]   Puccetti P, Bianchi R, Fioretti MC, *et al.* Use of a skin test assay to determine tumor-specific CD8+ T cell reactivity. Eur J Immunol 1994; 24(6): 1446-52.
       [http://dx.doi.org/10.1002/eji.1830240631] [PMID: 8206103]

[7]   Simons JW, Mikhak B, Chang JF, *et al.* Induction of immunity to prostate cancer antigens: results of a clinical trial of vaccination with irradiated autologous prostate tumor cells engineered to secrete granulocyte-macrophage colony-stimulating factor using *ex vivo* gene transfer. Cancer Res 1999; 59(20): 5160-8.
       [PMID: 10537292]

[8]   McNeel DG, Schiffman K, Disis ML. Immunization with recombinant human granulocyte-macrophage colony-stimulating factor as a vaccine adjuvant elicits both a cellular and humoral response to recombinant human granulocyte-macrophage colony-stimulating factor. Blood 1999; 93(8): 2653-9.
       [http://dx.doi.org/10.1182/blood.V93.8.2653] [PMID: 10194445]

[9]   Paul WE, Seder RA. Lymphocyte responses and cytokines. Cell 1994; 76(2): 241-51.
       [http://dx.doi.org/10.1016/0092-8674(94)90332-8] [PMID: 7904900]

[10]   Maino VC, Picker LJ. Identification of functional subsets by flow cytometry: intracellular detection of cytokine expression. Cytometry 1998; 34(5): 207-15.
[http://dx.doi.org/10.1002/(SICI)1097-0320(19981015)34:5<207::AID-CYTO1>3.0.CO;2-J] [PMID: 9822306]

[11]   Tayebi H, Lienard A, Billot M, Tiberghien P, Hervé P, Robinet E. Detection of intracellular cytokines in citrated whole blood or marrow samples by flow cytometry. J Immunol Methods 1999; 229(1-2): 121-30.
[http://dx.doi.org/10.1016/S0022-1759(99)00110-6] [PMID: 10556696]

[12]   Czerkinsky C, Andersson G, Ekre HP, Nilsson LA, Klareskog L, Ouchterlony O. Reverse ELISPOT assay for clonal analysis of cytokine production. I. Enumeration of gamma-interferon-secreting cells. J Immunol Methods 1988; 110(1): 29-36.
[http://dx.doi.org/10.1016/0022-1759(88)90079-8] [PMID: 3131436]

[13]   Khleif SN, Abrams SI, Hamilton JM, *et al.* A phase I vaccine trial with peptides reflecting ras oncogene mutations of solid tumors. J Immunother 1999; 22(2): 155-65.
[http://dx.doi.org/10.1097/00002371-199903000-00007] [PMID: 10093040]

[14]   Rucker R, Bresler HS, Heffelfinger M, Kim JA, Martin EW Jr, Triozzi PL. Low-dose monoclonal antibody CC49 administered sequentially with granulocyte-macrophage colony-stimulating factor in patients with metastatic colorectal cancer. J Immunother 1999; 22(1): 80-4.
[http://dx.doi.org/10.1097/00002371-199901000-00011] [PMID: 9924703]

[15]   Möller P, Sun Y, Dorbic T, *et al.* Vaccination with IL-7 gene-modified autologous melanoma cells can enhance the anti-melanoma lytic activity in peripheral blood of patients with a good clinical performance status: a clinical phase I study. Br J Cancer 1998; 77(11): 1907-16.
[http://dx.doi.org/10.1038/bjc.1998.317] [PMID: 9667667]

[16]   Sun Y, Jurgovsky K, Möller P, *et al.* Vaccination with IL-12 gene-modified autologous melanoma cells: preclinical results and a first clinical phase I study. Gene Ther 1998; 5(4): 481-90.
[http://dx.doi.org/10.1038/sj.gt.3300619] [PMID: 9614572]

[17]   D'Souza S, Rimoldi D, Líenard D, Lejeune F, Cerottini JC, Romero P. Circulating Melan-A/Mart-1 specific cytolytic T lymphocyte precursors in HLA-A2+ melanoma patients have a memory phenotype. Int J Cancer 1998; 78(6): 699-706.
[http://dx.doi.org/10.1002/(SICI)1097-0215(19981209)78:6<699::AID-IJC6>3.0.CO;2-U] [PMID: 9833762]

[18]   Terabe M, Berzofsky JA. Tissue-Specific Roles of NKT Cells in Tumor Immunity. Front Immunol 2018; 9: 1838.
[http://dx.doi.org/10.3389/fimmu.2018.01838] [PMID: 30158927]

[19]   Casalegno-Garduño R, Schmitt A, Yao J, *et al.* Multimer technologies for detection and adoptive transfer of antigen-specific T cells. Cancer Immunol Immunother 2010; 59(2): 195-202.
[http://dx.doi.org/10.1007/s00262-009-0778-4] [PMID: 19847424]

[20]   Yajima T, Hoshino K, Muranushi R, *et al.* Fas/FasL signaling is critical for the survival of exhausted antigen-specific CD8$^+$ T cells during tumor immune response. Mol Immunol 2019; 107: 97-105.
[http://dx.doi.org/10.1016/j.molimm.2019.01.014] [PMID: 30711908]

[21]   Yamshchikov G, Thompson L, Ross WG, *et al.* Analysis of a natural immune response against tumor antigens in a melanoma survivor: lessons applicable to clinical trial evaluations. Clin Cancer Res 2001; 7(3) (Suppl.): 909s-16s.
[PMID: 11300491]

[22]   Armstrong KM, Insaidoo FK, Baker BM. Thermodynamics of T-cell receptor-peptide/MHC interactions: progress and opportunities. J Mol Recognit 2008; 21(4): 275-87.
[http://dx.doi.org/10.1002/jmr.896] [PMID: 18496839]

[23]   Jackson KJ, Kidd MJ, Wang Y, Collins AM. The shape of the lymphocyte receptor repertoire: lessons

from the B cell receptor. Front Immunol 2013; 4: 263.
[http://dx.doi.org/10.3389/fimmu.2013.00263] [PMID: 24032032]

[24]   Armstrong KM, Piepenbrink KH, Baker BM. Conformational changes and flexibility in T-cell receptor recognition of peptide-MHC complexes. Biochem J 2008; 415(2): 183-96.
[http://dx.doi.org/10.1042/BJ20080850] [PMID: 18800968]

[25]   Lai WS, Wells ML, Perera L, Blackshear PJ. The tandem zinc finger RNA binding domain of members of the tristetraprolin protein family. Wiley Interdiscip Rev RNA 2019; 10(4)e1531
[http://dx.doi.org/10.1002/wrna.1531] [PMID: 30864256]

[26]   Maker AV, Hu V, Kadkol SS, *et al.* Cyst Fluid Biosignature to Predict Intraductal Papillary Mucinous Neoplasms of the Pancreas with High Malignant Potential. J Am Coll Surg 2019; 228(5): 721-9.
[http://dx.doi.org/10.1016/j.jamcollsurg.2019.02.040] [PMID: 30794864]

[27]   Qin J, Zeng N, Yang T, *et al.* Diagnostic Value of Autoantibodies in Lung Cancer: a Systematic Review and Meta-Analysis. ell Physiol Biochem 2018; 51: 2631-46.

[28]   Zhang J, Larrocha PS, Zhang B, Wainwright D, Dhar P, Wu JD. Antibody targeting tumor-derived soluble NKG2D ligand sMIC provides dual co-stimulation of CD8 T cells and enables sMIC$^+$ tumors respond to PD1/PD-L1 blockade therapy. J Immunother Cancer 2019; 7(1): 223.
[http://dx.doi.org/10.1186/s40425-019-0693-y] [PMID: 31446896]

[29]   Kaur A, Doberstein T, Amberker RR, Garje R, Field EH, Singh N. Immune-related adverse events in cancer patients treated with immune checkpoint inhibitors: A single-center experience. Medicine (Baltimore) 2019; 98(41)e17348
[http://dx.doi.org/10.1097/MD.0000000000017348] [PMID: 31593084]

[30]   Isitmangil G, Gurleyik G, Aker FV, *et al.* Association of CTLA4 and CD28 Gene Variants and Circulating Levels of Their Proteins in Patients with Breast Cancer. *In Vivo* 2016; 30(4): 485-93.
[PMID: 27381613]

[31]   Ng Kee Kwong F, Laggner U, McKinney O, Croud J, Rice A, Nicholson AG. Expression of PD-L1 correlates with pleomorphic morphology and histological patterns of non-small-cell lung carcinomas. Histopathology 2018; 72(6): 1024-32.
[http://dx.doi.org/10.1111/his.13466] [PMID: 29323731]

[32]   Janzic U, Kern I, Janzic A, Cavka L, Cufer T. PD-L1 expression in squamouscell carcinoma and adenocarcinoma of the lung. Radiol Oncol 2017; 51(3): 357-62.
[http://dx.doi.org/10.1515/raon-2017-0037] [PMID: 28959173]

[33]   Rodić N, Anders RA, Eshleman JR, *et al.* PD-L1 expression in melanocytic lesions does not correlate with the BRAF V600E mutation. Cancer Immunol Res 2015; 3(2): 110-5.
[http://dx.doi.org/10.1158/2326-6066.CIR-14-0145] [PMID: 25370533]

[34]   Topalian SL, Taube JM, Anders RA, Pardoll DM. Mechanism-driven biomarkers to guide immune checkpoint blockade in cancer therapy. Nat Rev Cancer 2016; 16(5): 275-87.
[http://dx.doi.org/10.1038/nrc.2016.36] [PMID: 27079802]

[35]   Li B, Yang J, Tao M, *et al.* Poor prognosis acute myelogenous leukemia 2--biological and molecular biological characteristics and treatment outcome. Leuk Res 2000; 24(9): 777-89.
[http://dx.doi.org/10.1016/S0145-2126(00)00035-7] [PMID: 10978783]

[36]   Nomizo T, Ozasa H, Tsuji T, *et al.* Clinical Impact of Single Nucleotide Polymorphism in PD-L1 on Response to Nivolumab for Advanced Non-Small-Cell Lung Cancer Patients. Sci Rep 2017; 7: 45124.
[http://dx.doi.org/10.1038/srep45124] [PMID: 28332580]

[37]   Kraaijeveld R, de Graav GN, Dieterich M, Litjens NHR, Hesselink DA, Baan CC. Co-inhibitory profile and cytotoxicity of CD57$^+$ PD-1$^-$ T cells in end-stage renal disease patients. Clin Exp Immunol 2018; 191(3): 363-72.
[http://dx.doi.org/10.1111/cei.13070] [PMID: 29027667]

[38]   Amiri MM, Bahadori T, Soltantoyeh T, *et al.* Development of a Novel Inhibitory Chimeric Anti-HER2

Monoclonal Antibody. Iran J Immunol 2019; 16(1): 26-42.
[PMID: 30864553]

[39]   Ben Hassine I, Gharbi H, Soltani I, *et al.* hOCT1 gene expression predict for optimal response to Imatinib in Tunisian patients with chronic myeloid leukemia. Cancer Chemother Pharmacol 2017; 79(4): 737-45.
[http://dx.doi.org/10.1007/s00280-017-3266-0] [PMID: 28286932]

[40]   Mascia F, Schloemann DT, Cataisson C, *et al.* Cell autonomous or systemic EGFR blockade alters the immune-environment in squamous cell carcinomas. Int J Cancer 2016; 139(11): 2593-7.
[http://dx.doi.org/10.1002/ijc.30376] [PMID: 27509256]

[41]   Razazan A, Behravan J, Arab A, *et al.* Conjugated nanoliposome with the HER2/neu-derived peptide GP2 as an effective vaccine against breast cancer in mice xenograft model. PLoS One 2017; 12(10)e0185099
[http://dx.doi.org/10.1371/journal.pone.0185099] [PMID: 29045460]

[42]   Li BR, Tong SQ, Zhang XH, Lu J, Gu QL, Lu DY. A new experimental and clinical approach of combining usage of highly active tumor-infiltrating lymphocytes and highly sensitive antitumor drugs for the advanced malignant tumor. Chin Med J (Engl) 1994; 107(11): 803-7.
[PMID: 7867384]

CHAPTER 4

Tumor Microenvironment, ADO/IDO Pathway-Foundation of Personalized Immunotherapy

Xiao Zhu[1], Li-Hua Jiang[2] and Biaoru Li[2,3,*]

[1] *Guangdong Key Laboratory for Research and Development of Natural Drugs, Guangdong Medical University, Zhanjiang 524023, PRC, China*

[2] *Departments of Immunology and Microbiology, Shanghai Second Medical University, Shanghai, 200003, PRC, China*

[3] *Georgia Cancer Center and Department of Pediatrics, Medical College at GA, Augusta, GA 30912, USA*

Abstract: Immune cells and antibodies respectively play a role in the cell-mediated and humorous-mediated immune response to tumor cells, while tumor microenvironment (TME) and tumor cells in tumor tissue take many strategies to evade the host immune response by creating many immune-suppressive factors, and thus, we should understand the knowledge of TME before performing personalized immunotherapy. TME consists of tissues, cells, and signaling molecules in tumor tissue, affecting the immune response to tumor cells. Furthermore, TME will be quickly changed by inflammation, hypoxia, and tumor growth *in vivo* so that its highly dynamic alteration must be considered for treatment selection for personalized immunotherapy. All TME elements of tissues, cells, and molecule factors interact with each other, including those during the early period of tumor tissues and those in an aggressive period in tumor tissues. Before human genomics decode in 2004, studying TME components with their genomic profiles of patients is a rare possibility. After human genomics decoded with research and development (R&D) of their techniques, TME is going to be increasingly considered by personalized immunotherapy of tumor diseases. Now, identifying regulating TME cells and regulating molecules with their therapeutic agents is largely reported. A few reports have outlined some networks such as extracellular matrix (ECM) and pathways such as adenosine (ADO) and indole-2,-dioxygenase (IDO) with their therapeutic agents that may guide a new generation of immunotherapy.

Keywords: Adenosine (ADO), Carcinoma-associated fibroblasts (CAFs), Extracellular matrix (ECM), Indole 2,3-dioxygenase (IDO), Myeloid-derived suppressor cells (MDSC), Tumor microenvironment (TME), Tumor-associated macrophage (TAM), Tumor-associated neutrophil (TAN).

* **Corresponding author Biaoru Li:** Georgia Cancer Center and Department of Pediatrics, Medical College at GA, Augusta, GA 30912, USA; Tel: 440-317-1443; E-mail: bli@augusta.edu

Biaoru Li, Alan Larson & Shen Li (Eds.)

INTRODUCTION

Tumor microenvironment (TME) around a tumor cell in tumor tissue plays an essential role in personalized immunotherapy, personalized chemotherapy, and targeted therapy [1]. TME contains three components as Fig. (**1**). (I) a tissue called extracellular matrix (ECM) with epithelium, basement, and endothelium (Fig. **1A**); (II) regulating cells including tumor-associated macrophages (TAM), neutrophils, carcinoma-associated fibroblasts (CAFs), myeloid-derived suppressor cells (MDSC) (Fig. **1B**); (III) signaling molecules affecting tumor growth by releasing extracellular signals, promoting tumor angiogenesis, inducing immune quiescence and increasing the growth of tumor cells [2 - 4]. Before decoding human genomics, TME components with TME profiles is not easy to be applied for patients. After human genomics decoded with research and development (R&D) of their techniques, TME components are going to be largely studied, and therefore, identifying new targets in TME components with discovering their therapeutic agents may guide a new generation of immunotherapy.

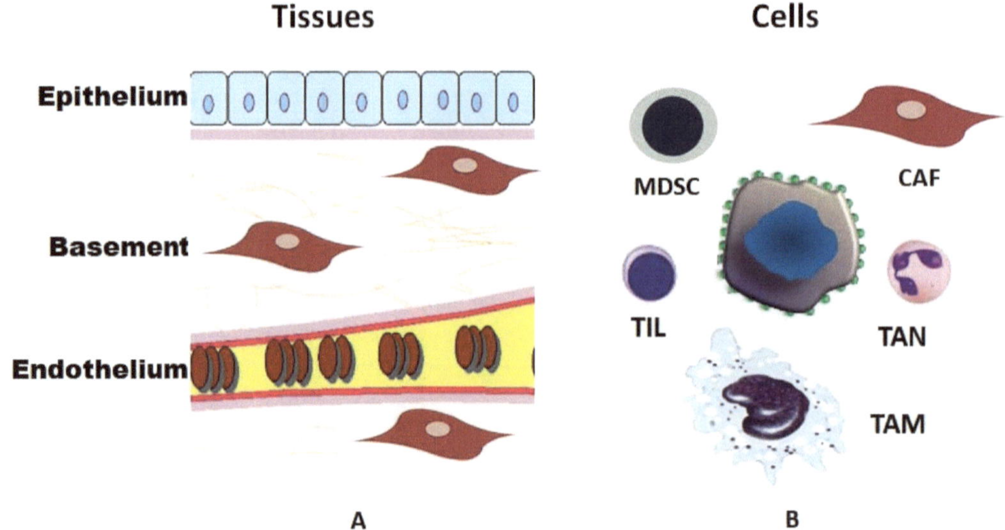

Fig. (1). Tumor cells and TME. Extracellular matrix (ECM) with epithelium, basement, and endothelium as Fig. (**1A**); Fig. (**1B**) demonstrates regulating cells including MDSC, tumor-associated macrophages, tumor-infiltrating lymphocyte and neutrophils with their signaling molecules by releasing extracellular signals for promoting tumor angiogenesis, inducing immune tolerance and affecting the growth of tumor cells.

However, TME should be quickly developed for clinical application once these TME techniques related to high throughput platforms with multiple cells and factors in TME are grown-up from genomic profiles. For example, at present, pathologists are attempting to identify the multiplex gene panel or proteins array by immunocytochemistry techniques. Moreover, genomics techniques can use different barcodes to identify cells, and then, define genomics expression of different cells in TME for their specific therapeutic agents. In the chapter, following sections will introduce fundamental of TME: (I) tissue called extracellular matrix (ECM) regarding epithelium, basement, and endothelium; (II) regulating cells including carcinoma-associated fibroblasts (CAF), myeloid-derived suppressor cells (MDSC), tumor-associated macrophages (TAM), tumor-infiltrating lymphocyte (TIL), neutrophils; (III) signaling molecules affecting tumor growth, promoting tumor angiogenesis and inducing immune tolerance, especially, some hot signaling molecules such as ADO and IDO. In the conclusion part, we present several checkpoint targets with their therapeutic agents to support personalized molecular therapy and personalized immunotherapy.

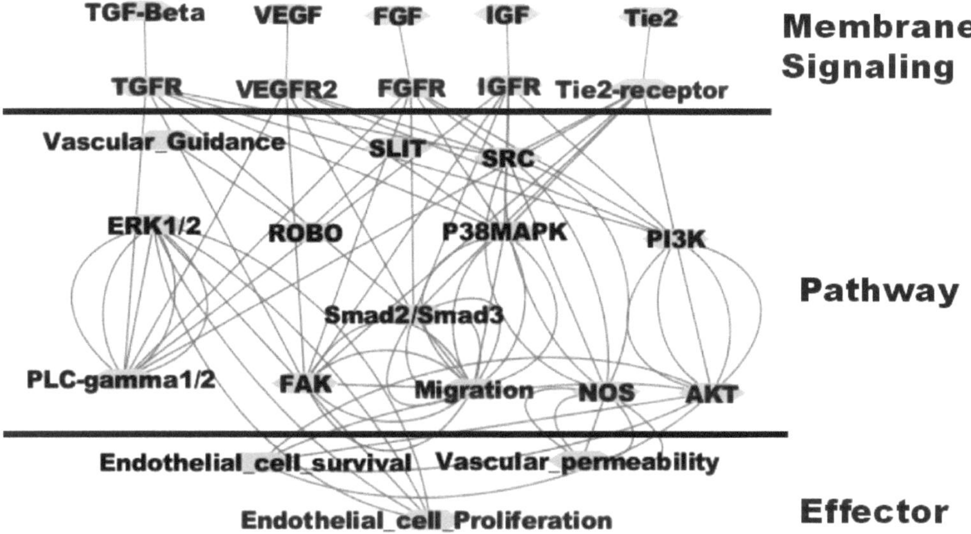

Fig. (2). ECM network.

EXTRACELLULAR MATRIX WITH NETWORK

Extracellular matrix (ECM) comprises epithelium, basement, and endothelium. Fibroblasts in the basement are vital components in the ECM [5]. A normal fibroblast can be transformed into CAFs during carcinogenesis, and thus, CAFs decrease normal ECM production and increase abnormal ECM, which will be altered into malformation. Finally, collagen in the basement may be loosely woven and even curved, resulting in CAF producing matrix metalloproteinases (MMP) and cleaving proteins within the ECM and disrupting normal ECM [6].

CAFs also release cytokines and growth factors such as VEGF, EGF, FGF, PDGF, IGF, and TGF-β to increase tumor growth. In the ECM, the endothelium is stimulated by these signal molecules as described above, and then, tumor vasculature will be formed. Finally, tumor ECM will produce abnormal networks regarding the VEGF signaling pathway, FGF signaling pathway, PDGF signaling pathway, EGFR signaling pathway as Fig. (**2**).

REGULATING CELLS

Several cells in a tumor tissue include tumor-associated macrophages (TAM), tumor-associated neutrophil-2 (TAN-2), carcinoma-associated fibroblasts (CAF) and myeloid-derived suppressor cells (MDSC) to stimulating tumor growth whereas several other cells in tumor location including M-1 macrophage, TAN-1, tumor-infiltrating lymphocyte (TIL) and normal fibroblast will inhibit tumor cell growth.

1. Tumor-Associated Macrophages

Macrophages are a significant component infiltrating into TME [7]. During tumorigenesis and tumor progression, macrophages are attracted to the tumor site, initiating the immune response against tumor cells. Activated macrophage presents tumor Ag to T-cell, which is then activated to kill tumor cells. However, tumor cells are often capable of escaping the immune function because macrophage in tumor tissue also contributes to tumor progression by growth factors and neovascularization. After several years' study, macrophages in tumor sites have been discovered as two groups, M1-macrophages exposed in IFN-γ have antitumor activity, and M2-macrophages (TAM) activated by IL-4 or IL-13 have oriented to tissue remodeling to support tumor cells [8]. Most of the evidence has supported M1 switch to M2 under local hypoxia, low glucose level, and low pH with regulating by CCL families, TGF-β, VEGF, PDGF, and M-CSF. This switch eventually appears in tumor dissemination and invasion characteristics. An increased TAMs is associated with worse prognosis *in vivo*, and thus, TAMs represent a potential target for novel cancer therapies.

2. Neutrophils

Neutrophils are polymorphonuclear immune cells that are critical components of the innate immune system. In tumor site, neutrophils can be divided into two types, TAN1 (tumor-associated neutrophils-1) with an antitumor function and tumor-associated neutrophils-2 (TAN2) with a pro-tumorigenic function [9, 10]. Antitumor activities of TAN1 include the expression of more immuno-activating cytokines and chemokines with lower levels of arginase and lower levels of TGF-β to killing tumor cells *in vitro*. Therapeutic targeting identification from a quantitative network with its genomic analysis is a very good tool to block TGF-β for molecular therapy *in vitro* and *in vivo*, and therefore, agents inducing TAN1 or inhibiting TAN2 may have a possibility to use as therapeutic targets.

3. Tumor-Infiltrating Lymphocytes

Tumor-infiltrating lymphocytes (TILs) are lymphocytes that penetrate into tumor tissue. Previously, TILs are only to achieve successful adoptive immunotherapy of patients with melanoma, whereas now more and more pieces of evidence have shown that TILs have a good response for solid tumors after we reported modified techniques to active TILs confirmed by CTL assay [11, 12].

4. Carcinoma Associated Fibroblasts

Fibroblasts are a heterogeneous group with normal fibroblasts coming from pericytes, smooth muscle cells, fibrocytes, mesenchymal stem cells epithelial-mesenchymal transition or endothelial-mesenchymal transition while carcinoma-associated fibroblasts (CAFs) coming from normal fibroblasts perform several functions supporting tumor growth by secreting vascular endothelial growth factor (VEGF), fibroblast growth factors (FGFs), platelet-derived growth factor (PDGF), and other pro-angiogenic signals to induce angiogenesis [13, 14]. CAF can also secrete transforming growth factor-beta (TGF-β) is associated with inhibiting CD8+ T-cells and NK T-cells. CAFs are also associated with the Reverse Warburg Effect for aerobic glycolysis to produce lactate resulting in tumor growth. At present, several markers can be used to identify CAFs, including expression of α smooth muscle actin (αSMA), vimentin, platelet-derived growth factor receptor α (PDGFR-α), platelet-derived growth factor receptor β (PDGFR-β), fibroblast specific protein 1 (FSP-1) and fibroblast activation protein (FAP).

Myeloid-Derived Suppressor Cells (MDSC)

MDSC is a heterogeneous group of immune cells from the myeloid lineage in the bone marrow. MDSCs are distinct from other myeloid cell types, playing a robust immunosuppressive activity of T-cells, dendritic cells, macrophages, and NK cells [15, 16]. Although their mechanisms are unknown, clinical evidence has shown that high infiltration of MDSCs in tumor tissues is related to the poor prognosis of patients.

Regulating cells, including TAM, TAN-2, and CAFs, have some particular networks to stimulate the growth of tumor cells regarding IL-6/JAK/STAT3 signaling pathway, NF-κB signaling pathway, TNF-α signaling pathway, COX2 signaling pathway, TGF-β signaling pathway as Fig. (**3**).

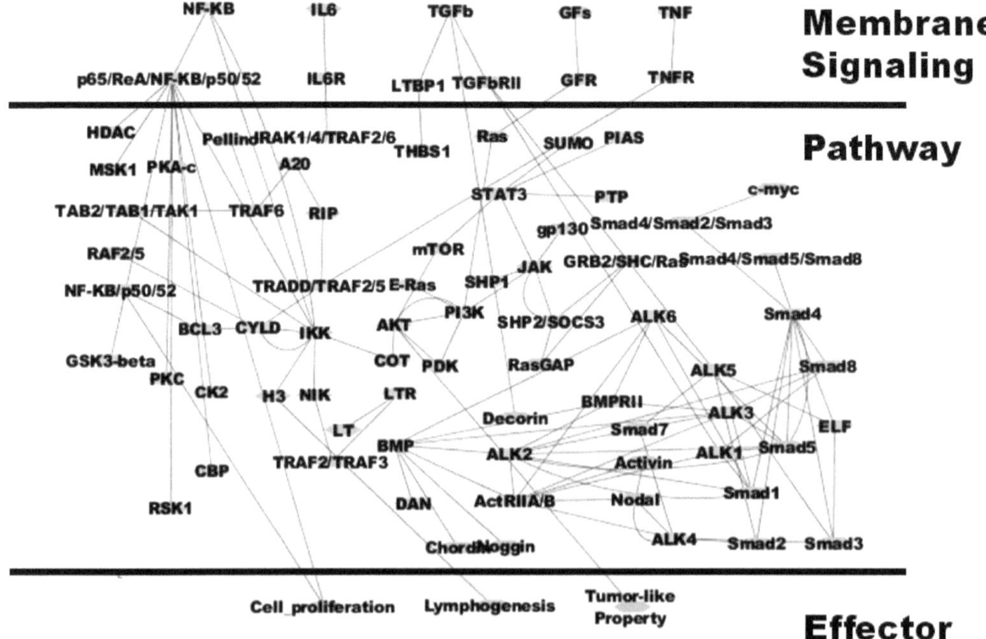

Fig. (3). TAM and TAN-2 network. TAM and TAN-2 will produce abnormal network regarding IL-6/JAK/STAT3 signaling pathway, NF-κB signaling pathway, TNF-α signaling pathway, COX2 signaling pathway, TGF-β signaling pathway.

REGULATING MOLECULES

As reported above, signaling molecules can influence tumor growth by releasing extracellular signals, promoting tumor angiogenesis, inducing the growth of tumor cells. At present, some special pathways in TME are going to be largely reported, for example, ADO regulating pathway and IDO regulating pathways.

1. ADO Regulating Pathways

As shown in Fig. (4), Adenosine triphosphate (ATP) is a popular molecule playing a vital role as the universal energy currency within the cell [17, 18]. However, within TME, extracellular ATP levels increase due to release from inflammatory, apoptotic, or necrotic cells, involved in multiple pathological processes. Extracellular ATP signal pathway through receptors (A2R) are widely expressed on immune and non-immune cells within the body.

During tumor progression, signaling on the immune cells and TME is unbalanced between extracellular ATP and adenosine (ADO). ATP can induce a form of immunogenic cell death (ICD) to tumor cells in tumor sites, promoting immunosurveillance in the TME, while increased ADO is playing the role of

ADO immune dysfunction of T cells, NK cells, and B cells. Due to high concentrations of ADO within the TME with their high expression of ADO receptors on tumor and immune cells, the role of ADO in cancer progression and antitumor immune responses have led to the clinical development of antibodies and small-molecule inhibitors to target ADO pathway including CD39, CD38, CD73, A2AR, and A2BR [19, 20].

2. IDO Regulating Pathways

Secondary regulating pathways, as in Fig. (**5**), is to impede T-cell proliferation in TME, called as indole 2,3-dioxygenase (IDO) pathway [21, 22]. DCs, MDSCs, and tumor cells can produce IDO, allowing to be catabolizing tryptophan, and generating kynurenine, resulting in the deprivation of tryptophan and the generation of its metabolic product to inhibit clonal T-cell expansion. IDO also promotes the conversion of T cells to Treg cells and increases IL-6 expression, which augments MDSC functions. Inhibiting IDO has demonstrated some therapeutic potential.

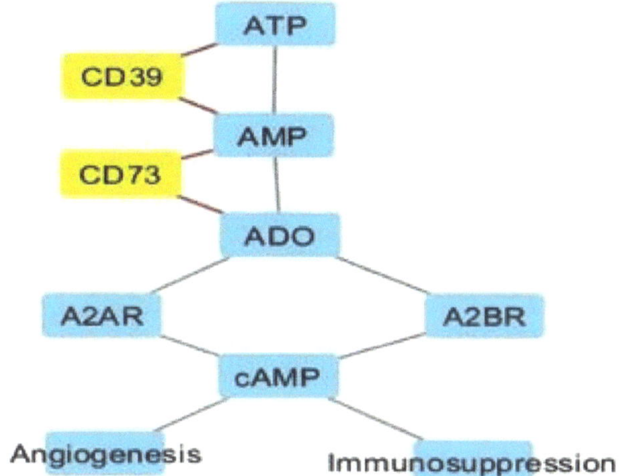

Fig. (4). ADO pathway. CD39 and CD73 cells as yellow color are targeting cells with their pathway and targeting agents.

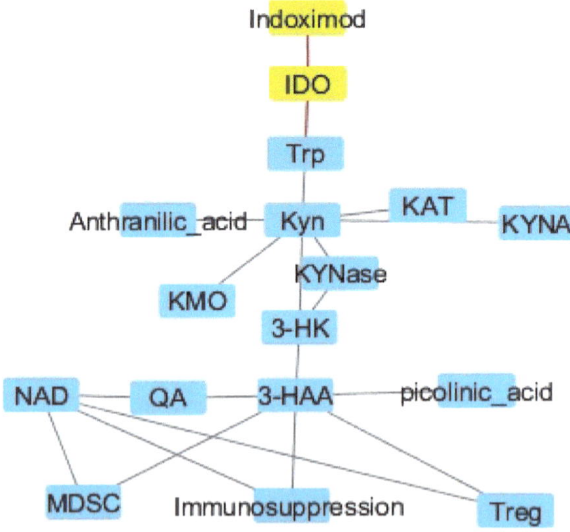

Fig. (5). IDO pathway. Indoximod as yellow color can inhibit IDO to block MDSC, Treg, and other immunosuppression cells.

THERAPEUTIC TARGETS WITH THEIR AGENTS

1. Therapies Antibodies and Kinase Inhibitors

Tumor ECM with their regulating cells and molecules can produce abnormal networks regarding the VEGF signaling pathway, FGF signaling pathway, PDGF signaling pathway, and EGFR signaling pathway [23, 24]. As Table **1**, monoclonal antibody and kinase inhibitor have been used to clinical trials or treatment approved by the FDA. For example, Bevacizumab is clinically approved by the FDA in the US to targeting VEGF-A, which is produced by both CAFs and TAMs, thus slowing down tumor angiogenesis. Many other small molecule kinase inhibitors in Table **1** block the receptors for the growth factors produced by CAFs and TAMs, making tumor cells to die. These inhibitors include Sunitinib, Pazopanib, Sorafenib to PDGFR, and VEGFR.

Table 1. Antibodies and Kinase Inhibitors for TME.

Therapies Antibodies and Kinase Inhibitors	Targets
Gefitinib	EGFR
Afatinib	EGFR
Cetuximab	EGFR
Matuzamab	EGFR

(Table 1) cont.....

Panitumumab	EGFR
Nimotuzumab	EGFR
Erlotinib	EGFR
Ponatinib	FGFR1
Dovitinib	FGFR2
Dovitinib	PDGFR
Sunitinib	PDGFR
Sorafenib	PDGFR
Ponatinib	PDGFRα
Aflibercept	VEGF-A
Bevacizumab	VEGFR
Ramucirumab	VEGFR2

2. Therapeutic Targets of ADO Pathway

As described above, adenosine (ADO) is produced by the ADO pathway by which adenosine triphosphate (ATP) is transformed into ADP on the surface of CD39 and further into AMP on the surface of CD73 under hypoxia with HIF-1. The high concentrations of ADO within the TME with their high ADO receptors can stimulate tumor cells and inhibit immune cells [25, 26]. As Table **2**, the role of ADO in tumor progression and antitumor immune responses have been studied by small molecule inhibitors for clinical trials to block the ADO pathway, including therapeutic targets of HIF-1, CD39, CD38, CD73, A2AR, and A2BR.

3. Therapeutic Targets of IDO Pathway

Indole 2,3-dioxygenase (IDO) is also a crucial target because IDO impedes T-cell proliferation and stimulates MDSCs and tumor cells, allowing to be catabolizing tryptophan and generating kynurenine, resulting in the deprivation of tryptophan and the generation of its metabolic product to inhibit clonal T cell expansion. IDO pathway blocked as Table **3** is going to be increasingly researched in experimental and clinical fields [27, 28].

Table 2. ADO therapeutic targets within TME.

Target	Drug	Company	Study Phase	Cancer Type
HIF-1	HSP90 inhibitor	developing	0/I	underway
$A_{2B}R$ (Antagonist)	PBF-1129	Palobiofarma	I	NSCLC

(Table 2) cont.....

			I/Ib	Solid cancers
$A_{2A}R$ (Antagonist)	CPI-444	Corvus	I/II	Carcinoma, NSCLC
	PBF-509	Palobiofarma	I/II	NSCLC
	NIR-178	Novartis	II	Solid cancers and DLBCL
	AZD-4635	Heptares	I	Solid cancers
A_3R (Agonist)	CF-102	CanFite BioPharma	II	Hepatocellular carcinoma
CD73	MEDI-9447	MedImmune	I	Solid cancers
			II	Ovarian cancer
			I/II	TNBC
			I/II	Carcinoma, NSCLC
	CPI-006	Corvus	I	Solid cancers
	NZV-930	Norvatis	I	Solid cancers
	BMS-986179	Bristol-Meyers-Squibb	I/II	Solid cancers

Table 3. IDO therapeutic targets for TME.

Agent	Indication(s)	Phase
Indoximod (D-1-MT)	solid tumor, GBM, Melanoma	I/II
INCB024360	solid tumor, MDS, Reproductive tract tumor, melanoma	I/II
GDC-0919	Solid tumors	I
IDO1 peptide	NSCLC/Melanoma	I
PF-06840003	GBM or grade III anaplastic glioma	I
BMS986205	Cervical,DLBCL, SCCHN, UC, pancreatic, melanoma, NSCLC	I

4. Other Ways of TME Therapy

1. High throughput therapeutics screens can reveal interesting therapeutic targets in TME. Currently, pathologists are developing some multiplex gene panel or proteins array by immunocytochemistry (ICH) techniques to define therapeutic targets. Moreover, some genomics techniques, for example, the 10x Genomics platform can use different barcodes to screen calls, and then, identify genomics expression from screen cells in TME [29].

2. The nanoparticle can transport drugs and other therapeutic molecules by a function of enhanced permeability and retention (EPR). These therapies can be selectively targeted to tumor vasculature in TME by the EPR effect [30]. Nanoparticles are now studied for tumor cells and cells in TME because it can target tumors and cells in TME that are hypovascularized, such as prostate and

pancreatic tumors.

3. Liposome formulations encapsulate anti-cancer drugs for selective uptake to tumors and TME by the EPR effect, including DNA intercalator for doxorubicin and albumin-bound paclitaxel to increase therapeutic targets to TME and tumor cells [31].

4. TME is going to be increasingly studied to personalized immunotherapy, personalized chemotherapy, and personalized targeting therapy of tumor diseases. Now, identifying new targets and discovering therapeutic agents such as new antibody and small molecules related to their networks (such as ECM, TAM, TAN, MDSC, and CAFs) and their pathways (such as ADO and IDO) can guide a new generation of treatments.

CONSENT FOR PUBLICATION

The authors declare no financial interests.

CONFLICT OF INTEREST

The authors declare no financial interests.

ACKNOWLEDGEMENTS

XZ and his colleagues are going to study therapeutic targets, and XHJ has studied therapeutic targets in immunotherapy. Both are co-first authors; BL, with their colleagues, studied biobanks of TME and set up genomics and bioinformatics platform to support specific targets.

The mention of trade names or commercial products in this article is solely to provide specific information and does not imply recommendation.

REFERENCES

[1]   Toor SM, Sasidharan Nair V, Decock J, Elkord E. Immune checkpoints in the tumor microenvironment. Semin Cancer Biol 2019; 1044-579X(19): 3-30123.

[2]   Horiuchi H, Tamai N, Kamba S, Inomata H, Ohya TR, Sumiyama K. Real-time computer-aided diagnosis of diminutive rectosigmoid polyps using an auto-fluorescence imaging system and novel color intensity analysis software. Scand J Gastroenterol 2019; 54(6): 800-5.
[http://dx.doi.org/10.1080/00365521.2019.1627407] [PMID: 31195905]

[3]   Park D, Son K, Hwang Y, *et al.* High-Throughput Microfluidic 3D Cytotoxicity Assay for Cancer Immunotherapy (CACI-IMPACT Platform). Front Immunol 2019; 10: 1133.
[http://dx.doi.org/10.3389/fimmu.2019.01133] [PMID: 31191524]

[4]   Neal JT, Li X, Zhu J, *et al.* Organoid Modeling of the Tumor Immune Microenvironment. Cell 2018; 175(7): 1972-1988.e16.
[http://dx.doi.org/10.1016/j.cell.2018.11.021] [PMID: 30550791]

[5]   Bai Y, Wang Y, Zhang X, *et al.* Potential applications of nanoparticles for tumor microenvironment remodeling to ameliorate cancer immunotherapy. Int J Pharm 2019; 570: 118636.
[http://dx.doi.org/10.1016/j.ijpharm.2019.118636] [PMID: 31446027]

[6]   Brooks EA, Galarza S, Gencoglu MF, *et al.* Applicability of drug response metrics for cancer studies using biomaterials. Philos Trans R Soc Lond B Biol Sci 2019; 374(1779)
[http://dx.doi.org/10.1098/rstb.2018.0226]

[7]   Mehla K, Singh PK. Metabolic Regulation of Macrophage Polarization in Cancer. Trends Cancer 2019; 5(12): 822-34.
[http://dx.doi.org/10.1016/j.trecan.2019.10.007] [PMID: 31813459]

[8]   Alame M, Pirel M, Costes-Martineau V, *et al.* Characterisation of tumour microenvironment and immune checkpoints in primary central nervous system diffuse large B cell lymphomas. Virchows Arch 2019.
[http://dx.doi.org/10.1007/s00428-019-02695-6] [PMID: 31811434]

[9]   Lecot P, Sarabi M, Pereira Abrantes M, *et al.* Neutrophil Heterogeneity in Cancer: From Biology to Therapies. Front Immunol 2019; 10: 2155.
[http://dx.doi.org/10.3389/fimmu.2019.02155] [PMID: 31616408]

[10]   Ferrari SM, Fallahi P, Galdiero MR, *et al.* Immune and Inflammatory Cells in Thyroid Cancer Microenvironment. Int J Mol Sci 2019; 20(18): E4413.
[http://dx.doi.org/10.3390/ijms20184413] [PMID: 31500315]

[11]   Li BR, Tong SQ, Zhang XH, Lu J, Gu QL, Lu DY. A new experimental and clinical approach of combining usage of highly active tumor-infiltrating lymphocytes and highly sensitive antitumor drugs for the advanced malignant tumor. Chin Med J (Engl) 1994; 107(11): 803-7.
[PMID: 7867384]

[12]   Li BR, Tong SQ, Hu BY, *et al.* [Study on the influence of enzymatic digestion upon tumor-infiltrating lymphocytes]. Shi Yan Sheng Wu Xue Bao 1994; 27(1): 103-7.
[PMID: 8042406]

[13]   Yin Z, Dong C, Jiang K, *et al.* Heterogeneity of cancer-associated fibroblasts and roles in the progression, prognosis, and therapy of hepatocellular carcinoma. J Hematol Oncol 2019; 12(1): 101.
[http://dx.doi.org/10.1186/s13045-019-0782-x] [PMID: 31547836]

[14]   Baglieri J, Brenner DA, Kisseleva T. The Role of Fibrosis and Liver-Associated Fibroblasts in the Pathogenesis of Hepatocellular Carcinoma. Int J Mol Sci 2019; 20(7): E1723.
[http://dx.doi.org/10.3390/ijms20071723] [PMID: 30959975]

[15]   Tian X, Shen H, Li Z, Wang T, Wang S. Tumor-derived exosomes, myeloid-derived suppressor cells, and tumor microenvironment. J Hematol Oncol 2019; 12(1): 84.
[http://dx.doi.org/10.1186/s13045-019-0772-z] [PMID: 31438991]

[16]   Won WJ, Deshane JS, Leavenworth JW, Oliva CR, Griguer CE. Metabolic and functional reprogramming of myeloid-derived suppressor cells and their therapeutic control in glioblastoma. Cell Stress 2019; 3(2): 47-65.
[http://dx.doi.org/10.15698/cst2019.02.176] [PMID: 31225500]

[17]   Masson N, Keeley TP, Giuntoli B, *et al.* Conserved N-terminal cysteine dioxygenases transduce responses to hypoxia in animals and plants. Science 2019; 365(6448): 65-9.
[http://dx.doi.org/10.1126/science.aaw0112] [PMID: 31273118]

[18]   Shi L, Yang L, Wu Z, Xu W, Song J, Guan W. Adenosine signaling: Next checkpoint for gastric cancer immunotherapy? Int Immunopharmacol 2018; 63: 58-65.
[http://dx.doi.org/10.1016/j.intimp.2018.07.023] [PMID: 30075429]

[19]   Whiteside TL. Targeting adenosine in cancer immunotherapy: a review of recent progress. Expert Rev Anticancer Ther 2017; 17(6): 527-35.
[http://dx.doi.org/10.1080/14737140.2017.1316197] [PMID: 28399672]

[20]   Bátori R, Kumar S, Bordán Z, *et al.* Differential mechanisms of adenosine- and ATPγS-induced microvascular endothelial barrier strengthening. J Cell Physiol 2019; 234(5): 5863-79.
[http://dx.doi.org/10.1002/jcp.26419] [PMID: 29271489]

[21]   Sforzini L, Nettis MA, Mondelli V, Pariante CM. Inflammation in cancer and depression: a starring role for the kynurenine pathway. Psychopharmacology (Berl) 2019; 236(10): 2997-3011.
[http://dx.doi.org/10.1007/s00213-019-05200-8] [PMID: 30806743]

[22]   Labadie BW, Bao R, Luke JJ. Reimagining IDO Pathway Inhibition in Cancer Immunotherapy *via* Downstream Focus on the Tryptophan-Kynurenine-Aryl Hydrocarbon Axis. Clin Cancer Res 2019; 25(5): 1462-71.
[http://dx.doi.org/10.1158/1078-0432.CCR-18-2882] [PMID: 30377198]

[23]   Muller AJ, Manfredi MG, Zakharia Y, Prendergast GC. Inhibiting IDO pathways to treat cancer: lessons from the ECHO-301 trial and beyond. Semin Immunopathol 2019; 41(1): 41-8.
[http://dx.doi.org/10.1007/s00281-018-0702-0] [PMID: 30203227]

[24]   Deng YT, Zhao MG, Xu TJ, Jin-Hou , Li XH. Gentiopicroside abrogates lipopolysaccharide-induced depressive-like behavior in mice through tryptophan-degrading pathway. Metab Brain Dis 2018; 33(5): 1413-20.
[http://dx.doi.org/10.1007/s11011-018-0246-y] [PMID: 29948656]

[25]   Wang Y, Liu X, Wang Y, *et al.* Attenuation of pentylenetrazole-induced acute status epilepticus in rats by adenosine involves inhibition of the mammalian target of rapamycin pathway. Neuroreport 2017; 28(15): 1016-21.
[http://dx.doi.org/10.1097/WNR.0000000000000878] [PMID: 28902712]

[26]   Stellrecht CM, Vangapandu HV, Le XF, Mao W, Shentu S. ATP directed agent, 8-chloro-adenosine, induces AMP activated protein kinase activity, leading to autophagic cell death in breast cancer cells. J Hematol Oncol 2014; 7: 23.
[http://dx.doi.org/10.1186/1756-8722-7-23] [PMID: 24628795]

[27]   Günther J, Däbritz J, Wirthgen E. Limitations and Off-Target Effects of Tryptophan-Related IDO Inhibitors in Cancer Treatment. Front Immunol 2019; 10: 1801.
[http://dx.doi.org/10.3389/fimmu.2019.01801] [PMID: 31417567]

[28]   Nahomi RB, Sampathkumar S, Myers AM, *et al.* The Absence of Indoleamine 2,3-Dioxygenase Inhibits Retinal Capillary Degeneration in Diabetic Mice. Invest Ophthalmol Vis Sci 2018; 59(5): 2042-53.
[http://dx.doi.org/10.1167/iovs.17-22702] [PMID: 29677366]

[29]   Pan Y, Lu F, Fei Q, *et al.* Single-cell RNA sequencing reveals compartmental remodeling of tumor-infiltrating immune cells induced by anti-CD47 targeting in pancreatic cancer. J Hematol Oncol 2019; 12(1): 124.
[http://dx.doi.org/10.1186/s13045-019-0822-6] [PMID: 31771616]

[30]   Huang X, Wu B, Li J, *et al.* Anti-tumour effects of red blood cell membrane-camouflaged black phosphorous quantum dots combined with chemotherapy and anti-inflammatory therapy. Artif Cells Nanomed Biotechnol 2019; 47(1): 968-79.
[http://dx.doi.org/10.1080/21691401.2019.1584110] [PMID: 30880468]

[31]   Sesarman A, Tefas L, Sylvester B, *et al.* Co-delivery of curcumin and doxorubicin in PEGylated liposomes favored the antineoplastic C26 murine colon carcinoma microenvironment. Drug Deliv Transl Res 2019; 9(1): 260-72.
[http://dx.doi.org/10.1007/s13346-018-00598-8] [PMID: 30421392]

CHAPTER 5

Molecular Targeting Checkpoint in Cancer-Foundation of Personalized Immunotherapy

Shuzhen Tan[1] and Xiao Zhu[2,*]

[1] *The Marine Biomedical Research Institute, Southern Marine Science and Engineering Guangdong Laboratory Zhanjiang, Guangdong Medical University, Zhanjiang 524023, China*

[2] *Guangdong Key Laboratory for Research and Development of Natural Drugs, Guangdong Medical University, Zhanjiang 524023, PRC*

Abstract: Currently, in the study of new anti-tumor therapies, the suppression of tumor growth through target checkpoints is a breakthrough in this treatment method. Now, this has gradually become the focus of in-depth research. By acting on specific molecular targets, tumor cells can be inhibited through information transmission in the human immune pathway, thereby inhibiting their growth and proliferation. Molecularly targeted checkpoint inhibitors can specifically kill tumors within the tumor microenvironment (TME), inhibiting the occurrence and development of tumors. On the other hand, they can target and inhibit other molecules, so that they can restore immune cell activity, and improve the body's anti-tumor immune function, namely the tumor immune microenvironment (TIME). At present, molecular target checkpoints that have been increasingly studied within TIME include PD-1, PD-L1, CTLA-4, TIM-3, LAG-3, and Siglec-15. Corresponding molecular target inhibitors have been prepared for these molecular targets, and thus they have been increasingly applied to the clinic. Although these inhibitors have unavoidable adverse reactions and limitations in their scope of application in certain types of tumors, they still offer hope for the successful elimination of tumors.

Keywords: Hepatocellular Carcinoma (HCC), Immune checkpoint inhibitor (ICI), Major histocompatibility complex (MHC), Mutation allele frequency (MAF), Non-small cell lung cancer (NSCLC), Regulatory T-cells (Treg), Small cell lung cancer (SCLC), T-cell receptor (TCR), Tumor immune microenvironment (TIME).

INTRODUCTION

In recent years, due to pollution of the ecological environment and changes in people's lifestyles, the incidence of cancer worldwide is increasing. At the same

* **Corresponding author Xiao Zhu:** Guangdong Key Laboratory for Research and Development of Natural Drugs, Guangdong Medical University, Zhanjiang 524023, PRC; E-mails: xzhu@gdmu.edu.cn & bioxzhu@yahoo.com

time, the specific and effective lack of cancer therapies requires the development of a new generation of therapies, such as personalized immunotherapy. As breakthroughs have been made in the treatment of cancer, immunotherapy has gradually become a concern and a hot topic. Unlike traditional therapies, some immunotherapies do not directly kill tumor cells but mobilizes and enhances the ability of immune cells in the body to recognize and attack tumor cells, which makes it difficult for tumor cells to escape from host defense. Finally, the tumor cells are specifically cleared by the immune system. Beyond that, memory immune cells are capable of identifying and killing specific tumor cells for a long time, effectively improving the survival of patients. Consequently, immunotherapy has more accurate anticancer effects and fewer side effects than radiotherapy and chemotherapy. Immune therapy can be divided into six parts: the immune checkpoint inhibitors, cellular immunotherapy, cancer vaccine, oncolytic therapy, targeted bispecific antibodies, and immune modulators, among which the most rapidly growing and most popular is the molecular target checkpoint inhibitors.

There are two types of checkpoint inhibitors: one is an immune checkpoint inhibitor, which focuses on immune checkpoint inhibitors (ICI) related to treatment for disorders in the tumor immune microenvironment (TIME). The second is a molecular target checkpoint inhibitor, as described in Chapter 4, which studies checkpoint inhibitors related to therapeutic inhibitors for disorders of the tumor microenvironment (TME). This chapter addresses immune checkpoint inhibitors (ICIs) related to therapeutic targets for disorders in the tumor immune microenvironment (TIME).

MOLECULAR TARGETING CHECKPOINT INHIBITORS

Under normal circumstances can T cells bind to tumor-specific antigen on the surface of the cell-major histocompatibility complex (MHC) to identify tumor cells and attack them. In contrast, the surface of healthy cells with inhibition of checkpoint proteins prevents immune cells from attacking, which results in autoimmune diseases. Nevertheless, tumor cells can also be affected by interferon released by T-cells and produce inhibition checkpoint proteins similar to healthy cells, which transmit immunosuppressive signals and achieve immune evasion. Molecular targeting checkpoint inhibitors are designed to block the immunosuppressive target of T cells, reactivate the anti-tumor immune response, as well as achieving the purpose of killing tumors accurately. At present, molecular targeting checkpoint inhibitors have a particular effect on many tumors, but some tumors have been discovered to be resistant to them [1]. The most common molecular targeting checkpoint inhibitors were PD-1 ICI, PD-L1 ICI, and CTLA-4 ICI.PD-1/PD-L1.

PD-1/PD-L1

PD-1 is an immunosuppressive molecule that exists on the surface of T-cells, being capable of binding to normal cells to prevent T-cell activation and reducing the occurrence of autoimmune diseases. The two ligands of PD-1 are PD-L1 and PD-L2 [2]. As the primary ligand, PD-L1 is only expressed in tonsils, placenta, and macrophages, while other normal cells are hardly expressed. In the tumor microenvironment, IFN-γ secreted by effector T-cells, and NK cells induce PD-L1 expression in tumor cells. PD-L2 is induced by IL-4 and expressed in leukocytes. Protein antibody drugs targeting PD-1 or PD-L1 can block the inhibitory signaling pathway of PD-1/PD-L1, activate T-cells, restore the function of T-cells to recognize and kill tumor cells, and enhance the anti-tumor immune effect (Fig. **1**). The anti-tumor response of PD-1/PD-L1 receptor antagonists is higher than that of CTLA-4 receptor inhibitors, and the incidence of side effects is less, so it is safer to apply. At present, this inhibitor has been used in the treatment of a variety of tumors, such as non-small cell lung cancer, malignant melanoma, gastric cancer, kidney cancer, liver cancer, and the like. Clinical representative drugs include Keytruda (Pembrolizumab), Tecentriq (Atezolizumab), Bavencio(Avelumab), and Opdivo (Nivolumab).

The expression level of PD-L1 in the tumor microenvironment and the mutation load of the tumor are the main factors affecting the efficacy. When the expression level of PD-L1 is higher, or the mutation load of the tumor is higher [3, 4], the tumor is more likely to be recognized by immune cells, and the immune checkpoint treatment effect is better [5]. As a result, the expression degree of pd-l1 and tumor mutation load can be used as predictors of ICI treatment. In addition, the curative effect is subject to mutation allele frequency (MAF), LDH content, smoking status, and physical state.

CTLA-4

CTLA-4 is a protein that is widely distributed on the surface of T cells. In general, activation of T-cells requires the antigen information presented by MCH II to combine with T-cell receptor (TCR), at the same time B7 protein combined with another receptor CD28 [6 - 8]. Nonetheless, CTLA-4 has a high affinity with B7, preventing B7 from binding to CD28 and inhibiting T-cell activation. The use of CTLA-4 receptor inhibitors can not only restore the activity of effector T-cells but also inhibit the immunosuppressive function of regulatory T-cells (Treg) and restore the anti-tumor immune function (Fig. **1**). Yet, blocking CTLA-4 activates the immune system and can lead to serious reactions, such as hepatitis, colitis, and thyroiditis. Clinically related drugs are Yervoy (Ipilimumab) and Tremelimumab, which are mostly used for advanced or metastatic lung cancer, Merkel cell carcinoma, melanoma, *etc.*

TIM-3

Tim-3 is a novel immunosuppressive target [9, 10], expressed in T-cells, NK cells, and monocytes. When TIM-3 binds to ligand galectin-9, the activity of Th1 and CTL1 cells can be inhibited [11 - 13], leading to T-cell failure and immune tolerance, and finally, poor prognosis in cancer patients (Fig. **1**). A recent study proclaimed that TIM-3 is associated with immune resistance during PD-1 immunotherapy, and TIM-3 expression can be measured up-regulated in some cancer patients [14]. Both mutations in the HAVCR2 gene [15] and taking advantage of TIM-3 inhibitors can inhibit TIM-3 expression so that the TIM-3 protein function is inactivated, and the immune system is activated. TIM-3 inhibitors are still under development.

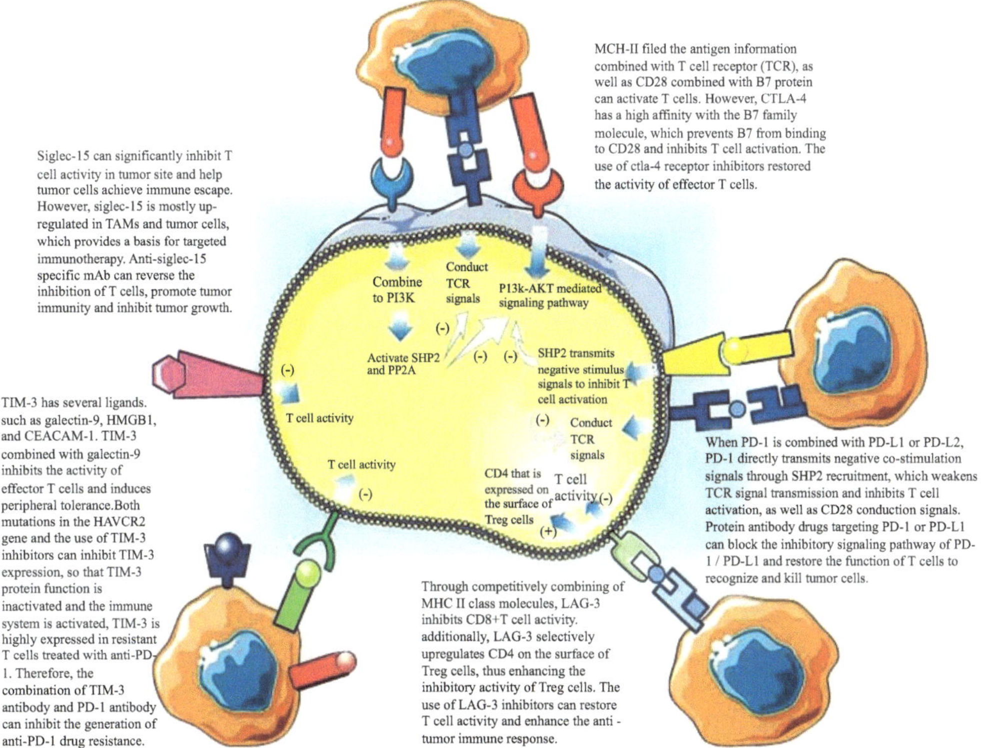

Fig. (1). T-cells targeting signaling.

LAG-3

LAG-3 [15] is an inhibitory receptor protein that is simultaneously expressed on the surface of immune cells, such as T-cells, NK cells, and plasma cells. With the combination of MHC II, LAG-3 can inhibit the activity of T cells, strengthen the regulatory T-cells (Treg) inhibitory. Consequently, making use of LAG-3 inhibitors can restore T-cell activity and enhance the anti-tumor immune response [16, 17] (Fig. **1**).

Inhibitory molecules such as CTLA-4, PD-1, TIM-3, and LAG-3 can be blocked to decrease T-cell exhaustion to kill tumor cells and activating molecules such as CD28 can be used to stimulate T-cell function for kill tumor cells.

Siglec-15

Siglec-15 can down-regulate the immune activity of T-cell so that the anti-tumor immune mechanism of the body is suppressed, and tumor cells can achieve immune escape. Siglec-15 is increased in a variety of tumor cells, such as bladder, kidney, liver, and lung cancer. By knocking out the siglec-15 or using the siglec-15 inhibitor, we can relieve immunosuppression and achieve specific killing of the tumor (Fig. **1**). Some studies have pointed out that the combination of siglec-15 inhibitor and PD-1/PD-L1 inhibitor can eliminate the resistance of tumors to PD-1/PD-L1 inhibitor, improving the success rate of treatment [18].

APPLICATION OF MOLECULAR TARGETING CHECKPOINT INHIBITORS

Small Cell Lung Cancer

SCLC has the characteristics of high malignancy, high mutation load [19], high incidence of drug resistance, easy recurrence, short doubling time, and early and extensive metastasis. CheckMate 032 study used PD-1 inhibitor (Nivolumab) alone or in combination with CTLA-4 inhibitor (Ipilimumab) to treat recurrent SCLC [20]. The study found that N1 mg/kg plusing I 3 mg/kg had a better therapeutic effect, and the toxicity increase was not very obvious, which became the optimal dose plan for phase III studies. In the latest IMpower 133 study, both overall survival and Progression-free survival were positive for extensive small-cell lung cancer treated with molecular targeting checkpoint inhibitors combined with chemotherapy [21]; thus, they become I class recommended for the treatment of extensive period of SCLC.

Non-Small Cell Lung Cancer (NSCLC)

In early-stage NSCLC, CD8+ tumor-infiltrating lymphocyte has a significant immune response to clonogenic neoantigen and a higher expression of PD-1; consequently, it is more conducive to the treatment of PD-1 inhibitor [22]. PFS rates in NSCLC patients treated with durvalumab in combination with radiotherapy were approximately 20% higher than with chemotherapy alone [23].

Current clinical data manifests that PD-1/PD-L1 inhibitors are less effective in treating NSCLC patients with EGFR mutation /ALK rearrangement than patients without these driver genes [24].

Hepatocellular Carcinoma (HCC) (for PDL1)

Aggressive HCC cells inhibit the immune response by expressing the PD-L1 immune checkpoint protein, which binds to the PD-1 receptor in the immune cells [25]. Professor David Ruggero *et al.* discovered that eFT508 could restrain ribosomal binding to RNA to halve the PD-L1 protein level of tumor cells and inhibit the synthesis of immune checkpoint protein. Finally, the survival rate of liver cancer mice was dramatically improved [26].

Melanoma

Melanoma is surrounded by a large number of infiltrating CD4+ and CD8+T cells, which are specific killer T cells that can recognize mutant peptides [27]. Some studies suggest that the effect could be even more dramatic by stimulating these T-cells and clustering them around the edges of tumors and then using molecular targeting checkpoint inhibitors [28]. Simultaneously, adopting the method of combining the use of checkpoint inhibitors, such as I and N (Nivolumab), increased the effectiveness of treatment in patients from 19% to 58%. However, it also aggravated the side effects of treatment [29]. How to reduce side effects while improving the efficiency of treatment still needs active exploration. In addition, through combining radiotherapy and chemotherapy to kill the melanoma, tumor cells release antigens, such as MAGE-A3, so that the remaining tumor cells are easier to identify and kill [30].

Kidney Cancer

In this study, nivolumab and ipilimumab combined therapy were found to have higher objective efficacy in metastatic renal cell carcinoma and advanced renal cell carcinoma at medium and high risk [31 - 33]. Another feasible dual-drug combination mode is PD1/PD-L1 inhibitor combined with the TKI drug. Preliminary results indicate that PD1/PD-L1 inhibitor associating with TKI is either rather effective in the treatment of advanced renal cancer [34, 35]. Clinical classification of renal clear cell carcinoma according to the changes of the tumor tissue genome is expected to predict the therapeutic effect of TKI on advanced renal cancer [36].

PROBLEM

Although immunotherapy has brought new hope to cancer, it is still in the early stage of development, and many issues need to be solved. The first is the personalized use of molecular targeting checkpoint inhibitors. The tumor microenvironment of different patients are inevitably different; accordingly, PD-L1 and tumor mutation load are different. Therefore, how to adjust the time and dose of inhibitor use is what we need to explore. Second, when using checkpoint inhibitors in association with other traditional treatments, such as chemotherapy, radiotherapy, and interventional therapy, different procedures need to be used in combination. The timing and dose of each application are the keys to improving efficacy. Third, molecular targeting checkpoint inhibitors tend to produce immune-related adverse events [37] during the use, such as allergic dermatitis, headache, fatigue, hepatitis, *etc.* It is urgent to reduce side effects while improving the curative effect. Only by closely monitoring the patient's physical condition and individualized adjustment of dose and treatment plan according to the patient's condition can adverse reactions be minimized.

CONCLUSION AND PERSPECTIVE

Nowadays, the treatment of the tumor has entered the era of immunity, and the treatment of molecular-targeted checkpoints has opened up a new field of anti-tumor therapy, which develops exceedingly rapidly. The discovery and application of various specific targets make immunotherapy more and more accurate and efficient, and it will have broad development prospects in the future. Nevertheless, there are still many issues worth discussing in the development of immunotherapy in China, such as the correlation between tumor mutation load in different populations and patient survival rates. Immunotherapy regimens in China still need to be adapted to the Chinese population, as the incidence of tumor-target mutations is higher in China than in the west. For the purpose of reducing the side effects of immunotherapy along with improving the safety and accuracy of treatment, we can select an accurate immune target and adjust the immune dose to maximize the patients' benefit. In addition, it is still open to debate on how to balance the advantages and disadvantages of combined use of this immune-targeted therapy and traditional therapy. In the future, the treatment of molecular-targeted checkpoints will make more breakthroughs in the selection of targets and the study of target information pathways, making contributions to the development of precision medicine

CONSENT FOR PUBLICATION

The authors declare no financial interests.

CONFLICT OF INTEREST

The authors declare no financial interests.

ACKNOWLEDGEMENTS

in order to support writing quality, two editors (Nancy Debry is editor in our America Society of Pediatrics) have been invited to modify some grammar in the writings.

The mention of trade names or commercial products in this article is solely to provide specific information and does not imply recommendation.

REFERENCES

[1]   Ribas A, Wolchok JD. Cancer immunotherapy using checkpoint blockade. Cancer immunotherapy using checkpoint blockade Science Mar 23 2018; 359(6382): 1350- 1355.
[http://dx.doi.org/10.1126/science.aar4060]

[2]   Pardoll DM. The blockade of immune checkpoints in cancer immunotherapy. Nat Rev Cancer 2012; 12(4): 252-64.
[http://dx.doi.org/10.1038/nrc3239] [PMID: 22437870]

[3]   Snyder A, Wolchok JD, Chan TA. Genetic basis for clinical response to CTLA-4 blockade. N Engl J Med 2015; 372(8): 783.
[http://dx.doi.org/10.1056/NEJMc1415938] [PMID: 25693024]

[4]   Rizvi NA, Hellmann MD, Snyder A, *et al.* Cancer immunology. Mutational landscape determines sensitivity to PD-1 blockade in non-small cell lung cancer. Science 2015; 348(6230): 124-8.
[http://dx.doi.org/10.1126/science.aaa1348] [PMID: 25765070]

[5]   Yarchoan M, Albacker LA, Hopkins AC, *et al.* PD-L1 expression and tumor mutational burden are independent biomarkers in most cancers. JCI Insight 2019; 4(6)126908
[http://dx.doi.org/10.1172/jci.insight.126908] [PMID: 30895946]

[6]   Sica GL, Choi IH, Zhu G, *et al.* B7-H4, a molecule of the B7 family, negatively regulates T cell immunity. Immunity 2003; 18(6): 849-61.
[http://dx.doi.org/10.1016/S1074-7613(03)00152-3] [PMID: 12818165]

[7]   Prasad DV, Richards S, Mai XM, Dong C. B7S1, a novel B7 family member that negatively regulates T cell activation. Immunity 2003; 18(6): 863-73.
[http://dx.doi.org/10.1016/S1074-7613(03)00147-X] [PMID: 12818166]

[8]   Marisa L, Svrcek M, Collura A, *et al.* The Balance Between Cytotoxic T-cell Lymphocytes and Immune Checkpoint Expression in the Prognosis of Colon Tumors. J Natl Cancer Inst 2018; 110(1)
[http://dx.doi.org/10.1093/jnci/djx136] [PMID: 28922790]

[9]   Zhang Y, Cai P, Liang T, Wang L, Hu L. TIM-3 is a potential prognostic marker for patients with solid tumors: A systematic review and meta-analysis. Oncotarget 2017; 8(19): 31705-13.
[http://dx.doi.org/10.18632/oncotarget.15954] [PMID: 28423646]

[10]   Du W, Yang M, Turner A, *et al.* TIM-3 as a Target for Cancer Immunotherapy and Mechanisms of Action. Int J Mol Sci Mar 16 2017; 18(3)

[11]   Golden-Mason L, Palmer BE, Kassam N, *et al.* Negative immune regulator Tim-3 is overexpressed on T cells in hepatitis C virus infection and its blockade rescues dysfunctional CD4+ and CD8+ T cells. J Virol 2009; 83(18): 9122-30.
[http://dx.doi.org/10.1128/JVI.00639-09] [PMID: 19587053]

[12]   Zhu C, Anderson AC, Kuchroo VK. TIM-3 and its regulatory role in immune responses. Curr Top Microbiol Immunol 2011; 350: 1-15.
[PMID: 20700701]

[13]   Anderson AC, Joller N, Kuchroo VK. Lag-3, Tim-3, and TIGIT: Co-inhibitory Receptors with Specialized Functions in Immune Regulation. Immunity 2016; 44(5): 989-1004.
[http://dx.doi.org/10.1016/j.immuni.2016.05.001] [PMID: 27192565]

[14]   Sakuishi K, Apetoh L, Sullivan JM, Blazar BR, Kuchroo VK, Anderson AC. Targeting Tim-3 and PD-1 pathways to reverse T cell exhaustion and restore anti-tumor immunity. J Exp Med 2010; 207(10): 2187-94.
[http://dx.doi.org/10.1084/jem.20100643] [PMID: 20819927]

[15]   Huang CT, Workman CJ, Flies D, *et al.* Role of LAG-3 in regulatory T cells. Immunity 2004; 21(4): 503-13.
[http://dx.doi.org/10.1016/j.immuni.2004.08.010] [PMID: 15485628]

[16]   Long L, Zhang X, Chen F, *et al.* The promising immune checkpoint LAG-3: from tumor microenvironment to cancer immunotherapy. Genes Cancer 2018; 9(5-6): 176-89.
[http://dx.doi.org/10.18632/genesandcancer.180] [PMID: 30603054]

[17]   Marin-Acevedo JA, Dholaria B, Soyano AE, Knutson KL, Chumsri S, Lou Y. Next generation of immune checkpoint therapy in cancer: new developments and challenges. J Hematol Oncol 2018; 11(1): 39.
[http://dx.doi.org/10.1186/s13045-018-0582-8] [PMID: 29544515]

[18]   Wang J, Sun J, Liu LN, *et al.* Siglec-15 as an immune suppressor and potential target for normalization cancer immunotherapy. Nat Med 2019; 25(4): 656-66.
[http://dx.doi.org/10.1038/s41591-019-0374-x] [PMID: 30833750]

[19]   Peifer M, Fernández-Cuesta L, Sos ML, *et al.* Integrative genome analyses identify key somatic driver mutations of small-cell lung cancer. Nat Genet 2012; 44(10): 1104-10.
[http://dx.doi.org/10.1038/ng.2396] [PMID: 22941188]

[20]   Antonia SJ, López-Martin JA, Bendell J, *et al.* Nivolumab alone and nivolumab plus ipilimumab in recurrent small-cell lung cancer (CheckMate 032): a multicentre, open-label, phase 1/2 trial. Lancet Oncol 2016; 17(7): 883-95.
[http://dx.doi.org/10.1016/S1470-2045(16)30098-5] [PMID: 27269741]

[21]   Pacheco J, Bunn PA. Advancements in Small-cell Lung Cancer: The Changing Landscape Following IMpower-133. Clin Lung Cancer 2019; 20(3): 148-160.e2.
[http://dx.doi.org/10.1016/j.cllc.2018.12.019] [PMID: 30686680]

[22]   Reck M, Heigener D, Reinmuth N. Immunotherapy for small-cell lung cancer: emerging evidence. Future Oncol 2016; 12(7): 931-43.
[http://dx.doi.org/10.2217/fon-2015-0012] [PMID: 26882955]

[23]   Antonia SJ, Villegas A, Daniel D, *et al.* Durvalumab after Chemoradiotherapy in Stage III Non-Smal--Cell Lung Cancer. N Engl J Med 2017; 377(20): 1919-29.
[http://dx.doi.org/10.1056/NEJMoa1709937] [PMID: 28885881]

[24]   Gainor JF, Shaw AT, Sequist LV, *et al.* EGFR Mutations and ALK Rearrangements Are Associated with Low Response Rates to PD-1 Pathway Blockade in Non-Small Cell Lung Cancer: A Retrospective Analysis. Clin Cancer Res 2016; 22(18): 4585-93.
[http://dx.doi.org/10.1158/1078-0432.CCR-15-3101] [PMID: 27225694]

[25]   Xu Y, Poggio M, Jin HY, *et al.* Translation control of the immune checkpoint in cancer and its therapeutic targeting. Nat Med 2019; 25(2): 301-11.
[http://dx.doi.org/10.1038/s41591-018-0321-2] [PMID: 30643286]

[26]   Qiao R, Zhong R, Xu J, *et al.* Prediction of lymph node status in completely resected IIIa/N2 small cell lung cancer: importance of subcarinal station metastases. J Cardiothorac Surg 2019; 14(1): 63.

[http://dx.doi.org/10.1186/s13019-019-0886-y] [PMID: 30925891]

[27] Márquez-Rodas I, Cerezuela P, Soria A, *et al.* Immune checkpoint inhibitors: therapeutic advances in melanoma. Ann Transl Med 2015; 3(18): 267.
[PMID: 26605313]

[28] Kakavand H, Wilmott JS, Menzies AM, *et al.* PD-L1 Expression and Tumor-Infiltrating Lymphocytes Define Different Subsets of MAPK Inhibitor-Treated Melanoma Patients. Clin Cancer Res 2015; 21(14): 3140-8.
[http://dx.doi.org/10.1158/1078-0432.CCR-14-2023] [PMID: 25609064]

[29] Kurupati RK, Zhou X, Xiang Z, Keller LH, Ertl HCJ. Safety and immunogenicity of a potential checkpoint blockade vaccine for canine melanoma. Cancer Immunol Immunother 2018; 67(10): 1533-44.
[http://dx.doi.org/10.1007/s00262-018-2201-5] [PMID: 30051333]

[30] Lu YC, Parker LL, Lu T, *et al.* Treatment of Patients With Metastatic Cancer Using a Major Histocompatibility Complex Class II-Restricted T-Cell Receptor Targeting the Cancer Germline Antigen MAGE-A3. J Clin Oncol 2017; 35(29): 3322-9.
[http://dx.doi.org/10.1200/JCO.2017.74.5463] [PMID: 28809608]

[31] Wan X, Zhang Y, Tan C, Zeng X, Peng L. First-line Nivolumab Plus Ipilimumab *vs* Sunitinib for Metastatic Renal Cell Carcinoma: A Cost-effectiveness Analysis. JAMA Oncol 2019; 5(4): 491-6.
[http://dx.doi.org/10.1001/jamaoncol.2018.7086] [PMID: 30789633]

[32] Gao X, McDermott DF. Ipilimumab in combination with nivolumab for the treatment of renal cell carcinoma. Expert Opin Biol Ther 2018; 18(9): 947-57.
[http://dx.doi.org/10.1080/14712598.2018.1513485] [PMID: 30124333]

[33] Hammers HJ, Plimack ER, Infante JR, *et al.* Safety and Efficacy of Nivolumab in Combination With Ipilimumab in Metastatic Renal Cell Carcinoma: The CheckMate 016 Study. J Clin Oncol 2017; 35(34): 3851-8.
[http://dx.doi.org/10.1200/JCO.2016.72.1985] [PMID: 28678668]

[34] Esther J, Hale P, Hahn AW, Agarwal N, Maughan BL. Treatment Decisions for Metastatic Clear Cell Renal Cell Carcinoma in Older Patients: The Role of TKIs and Immune Checkpoint Inhibitors. Drugs Aging 2019; 36(5): 395-401.
[http://dx.doi.org/10.1007/s40266-019-00644-1] [PMID: 30784023]

[35] Koshkin VS, Rini BI. Emerging therapeutics in refractory renal cell carcinoma. Expert Opin Pharmacother 2016; 17(9): 1225-32.
[http://dx.doi.org/10.1080/14656566.2016.1182987] [PMID: 27112171]

[36] Liu KG, Gupta S, Goel S. Immunotherapy: incorporation in the evolving paradigm of renal cancer management and future prospects. Oncotarget 2017; 8(10): 17313-27.
[http://dx.doi.org/10.18632/oncotarget.14388] [PMID: 28061473]

[37] Postow MA, Sidlow R, Hellmann MD. Immune-Related Adverse Events Associated with Immune Checkpoint Blockade. N Engl J Med 2018; 378(2): 158-68.
[http://dx.doi.org/10.1056/NEJMra1703481] [PMID: 29320654]

CHAPTER 6

Molecular Screening and Neoantigen Cloning-Fundamental of Adoptive T-cell Immunotherapy

Wei Zhang[1], George Liu[1], Emmanuelle Devemy[2] and Biaoru Li[1,2,3,*]

[1] Department of Biochemistry, Case Western Reserve University School of Medicine, Cleveland, OH, USA

[2] Rush Cancer Institute, Chicago, IL, USA

[3] Georgia Cancer Center and Department of Pediatrics, Medical College at GA, Augusta, GA 30912, USA

Abstract: Specific T-cells, TCR T-cells, and CAR-T-cells require to establish some techniques of molecular biology to support them, including screening tumor-associated antigen (TAA)/tumor specific antigen (TSA) and mutant proteins/peptides; constructing an expression system; packaging an expression vector. The molecular biology technique is a very important performance in targeting neoantigens for tumor-specific T-cells of adoptive T-cell immunotherapy. Since tumor cells often accumulate hundreds of mutations and harbor several immunogenic neoantigens, the repertoire of mutant protein or neoantigen from patient tumor cells might need to screen and discover the antigens for engineering specific T-cells, TCR T-cells, and CAR T-cells. In order to understand the procedures for T-cell adoptive immunotherapy based on molecular biology techniques for mutant proteins and neoantigens from an individual patient, in this chapter, we focus on streamlining of screening tumor antigens (TAA or TSA) and mutant proteins (proteins or peptides), constructing an expression and packaging system with the expression. Moreover, because the three T-cells are distinct from development and clinical application, we first introduce their research and Development (R&D). These methodologies are increasingly supporting clinical oncologists to apply to T-cell immunotherapy. The chapter aims to present fundamental of molecular biology for adoptive T-cell immunotherapy of clinical patients.

Keywords: CAR (chimeric antigen receptor) T-cells, Lentiviral, Monoclonal Ab, Phage display system, Retroviral vector, Specific T-cells, T-cell adoptive immunotherapy, TCR (T-cell receptors).

INTRODUCTION

Molecular biology-related comprehensive techniques are essential fundamentals

---

* **Corresponding author Biaoru Li:** Georgia Cancer Center and Department of Pediatrics, Medical College at GA, Augusta, GA 30912, USA; Tel: 440-317-1443; E-mail: bli@augusta.edu

to support adoptive immunotherapy for clinical patients with different tumor diseases. Moreover, the selection of the techniques of specific T-cells, CAR T-cells, and TCR T-cells also is essential for the efficacy of T-cell immunotherapy. According to early publication in 1989 [1], constructing chimeric molecules with some specific antigens or peptides recognized by immune cells is over 30 years.

First chimeric TCR was reported for T-cell specific affinity by anti-TNP mRNA cloning into TCR v-chain and c-chain to targeting cell in 1989 [2]. In the early period, we were involved in T-cell reconstructs, specifically recognizing tumor antigens. For example, we had planned DHBsAb from Duck Hepatitis B Virus (DHBV) to clone into CD3 of TIL to produce DHBsAb-CD3 TIL to kill hepatic cancer cells infected by HBV. As we know, DHBV from Chinese duck is the same family as the hepatitis B virus (HBV) from human HBV. The viral envelope has viral surface antigens (DHBsAg) which is almost same homologous sequences as those of HBsAg; Although we achieved a successful result for DHBV-LSP (Lipopolysaccharides) inducting hepatic necrosis as reported in 1989 [3] and successfully set up TIL culture and clone technique as reported in 1995 [4], we failed to achieve DHBsAb-CD3 chimeric TILs to specific affinity both DHBV and HBV infected HCC cells because unclear CD3 and TCR structure limited our study at that early time.

However, after 1989, some scientists reported the first synthetic immunoglobulin/TCR chimeric molecule with antibody-like specificity, some scientists discovered that CD8 and the CD3ζ chain could independently mediate T-cell activation of the endogenous TCR [5], so that specific chimeric T-cells begin to be extensively researched. Since then, specific T-cells, CAR, and TCR have been studied for more than 20 years. Now CAR constructs are very mature, including three domains' constructs: an ectodomain containing a scFv for recognition of specific antigen, a transmembrane domain, and signaling domains [6]. At present, these CAR T-cells are capable of on-target lymphocytic leukemia and lymphoma because these designs lead to producing autologous CD19 CAR-T cells to treat B-cell malignancies [7]. Recently, CAR T-cells are going to be involved in different hematological malignancies [8].

Although CAR T-cell immunotherapy demonstrated excellent response against B-cell hematological malignancies, its effect against solid tumors is unsatisfactory. After 20 years' effort, TCR engineered T-cells have demonstrated better responses against solid tumors than those of CAR engineering T-cells. The TCR constructs depend on complexes with peptide-major histocompatibility complex (MHC). The peptides bind MHC class I to CD8+cell and MHC class II to CD4+cells, allowing these peptide-MHCs binding or killing cancer cells [9].

Furthermore, even if CAR and TCR constructs demonstrated excellent response against hematological malignancies and tumor cells from solid tumors, their products are required a complicated performance. Some scientists developed a procedure of synthetic peptides, and thus, dendritic cell (DC) pulsed by specific peptides produces peptide-MHC complex [10]. The specific MHC-peptides in DC can be used by active immunotherapy as vaccines [11] or co-culture with PBMN T-cells to produce adoptive immunotherapy as specific T-cell to killing tumor cells [12].

Because three constructs, specific T-cells, CAR T-cells, and TCR T-cells are distinct, the constructs of full-length TCR have greater sensitivity while CAR constructs are expressed at higher densities. Furthermore, TCR T-cells are subject to studying killing tumor cells of solid tumors, while CAR T-cells are going to be involved in hematological malignancies [13]. The higher sensitivity of TCR T-cells can enable the quicker killing of tumor cells, although these increases the risk of "on-target, off-tumor" toxicity. TCR T-cells have shown the release of fewer amounts of cytokines after treatment [14], and therefore, cytokine release syndromes (CRS) of TCR T-cell therapy should be lower than those of CAR T-cell therapy. As described above, DC pulsed by specific peptides forming peptide-MHC complex can be easily used to produce active immunotherapy by DC vaccines or co-culture with T-cell to engage adoptive immunotherapy by specific T-cells as Table **1**.

After understanding the backgrounds with their R&D, the following sections will introduce fundamental in molecular biology: (I) screening specific or shared neoantigens or mutant proteins and peptides; (II) constructing an expression plasmid from the screened or shared products; (III) delivering and packaging expression systems.

Table 1. Different constructs for distinct functions.

Reconstructs	Cells Involved	Functions
Shared or specific peptides pulsed into DC	DC	Specific vaccine for active immunotherapy
	DC co-culture with T-cells from PBMN	Specific T-cells for adoptive immunotherapy
TCR constructs	T-cell from PBMN	TCR T-cells for solid malignant tumors
CAR constructs	T-cell from PBMN	CAR T-cells for hematological malignancies

MOLECULAR SCREENING NEOANTIGEN AND MUTANTS

Molecular screening techniques of shared or specific tumor antigen/peptides includes at least six platforms and strategies: (I) phage display screen system; (II) scFv molecular screening neoantigens or mutant proteins for CARs; (III) peptide-MHC complex screening neoantigens or mutant proteins for TCR; (IV) Yeast two-hybrid library screening tumor protein or peptides; (V) genomic library with molecular support; (VI) other techniques.

1. Phage Display Screen System

We initiated a phage display screening system for malignant myeloid cells under support of Drs. HD. Preisler and G Smiths in 1996. After we set up isolation and culture of malignant myeloid cells as Fig. (**1**) [15 - 20], our colleagues have experienced about 15 years to discover several peptides to recognize malignant myeloid cells as reports since then [21]. The system can discover specific biomarkers on malignant cells so that the peptides can directly use to bind biomarkers on the surface of malignant cells. A disadvantage is a distinct phenotype and genotype from different patients so that screening beginning of malignant cells require very pure single-cells. After more than twenty-years' effort. We have set up several single-cell culture techniques [22] to screen neoantigen or mutant from tumor cells, TILs, and cancer stem cells, allowing the pure cells to achieve specific protein or peptides. On the other hand, a phage display system has been often used to produce scFv for the CAR construct.

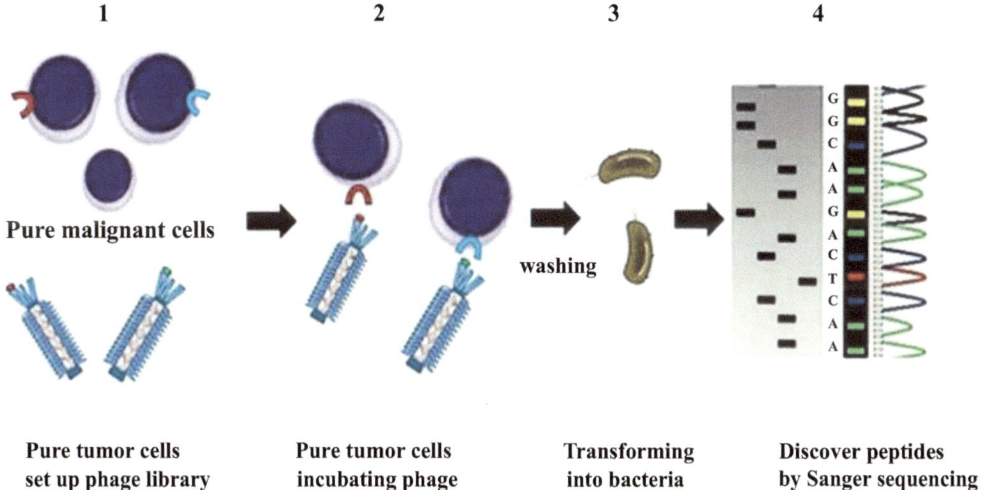

Fig. (1). Screening technique by a phage display system. Four steps: (**1**) set up phage display screening: (**2**) purifying malignant cells, incubating with random peptide phage, (**3**) phage transform after strict washing the binding, (**4**) Sanger sequence to discover peptide sequences with the specific bindings.

2. scFv Screening

Screening and generation of a single-chain variable fragment (scFv) are developed from hybridoma or phage display for the chimeric antigen receptor (CAR).

Although both techniques are feasible and services are available from companies, here we focus on CAR technique by hybridoma system. Mechanisms of CAR constructs is that an antigen recognizing molecule consists of a heavy chain variable region (VH) and a light chain variable region (VL), while an scFv consists typically of a VH and a VL connected *via* a peptide linker. scFv screening is performed by library techniques with their platform, allowing them to discover the desired scFv whose expression and function are correlated with T-cell activation. As published reports [23], the generations of specific scFv with their optimization of specific affinity include four steps of molecular and cellular biology as Fig. (**2**): antigen immunization, plasma cell fused into myeloma cell, mAbs production, and scFv screening and determining by PCR combined Sanger sequence. Without a doubt, a specific scFv can lead to specific CAR T-cell therapy. Generating scFv from hybridoma cell is as shown in Fig. (**2**), the techniques of molecular and cellular biology of scFv are demonstrated, in detail, as below:

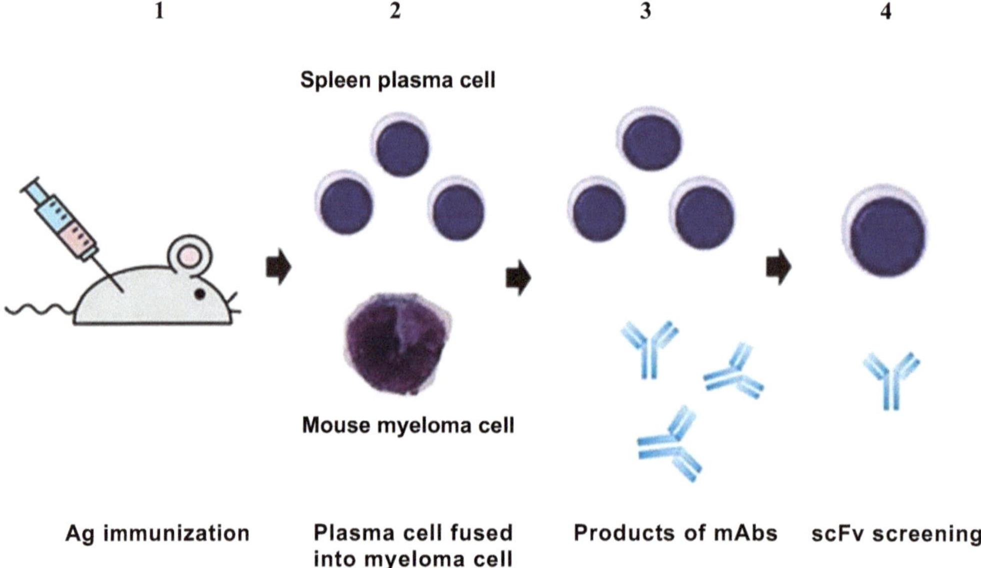

Fig. (2). Screening technique by scFv strategies.Four steps, including (**1**) antigen immunization; (**2**) plasma cells used into myeloma cell; (**3**) producing mAbs and (**4**) scFv screening by rtPCR with Sanger sequence.

a. Immunize mice with a shared or specific antigen, and then, remove the spleen to get splenocytes (plasma B cells);

b. Fuse the acquired splenocytes with the cultured myeloma cells to establish hybridoma cell lines following by the cell limited-dilution and affinity screen;

c. Produce mAb and convert the Fv from the discovered full monoclonal antibody into an scFv, which can target the tumor antigen;

d. Clone the superior scFv with sequencing and binding confirmation for future CAR components to construct a lentiviral/retroviral vector for the future steps.

3. TCR Screening

To increase efficiency and sensitivity to kill tumor cells from a solid tumor, the molecular design of the T-cell receptor (TCR) is a crucial step of TCR constructs. At present, at least three strategies are used to produce TCR screening systems with their molecular designs: TCR generated by patient TIL, TCR generated by phage display, and TCR generated by *in vivo*. Although all three strategies of TCR screening and generation are feasible, here we just introduce TCR construct generated from TIL.

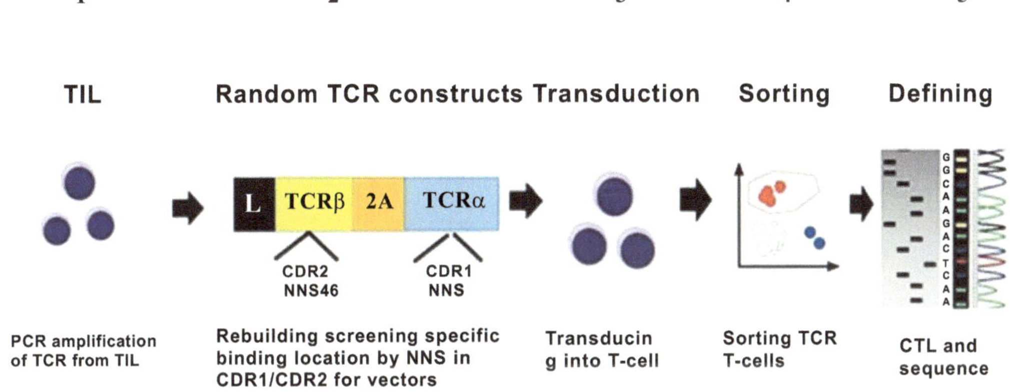

Fig. (3). Screening technique by TCR strategies.Five steps, including **(1)** TIL isolation with TCR cDNA fragment harvested by PCR; **(2)** reconstructing random binding sequences (NNS located CDR1 and CDR2 in TCR); **(3)** transducing into T-cell from PBMN; **(4)** sorting by FACS; **(5)** CTL assay-specific TCR T-cells with final sequencing confirmation.

As shown in Fig. (3), complementarity-determining regions (CDRs) [24] are part of the variable region in TCR generated by TILs. CDR2 located at TCR-β and CDR1 at TCR-α are some specific binding sites or codes so that NNS (*NNS* codons, where N=G or A or T or C and S = C or G) replacement can produce 20 different possibilities of amino acids with the random designed codes [25]. TCR produced by TILs are (I) to extract mRNA from TIL, (II) to produce TCR cDNA product by overlapping extension *PCR* for two *fragments* (TCRβ and TCRα) including 2A self-cleaving peptide, (III) to transduce the complex into T-cells, (IV) TCR biomarker identification & selection, (V) TCR generation by sequence. These random binding TCRs have been used to screen candidates and determine specific binding antigens that are expressed by tumor cells from patients.

4. Yeast Two-Hybrid Screening

In order to study binding DNA minor groove by DM domain, we have studied Yeast Two-Hybrid (Y2H) to screen specific binding systems since 2000 [26]. The first successful Y2H technique was reported to screen tumor cells for FHL2 related to gastrointestinal cancer in 2009 [27]. A screening scFv specific binding P53 proteins was reported in 2016 [28]. To construct a scFv library specific to human P53, some scientists used bait vector (pGBKT-p53 expressing P53 protein) and prey vector (pGADT7 with an scFv cDNA from p53 immunized mouse) to screen specific binding sites. After P53-immunized mouse spleen tissue, as Fig. (4), the single chain V(H)-linker-V(L) fragment is rebuilt by reverse transcription-PCR and overlapping PCR, and then, V(H)-linker-V(L) fragment is constructed on the vector pGADT7. They discovered that some regions of scFv have a good affinity for human P53 protein. The technique could be increasingly used for the identification of neoantigen/peptides.

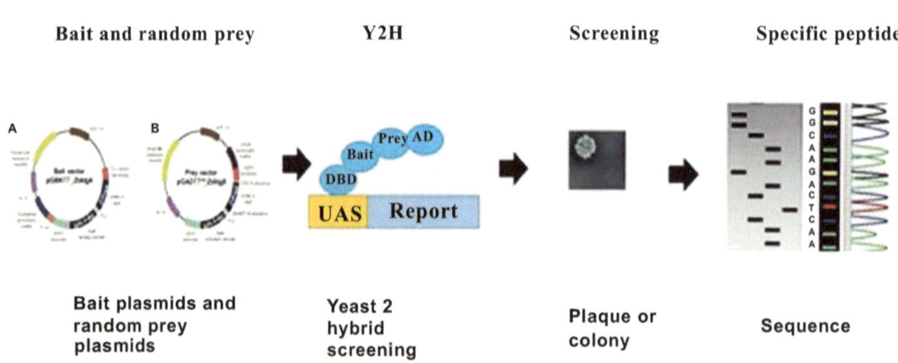

Fig. (4). Screening technique by Y2H.Four steps including **(1)** bait and prey constructs; **(2)** Y2H process; **(3)** screening and **(4)** discovering specific peptides.

5. Molecular Technique Supporting Genomics and Bioinformatics

After RNA-seq and DNA-seq are developed since 1995, most scientists working on screening techniques have often used genomic techniques to discover new candidates of neoantigens. For example, a group of scientists successfully set up a bioinformatics module to identify neoantigen-specific T-cells from epithelial ovarian cancer (EOC). They performed whole-exome sequence (WES) and transcriptome sequencing to 20 EOC patients. After both data were analyzed, they used immunogenicity prediction (NetMHC) combined with transcriptome from

RNA-seq to set up candidates of profiles, and then prioritize the tumor neoantigens. The genomics performance should be supported by molecular technique as Fig. (**5**). The molecular technique includes (1) synthesizing RNA or DNA to transfect DC to produce peptides by DNA/RNA transfection and (2) reconstructing TCR by overlapping PCR to define specific T-cells. The engineering T-cells with tumor antigen-specific TCR can be used to generate T-cells for personalized adoptive T-cell immunotherapy [29]. As described in another chapter, we have been going to study genomics with bioinformatics platform to study personalized TIL immunotherapy as publications since 2000 [30].

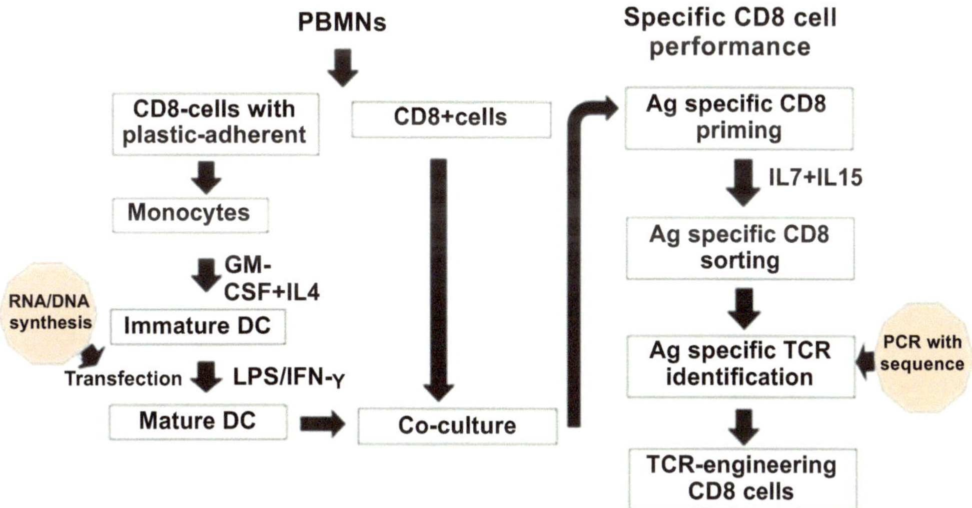

Fig. (5). Molecular technique support screening by genomics and bioinformatics. Two molecular techniques as pink support genomic files by related RNA and DNA transfection replacing to peptides synthesis and TCR rebuilding and PCR confirming TCR.

6. Other Screenings of Molecular Biology

Before microarray and NGS were available, most scientists had used Serial Analysis of Gene Expression (SAGE) and mRNA differential display to screen neoantigens or new biomarkers as Fig. (**6**) [31, 32]. In order to study quiescent genes from TIL CD8+T-cell, we have set up cloning-based mRNA differential display to discover several quiescent genes from CD8 cells of TILs as publications in 2000-2008 [33 - 35]. After microarray and NGS have emerged for a genomic platform, now only very few laboratories still use these techniques because both SAGE and mRNA display is not high throughput.

In general, the selection of screening techniques of shared or specific tumor antigen/peptides relies on the sources of screening molecules. Phage-display system, mRNA differential display, TCR, and genomics are often subject to a whole-cell level of tumor cells, while CAR and Y2H are often used to molecules from tumor cells. Based on different backgrounds of scientists and available techniques, different scientists select different strategies to discover neoantigen or mutant peptides. We have been working at the whole-cell level so that we are going to study single-cell techniques, including single-cell cloning, single-cell culture, and single genomics as our publications [36 - 38].

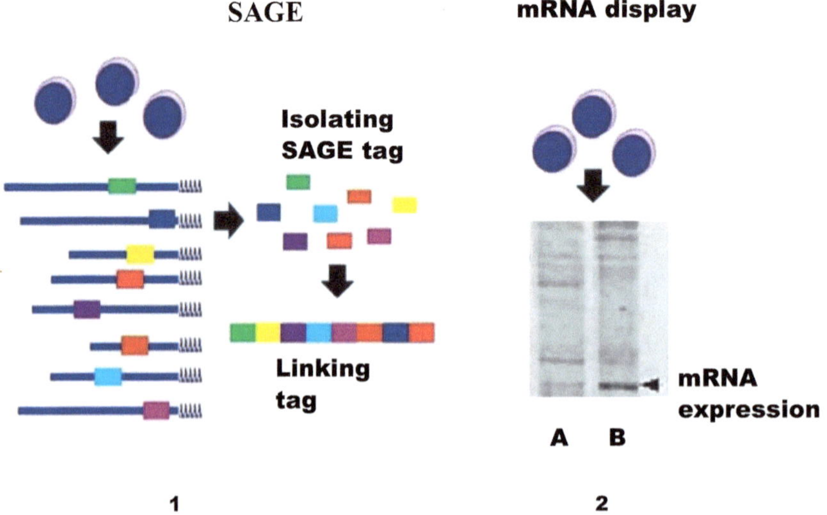

Fig. (6). Screening technique by other strategies. **(1)** Serial analysis of gene expression (SAGE). **(2)** Differential mRNA display A means control and B is specific mRNA expression

MOLECULAR CONSTRUCTS

According to research & development (R&D) of constructing techniques for T-cell immunotherapy, there are three constructing techniques and strategies are emerging in thirty years: (1) CAR construct for recognizing shared or specific neoantigen; (2) TCR construct for shared tumor antigen or specific neoantigen; (2) specific peptides pulsing dendritic cells or constructs of DNA or RNA as specific peptides transfecting into DC. The constructs are packaged by the viral vector and transduced into T-cells for engineering specific T-cells of T-cell immunotherapy.

1. CAR Design and Constructs

CAR stands for the chimeric antigen receptor, which is engineered for a T-cell with an arbitrary specificity *via* a monoclonal antibody. First-generation CAR constructs consist of an intracellular domain from the CD3ζ chain and a primary transmitter of signals from endogenous TCRs, which showed success in preclinical trials for neuroblastoma [39]. Second-generation CAR was designed to combine the intracellular signaling domains from various costimulatory protein receptors (CD28-41BB, ICOS) incorporated in the cytoplasmic tail of the CAR to enhance the signaling. For instance, the CD19-targeted CARs incorporated with CD28 or 4-1BB signaling domains manifested remarkable complete remission in patients with refractory B-cell malignancies [40]. Third-generation CAR combined multiple signaling domains (CD3 ζ-CD28-41BB, CD3 ζ-CD28-OX40) to acquire further enhanced activation signals, proliferation, production of cytokines, and effective function [41]. As Fig. (**7**), after overlapping PCR, a third-generation CAR is designed and constructed to produce CAR molecules. The α-CD19-TM-signaling co-stimulating (CD3ζ-4-1BB-CD28 or CD28-4-1BB-CD3ζ) CAR for chronic lymphocyte leukemia showed complete remission [42]. Although a few of companies are available to support kits or service to produce CAR, which is desired by laboratories, most laboratories still rebuild some CAR constructs for own purposes.

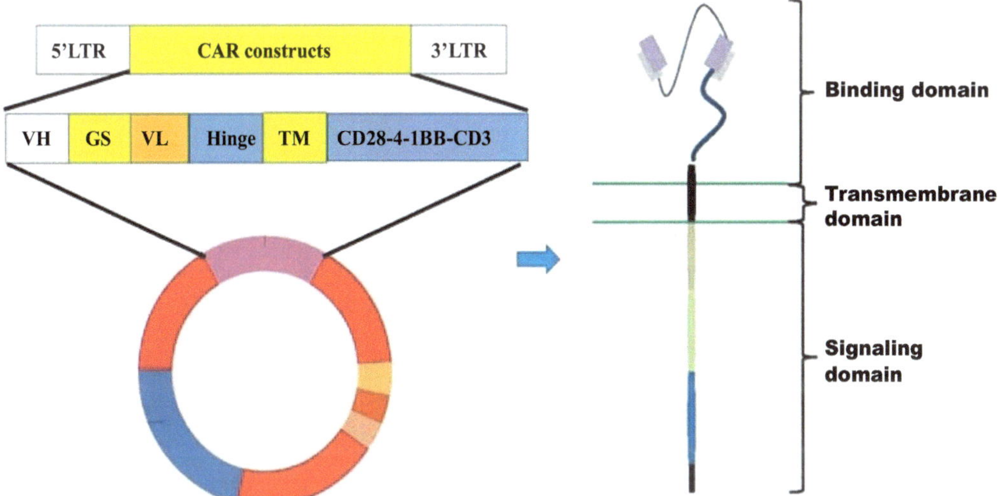

Fig. (7). Constructs of chimeric antigen receptor. Left is CAR construct by overlapping PCR and right is CAR products.

2. Specific TCR Design

The TCR is a molecule that existed on the surface of T cells. Its responsibility is to recognize fragments of antigen to provide peptides bound to major histocompatibility complex (MHC) molecules. The relationship between the TCRs is made up of two different protein chains with a 2A self-cleaving peptides as Fig. (**8**). If overlapping extension PCR achieves TCR complex from TIL, selective TCR domain can recognize and bind to a tumor-specific peptide target presented in the context of HLA class I receptor so that the TCR can be directly used to packaging viral vectors [43].

3. Specific T-cell and Constructs

In general, specific peptides can be produced by amino acid synthesis. Now microRNA techniques are going to be used to study an RNA sequence transfecting into DC to replace tumor specific-peptide pulsed into DC [44]. The RNA can be transfected into DC by lipofectamine or Nucleofector kit.

VECTOR SELECTION FOR GENE PACKAGE AND DELIVERY

After completing molecular constructs, gene transfer techniques have given scientists the possibility for clinical therapies in many genetic and tumor diseases since the late 1980s. A first clinical trial was initiated for children with severe combined immune deficiency (SCID) due to mutations in the adenosine deaminase (ADA) gene. Unfortunately, the child had the concurrent treatment of ADA

injections impairing the success of gene therapy, resulting in limit the development of viral vector technique [45]. After two decades' development, the gene transfer techniques have matured since 2009, named as the "return of gene therapy" [46]. Now, the concept of gene therapy is transferring the gene into cells, which had been removed from the patient and then reconstrued gene back *in vivo* patient, called gene therapy. Clinically, constructed vectors consist of viral vectors or non-viral vectors. For transferring techniques of clinical application, viral delivery utilizes a viral vector such as retrovirus, AAVs, lentiviruses, and adenoviruses to encapsulate a construct in RNA or DNA form, to facilitate efficient delivery [47]. Non-viral delivery includes physical methods (electroporation, micro-fluidic-based technologies), nanomaterial-based methods (cationic lipids, and cell-penetrating peptides), and self-assembled nanoparticle [48]. Now viral vector systems can provide useful tools to deliver the genetically modified gene for clinical applications. Retroviral and lentiviral vectors will be first considered *ex vivo* delivery systems into T-cells to stably express therapeutic genes with relatively high transfection efficiency as Fig. (**9**) [49].

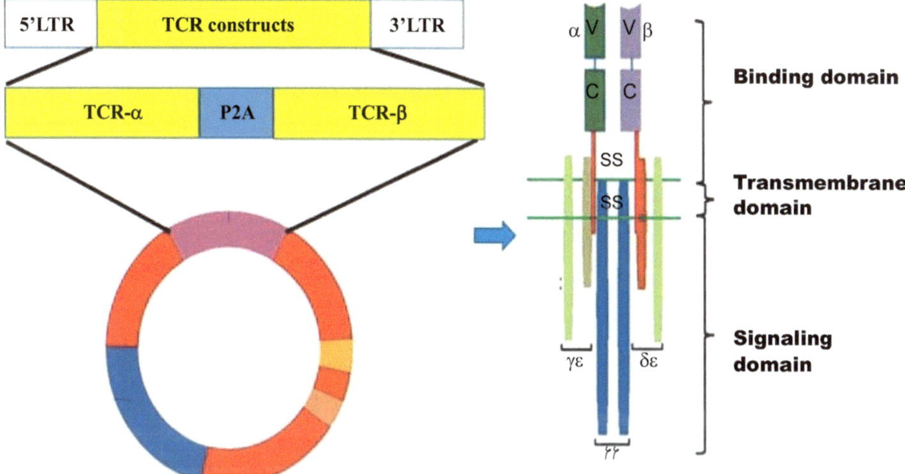

Fig. (8). Constructs of T-cell receptor. Left is a TCR construct by overlapping PCR and right is TCR products.

Retroviral (murine leukemia virus, MLV) transfection is a mainstay of genetically modified T-cells, which consists of reverse transcriptase in the packaging system to enable the integration of artificial constructs (genes) into the host genome in a stable status [50]. Following rebuilding plasmid with 8-10 kb length, CAR or TCR insertions into plasmids are capable of producing replication-defective viral vector and delivering the specific constructs into T-cells.

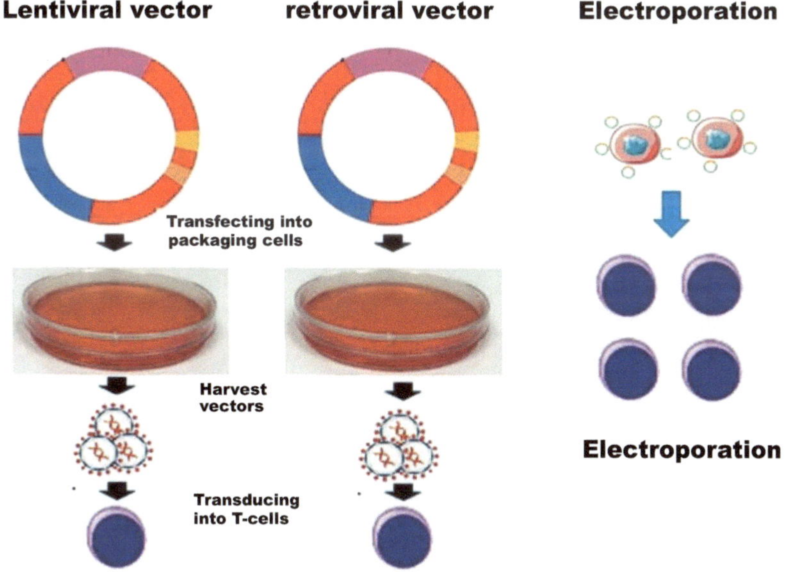

Fig. (9). Packaging and Delivering of constructs in the packaging system.

Lentiviral transfection is the second mainstay of genetically modified T-cells, which enable the integration of artificial genes into the host genome in a stable status for genetical modifications in T-cells as dividing cells and in CD34 cell as non-dividing cells [51].

In general, the virus-based transfections are comparatively time-consuming and expensive, which need excellent GMP laboratories to apply for a clinical purpose.

Electroporation comes out as a good strategy for genetic modification of diverse cell types based on the transient disruption of cell membranes *via* the electric field, allowing charged molecules into the desired cells. For instance, the Lonza Nucleofector II electroporation system demonstrated high efficiency in the genetic modification of T-cells with 80% of viability and 40-60% of expression in T-cells. The disadvantage is that electroporation can result in cell death with varied efficacy after electroporation for different cells [52].

CONCLUSION

Screening of tumor antigen and tumor mutant protein is essential to a target of tumor-specific T-cells such as TIL, TCR T-cells, and CAR-T-cells for adoptive T-cell immunotherapy. In order to discover specific mutant proteins and specific antigen or shared antigen with several immunogenic neoantigens from the tumor, at present, at least six platforms are going to be applied for the screening strategies of immunogenetic adoptive immunotherapy, including whole-cell level, complete molecules, and partial protein sequence. Now screening tumor antigens based on the whole-cell level is to apply for phage display, TCR, and genomic techniques, while molecular screening level based on protein sequence is often employing CAR and Y2H. Screening whole-cell requires very quality cells to initiate the procedure, while screening molecules or peptides is based on a few information such as known antigens/peptides or share antigens/peptides. After determining peptides or proteins from the tumor, constructs are rebuilt for CAR or TCR and specific peptides into DC as well. Manufacture of CAR T-cells or TCR T-cells is mostly dependent on viral vectors to gene transfer, so that the genetic transducing T-cells is one of the most critical steps to generate good QC TCR T-cells or CAR-T cells. RNA level techniques such as microRNA transfecting into DC for specific T-cells are going to developed. Nowadays, lipofectamine and nucleofector systems are available methods to perform non-viral transfection of immune cells.

CONSENT FOR PUBLICATION

The authors declare no financial interests.

CONFLICT OF INTEREST

The authors declare no financial interests.

ACKNOWLEDGEMENTS

During the early period, BL with his colleagues set up the first TIL polyclonal culture in China, as described in the chapter (1986-1993). BL further study for more than 25 years, including purified single tumor cells with ED to support phage display under the leaders of Drs. Preisler and Smith in Rush Cancer Institute (1996-2000), set up single-cell methods with WC, GL to analyze genomic profiles, including CD3+, CD3+CD8+ cells in Case Western Reserve University (1999-2007).

The mention of trade names or commercial products in this article is solely to provide specific information and does not imply recommendation.

REFERENCES

[1]   Gross G, Waks T, Eshhar Z. Expression of immunoglobulin-T-cell receptor chimeric molecules as functional receptors with antibody-type specificity. Proc Natl Acad Sci USA 1989; 86(24): 10024-8.
[http://dx.doi.org/10.1073/pnas.86.24.10024] [PMID: 2513569]

[2]   Irving BA, Weiss A. The cytoplasmic domain of the T cell receptor zeta chain is sufficient to couple to receptor-associated signal transduction pathways. Cell 1991; 64(5): 891-901.
[http://dx.doi.org/10.1016/0092-8674(91)90314-O] [PMID: 1705867]

[3]   Li B, Tong SQ, Lu DY, *et al*. DHBV induced acute hepatic cell necrosis in duck-An experimental model for fulminant hepatitis. Acta Shanghai Second Medical University 1990; 10(3): 189-93.

[4]   Li BR, Tong SQ, Zhang XH, Lu J, Gu QL, Lu DY. A new experimental and clinical approach of combining usage of highly active tumor-infiltrating lymphocytes and highly sensitive antitumor drugs for the advanced malignant tumor. Chin Med J (Engl) 1994; 107(11): 803-7.
[PMID: 7867384]

[5]   Siemionow M, Klimczak A. Immunodepletive anti-alpha/beta-TCR antibody in transplantation of composite tissue allografts: Cleveland Clinic research experience. Immunotherapy 2009; 1(4): 585-98.
[PMID: 20635989]

[6]   Dos Santos NR, Ghysdael J, Tran Quang C. The TCR/CD3 complex in leukemogenesis and as a therapeutic target in T-cell acute lymphoblastic leukemia. Adv Biol Regul 2019; 74100638
[http://dx.doi.org/10.1016/j.jbior.2019.100638] [PMID: 31378701]

[7]   Kershaw MH, Westwood JA, Parker LL, *et al*. A phase I study on adoptive immunotherapy using gene-modified T cells for ovarian cancer. Clin Cancer Res 2006; 12(20 Pt 1): 6106-15.
[http://dx.doi.org/10.1158/1078-0432.CCR-06-1183] [PMID: 17062687]

[8]   Jurcic JG. What happened to anti-CD33 therapy for acute myeloid leukemia? Curr Hematol Malig Rep 2012; 7(1): 65-73.
[http://dx.doi.org/10.1007/s11899-011-0103-0] [PMID: 22109628]

[9]   Uzhachenko RV, Shanker A, Shanker A. CD8$^+$ T Lymphocyte and NK Cell Network: Circuitry in the Cytotoxic Domain of Immunity. Front Immunol 2019; 10: 1906.
[http://dx.doi.org/10.3389/fimmu.2019.01906] [PMID: 31456803]

[10]   Celluzzi CM, Mayordomo JI, Storkus WJ, Lotze MT, Falo LD Jr. Peptide-pulsed dendritic cells

induce antigen-specific CTL-mediated protective tumor immunity. J Exp Med 1996; 183(1): 283-7.
[http://dx.doi.org/10.1084/jem.183.1.283] [PMID: 8551233]

[11]   Sayour EJ, Mitchell DA. Manipulation of Innate and Adaptive Immunity through Cancer Vaccines. J Immunol Res 2017; 20173145742
[http://dx.doi.org/10.1155/2017/3145742] [PMID: 28265580]

[12]   Stein JV. T Cell Motility as Modulator of Interactions with Dendritic Cells. Front Immunol 2015; 6: 559.
[http://dx.doi.org/10.3389/fimmu.2015.00559] [PMID: 26579132]

[13]   Xu Y, Yang Z, Horan LH, *et al.* A novel antibody-TCR (AbTCR) platform combines Fab-based antigen recognition with gamma/delta-TCR signaling to facilitate T-cell cytotoxicity with low cytokine release. Cell Discov 2018; 4(1): 62.
[http://dx.doi.org/10.1038/s41421-018-0066-6] [PMID: 30479831]

[14]   Rabinovich GA, Gabrilovich D, Sotomayor EM. Immunosuppressive strategies that are mediated by tumor cells. Annu Rev Immunol 2007; 25(1): 267-96.
[http://dx.doi.org/10.1146/annurev.immunol.25.022106.141609] [PMID: 17134371]

[15]   Yang J, Li BR, Nayini J, *et al.* Tyrosine phosphorylation of Shc proteins in normal CD34+ progenitor cells and leukemic cells. Blood 1999; 94(1): 373-4.
[http://dx.doi.org/10.1182/blood.V94.1.373.413a48b_373_374] [PMID: 10428548]

[16]   Li B, Yang J, Andrews C, *et al.* Telomerase activity in preleukemia and acute myelogenous leukemia. Leuk Lymphoma 2000; 36(5-6): 579-87.
[http://dx.doi.org/10.3109/10428190009148406] [PMID: 10784403]

[17]   Li B, Yang J, Tao M, *et al.* Poor prognosis acute myelogenous leukemia 2--biological and molecular biological characteristics and treatment outcome. Leuk Res 2000; 24(9): 777-89.
[http://dx.doi.org/10.1016/S0145-2126(00)00035-7] [PMID: 10978783]

[18]   Preisler HD, Perambakam S, Li B, *et al.* Alterations in IRF1/IRF2 expression in acute myelogenous leukemia. Am J Hematol 2001; 68(1): 23-31.
[http://dx.doi.org/10.1002/ajh.1144] [PMID: 11559933]

[19]   Preisler HD, Li B, Yang BL, *et al.* Suppression of telomerase activity and cytokine messenger RNA levels in acute myelogenous leukemia cells *in vivo* in patients by amifostine and interleukin 4. Clin Cancer Res 2000; 6(3): 807-12.
[PMID: 10741700]

[20]   Devemy E, Li B, Tao M, *et al.* Poor prognosis acute myelogenous leukemia: 3--biological and molecular biological changes during remission induction therapy. Leuk Res 2001; 25(9): 783-91.
[http://dx.doi.org/10.1016/S0145-2126(01)00032-7] [PMID: 11489472]

[21]   Galili N, Devemy E, Raza A. Isolation of specific and biologically active peptides that bind cells from patients with acute myeloid leukemia (AML). J Hematol Oncol 2008; 1(1): 8.
[http://dx.doi.org/10.1186/1756-8722-1-8] [PMID: 18616802]

[22]   Li B. strategy to identify genomic expression at single-cell level or a small number of cells. J Biotechnol 2005; 8(1): 71-81.
[PMID: 16290242]

[23]   Cohen AD, Raje N, Fowler JA, Mezzi K, Scott EC, Dhodapkar MV. How to Train your T cells: Overcoming Immune Dysfunction in Multiple Myeloma. Clin Cancer Res 2019; 10: 1078-0432.
[http://dx.doi.org/10.1158/1078-0432.CCR-19-2111] [PMID: 31672768]

[24]   Bhati M, Cole DK, McCluskey J, Sewell AK, Rossjohn J. The versatility of the αβ T-cell antigen receptor. Protein Sci 2014; 23(3): 260-72.
[http://dx.doi.org/10.1002/pro.2412] [PMID: 24375592]

[25]   Thaxton JE, Li Z. To affinity and beyond: harnessing the T cell receptor for cancer immunotherapy. Hum Vaccin Immunother 2014; 10(11): 3313-21.

[http://dx.doi.org/10.4161/21645515.2014.973314] [PMID: 25483644]

[26]   Zhang W, Li B, Singh R, Narendra U, Zhu L, Weiss MA. Regulation of sexual dimorphism: mutational and chemogenetic analysis of the doublesex DM domain. Mol Cell Biol 2006; 26(2): 535-47.
[http://dx.doi.org/10.1128/MCB.26.2.535-547.2006] [PMID: 16382145]

[27]   Qiao L, Wang Y, Pang R, *et al.* Oncogene functions of FHL2 are independent from NF-kappaBIalpha in gastrointestinal cancer. Pathol Oncol Res 2009; 15(1): 31-6.
[http://dx.doi.org/10.1007/s12253-008-9085-1] [PMID: 18752053]

[28]   Zheng M, Li M, Shen G, *et al.* [Screening of special scFv antibody against human p53 protein by yeast two-hybrid system]. Xibao Yu Fenzi Mianyixue Zazhi 2016; 32(1): 112-7.
[PMID: 26728386]

[29]   De Almeida CV, Zamame JA, Romagnoli GG, *et al.* Treatment of colon cancer cells with 5-fluorouracil can improve the effectiveness of RNA-transfected antitumor dendritic cell vaccine. Oncol Rep 2017; 38(1): 561-8.
[http://dx.doi.org/10.3892/or.2017.5692] [PMID: 28586072]

[30]   Li B, Chang T, Larson A, Ding J. Identification of mRNAs expressed in tumor-infiltrating lymphocytes by a strategy for rapid and high throughput screening. Gene 2000; 255(2): 273-9.
[http://dx.doi.org/10.1016/S0378-1119(00)00330-9] [PMID: 11024287]

[31]   Li B, Perabekam S, Liu G, Yin M, Song S, Larson A. Experimental and bioinformatics comparison of gene expression between T cells from TIL of liver cancer and T cells from UniGene. J Gastroenterol 2002; 37(4): 275-82.
[http://dx.doi.org/10.1007/s005350200035] [PMID: 11993511]

[32]   Wang Z, Hu H, Zheng J, Li B.

[33]   Li B, Hu HL, Ding JQ, Yan D, Yang LM. Functional cell proliferation and differentiation by system modeling for cell therapy. International Journal of Latest Research in Science and Technology 2015; 2: 180-7.

[34]   Li B, Shen DH. Preliminary Study on the Resting Status of Tumor-infiltrating Lymphocytes. Chinese Microbiology and Immunology 1994; 14(6): 399-402.

[35]   Li B, Liu G, Hu HL, Ding JQ, Zheng J, Tong A. A CLUE OF PERSONALIZED IMMUNOTHERAPY. Biom J 2015; 1: 3.

[36]   Zhang W, Ding J, Qu Y, *et al.* 2009.

[37]   Li B. Breakthroughs of 2015-Personalized Immunotherapy Based on Individual GWAS and Biomarkers. Biom J 2015; 1: 1-2.

[38]   Xu Y, Hu H, Zheng J, Li B. Feasibility of whole RNA sequencing from single-cell mRNA amplification. Genet Res Int 2013; 2013724124
[http://dx.doi.org/10.1155/2013/724124] [PMID: 24455282]

[39]   Handgretinger R, Schlegel P. Emerging role of immunotherapy for childhood cancers. Linchuang Zhongliuxue Zazhi 2018; 7(2): 14.
[http://dx.doi.org/10.21037/cco.2018.04.06] [PMID: 29764159]

[40]   Lamers CH, Sleijfer S, Vulto AG, *et al.* Treatment of metastatic renal cell carcinoma with autologous T-lymphocytes genetically retargeted against carbonic anhydrase IX: first clinical experience. J Clin Oncol 2006; 24(13): e20-2.
[http://dx.doi.org/10.1200/JCO.2006.05.9964] [PMID: 16648493]

[41]   Till BG, Jensen MC, Wang J, *et al.* Adoptive immunotherapy for indolent non-Hodgkin lymphoma and mantle cell lymphoma using genetically modified autologous CD20-specific T cells. Blood 2008; 112(6): 2261-71.
[http://dx.doi.org/10.1182/blood-2007-12-128843] [PMID: 18509084]

[42]   Finney HM, Lawson AD, Bebbington CR, Weir AN. Chimeric receptors providing both primary and costimulatory signaling in T cells from a single gene product. J Immunol 1998; 161(6): 2791-7.
[PMID: 9743337]

[43]   Friedmann-Morvinski D, Bendavid A, Waks T, Schindler D, Eshhar Z. Redirected primary T cells harboring a chimeric receptor require costimulation for their antigen-specific activation. Blood 2005; 105(8): 3087-93.
[http://dx.doi.org/10.1182/blood-2004-09-3737] [PMID: 15626734]

[44]   Golubovskaya V, Berahovich R, Xu S, Harto H, Wu L. Major Highlights of the CAR-TCR Summit, Boston, 2016. Anticancer Agents Med Chem 2017; 17(10): 1344-50.
[http://dx.doi.org/10.2174/1871520617666170110151900] [PMID: 28071584]

[45]   Sun ZJ, Kim KS, Wagner G, Reinherz EL. Mechanisms contributing to T cell receptor signaling and assembly revealed by the solution structure of an ectodomain fragment of the CD3 epsilon gamma heterodimer. Cell 2001; 105(7): 913-23.
[http://dx.doi.org/10.1016/S0092-8674(01)00395-6] [PMID: 11439187]

[46]   Uhlén M, Fagerberg L, Hallström BM, *et al.* Proteomics. Tissue-based map of the human proteome. Science 2015; 347(6220): 1260419-11260419.
[http://dx.doi.org/10.1126/science.1260419] [PMID: 25613900]

[47]   Gándara C, Affleck V, Stoll EA. Manufacture of Third-Generation Lentivirus for Preclinical Use, with Process Development Considerations for Translation to Good Manufacturing Practice. Hum Gene Ther Methods 2018; 29(1): 1-15.
[http://dx.doi.org/10.1089/hgtb.2017.098] [PMID: 29212357]

[48]   Schilz AJ, Kühlcke K, Fauser AA, Eckert HG. Optimization of retroviral vector generation for clinical application. J Gene Med 2001; 3(5): 427-36.
[http://dx.doi.org/10.1002/jgm.204] [PMID: 11601756]

[49]   Ruella M, Xu J, Barrett DM, *et al.* Induction of resistance to chimeric antigen receptor T cell therapy by transduction of a single leukemic B cell. Nat Med 2018; 24(10): 1499-503.
[http://dx.doi.org/10.1038/s41591-018-0201-9] [PMID: 30275568]

[50]   Scholler J, Brady TL, Binder-Scholl G, *et al.* Decade-long safety and function of retroviral-modified chimeric antigen receptor T cells. Sci Transl Med 2012; 4(132)132ra53
[http://dx.doi.org/10.1126/scitranslmed.3003761] [PMID: 22553251]

[51]   Naldini L, Blömer U, Gallay P, *et al.* *In vivo* gene delivery and stable transduction of nondividing cells by a lentiviral vector. Science 1996; 272(5259): 263-7.
[http://dx.doi.org/10.1126/science.272.5259.263] [PMID: 8602510]

[52]   Landi A, Babiuk LA, van Drunen Littel-van den Hurk S. High transfection efficiency, gene expression, and viability of monocyte-derived human dendritic cells after nonviral gene transfer. J Leukoc Biol 2007; 82(4): 849-60.
[http://dx.doi.org/10.1189/jlb.0906561] [PMID: 17626798]

CHAPTER 7

Primary Cell Culture and T-cell Cloning - Fundamental of Adoptive T-cell Immunotherapy

Biaoru Li[1,2,3,*], Supriya Perabekam[2], Alan Larson[2] and Hong-Liang Hu[1]

[1] *Department of Microbiology, Shanghai Second Medical University, Shanghai, 200003, PRC*

[2] *Rush Medical Center, Chicago, IL, USA*

[3] *Georgia Cancer Center and Department of Pediatrics, Medical College at GA, Augusta, GA 30912, USA*

Abstract: Tumor-associated antigen (TAA) or tumor-specific antigen (TSA) is essential for the target of tumor-specific T-cells such as tumor-infiltrating T cells (TIL), specific T-cells, TCR T-cells and CAR-T-cells for adoptive T-cell immunotherapy. The tumor cells often accumulate hundreds of mutations and harbor several immunogenic neoantigens, and thus, the repertoire of mutation or neoantigen from patient tumor cells might need the screen to uncover for engineering these T-cells. To understand the T-cell screening and determining tumor antigen-based on primary tumor cells from an individual patient, this chapter, we focus on streamlining the process of *ex vivo* T-cell culture and primary tumor cell culture, T-cell cloning for tumor neoantigen-specific T cells, allowing the patient to the benefit of downstream T-cell targets. Because T-cell engineering cultures are very important methods for TIL, TCR and CAR T-cells, moreover, because using primary tumor cells isolation and cultures is very important for screening and identifying tumor antigen of patients, we first introduce primary cell culture techniques, including those developed from two-dimensional (2-D) tumor cell cultures, three-dimensional (3-D) tumor cell culture and multiple dimensional tumor cell culture (4-D cultures). These methodologies are increasingly supporting clinical oncologists to apply to tumor therapeutic agents and Ag targets for patients in the clinical laboratory. Besides, we also conclude some growth factors for T-cell cloning cultures. The chapter aims to present a foundation to adoptive T cell immunotherapy of clinical patients.

Keywords: T-cell Adoptive immunotherapy, TIL (tumor-infiltrating lymphocyte), TCR (T-cell receptors), and CAR (chimeric antigen receptor) T-cells, T-cell cloning, personalized immunotherapy, three-dimensional *ex vivo* culture.

*** Corresponding author Biaoru Li**: Georgia Cancer Center and Department of Pediatrics, Medical College at GA, Augusta, GA 30912, USA; Tel: 440-317-1443; E-mail: bli@augusta.edu

INTRODUCTION

T-cell culture from patients is a very important process to support adoptive immunotherapy for clinical tumor diseases. Moreover, isolation and culture of primary tumor cells from patients also are critical to support the identification of tumor antigen or personalized medicines for most types of clinical tumor diseases as Fig. (**1**) [1]. These tumor cell cultures have contributed much information to evaluate tumor diseases, including drug sensitivity for personalized medicine and identification of tumor antigens for CAR T-cells and TCR T-cells [2]. After 40 years' development, now primary cell isolation and culture from tumor tissues have become an essential process to T-cell adoptive immunotherapy and tumor cells to determine the drug efficacy of anticancer drugs and identify tumor antigen.

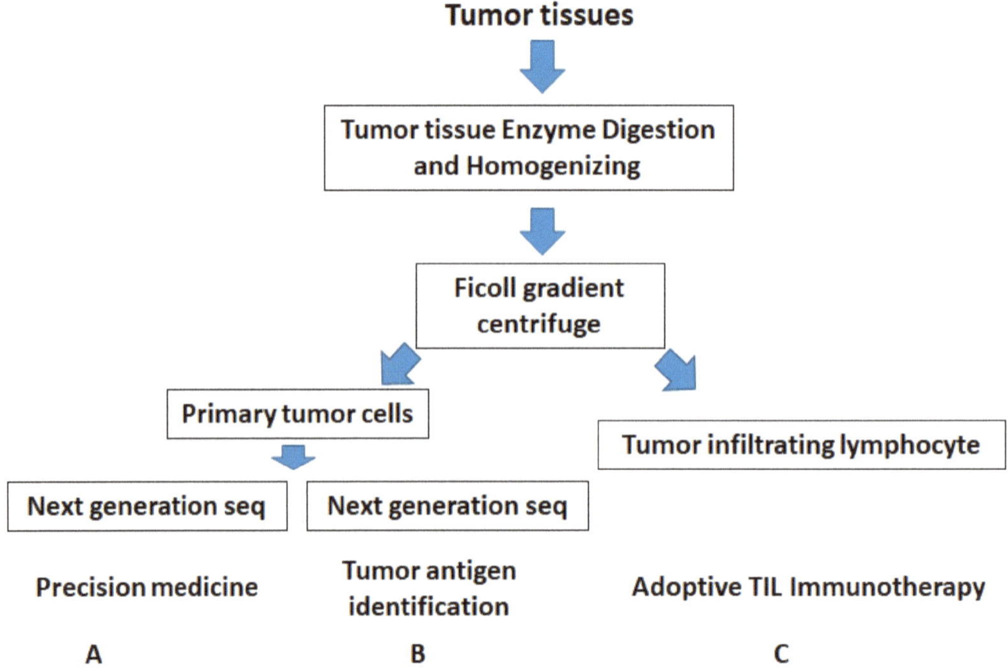

Fig. (1). Primary cells isolation and culture from tumor tissues.

In a preclinical trial, the primary tumor cell culture can support the efficacy of anticancer drugs; the primary cells have been used to screen and confirm new drugs by the guidelines of the FDA before humans are exposed to the potential therapeutic compounds [3] although some models of primary tumor-cell culture mislead to inaccuracies in efficacy due to loss of tumor growth microenvironments [4]. Moreover, isolation and culture of primary tumor-cells can support screening and identification of tumor antigen and SNPs for TCR T-cells. To understand the development of primary tumor-cell culture for personalized immunotherapy, we first introduce the development of these techniques, such as two-dimensional (2-D) primary tumor cell cultures, three-dimensional (3-D) model, and multiple dimensional models. The new culture methods from primary tumor-cells may play a decisive role in the development and establishment of successful personalized medicines and identification of the neoantigen of tumor antigens.

Furthermore, neoantigens with their mutant sequences are the main targets of tumor-specific T-cells so that, in this chapter, we further present workflow, including *ex vivo* priming of neoantigen-specific T-cells, isolating their T-cell receptors (TCRs) and identifying specific TCR T-cells, allowing the specific TCR T-cell engineering for the new T-cell immunotherapy. In T-cell culture, we will introduce TIL culture and functional TIL culture based on genomic profiles with their procedures for clinical application.

Finally, we briefly conclude interleukins and growth factors for specific T-cell cultures. Although we will link interleukins and growth factors to system biology, we discuss functional personalized immunotherapy in chapter 13.

PERSONALIZED MUILTIPLE DIMENSIONAL CULTURE SYSTEM

In general, new drug R&D should experience about 16 years from bench researches into the patient bedside. The average cost will be as high as 1.2-1.5 billion dollars [5]. Therefore, the primary cell culture model can shorten the time-course to confirm individual drugs for personalized applications. Moreover, neoantigen identification is required to use primary tumor-cells to screen SNP or neoantigens to identify TCR T-cells for personalized immunotherapy. In our early periods of TIL R&D, we had used TIL CTL assay to autogenous tumor cells to screen and determine TIL efficacy and chemosensitivity assay (CSA) to define drug efficacy by the autologous tumor cell culture. Now clinical scientists and physicians are making more considerable efforts to develop new culture models from primary tumor-cells for tumor Ag-specific identification and accurate determination of drug efficacy for clinical patients. Fortunately, after 40 years' effort, a few new culture techniques are developed, as listed in Table **1**. For example, special two-dimensional (2-D) tumor-cell cultures, humanized mice model, three--dimensional (3-D) bio-printed models, different artificial materials for three-dimensional (3-D) model, and multiple dimensional models have been successfully used for the culture of primary tumor-cells.

1. 2-D Primary Cell Culture

To predict drug efficacy and measure CD8+cell cytotoxicity (CTL) to tumor cells for clinical patients, we have often used traditional 2-D primary tumor-cell culture for drug sensitivity assay and CTL assay for thirty years [6]. Because the 2-D culture systems lack the important microenvironment, we only achieved about 27% efficacy from the bench researches into the patient bedside. At present, we understand 2-D culture systems not only lack the tumor microenvironment but also result in a loss of important genes and their genomic expression profiles. Now some clinical scientists are going to develop some specialized 2-D culture systems. For example, hematological malignant cells from clinical diseases (such as MDS,CML and AML) can be used by CFU-GEMM (colony-forming unit for granulocyte, erythrocyte, monocyte, megakaryocyte) for clinical application [7].

Table 1. Personalized multiple dimensional system.

Methods	Application	Advantage	Disadvantage
Basic 2-D Culture	Basic screening	Traditional method	non-tumor microenvironment
Unique 2-D (Clonogenic forming unit)	Hematological tumor	Commercially available	non-tumor microenvironment
Humanized animal model	Solid tumor	1. Similar tumor microenvironment	1. Not fit time-course
		2. Commercially available	2. Higher cost
Basic 3-D Culture	Solid tumor	1. Similar tumor microenvironment	Need experiences
		2. Commercially available	
3-D bio-printing culture	Solid tumor	1. Similar tumor microenvironment	On research
		2. Tumor 3-D imaging growth	
Multiple D culture (4-D)	Cancer stem cells	1. Similar tumor microenvironment	Need experiences
		2. Commercially available	

2. Humanized Animal Model by Primary Tumor Cells

To achieve a better microenvironment for the growth of primary tumor-cell, an animal model had become the main preclinical research models. The humanized mice model is to assay drugs as human-tumor grown conditions and detect neoantigens for T-cell adoptive immunotherapy. The humanized mice model is a single human tumor tissue or cells planted within the animal body; therefore, tumor cells lead to their behavior different from their human environment. Moreover, human tumor cells are commonly transplanted into the mice with an immunocompromised situation that needs a time-course to accept foreign human tumor cells grown up, so that the humanized mice model is very difficult to fit clinical application of individual patient [8]. All in all, now, some clinical oncologists have been studying modeling humanized mice models with good time-course for patients' applications.

3. Basic 3-D Primary Tumor Cell Culture

In human beings, almost all tumor cells in tissues reside in an extracellular matrix (ECM) consisting of a complex three-dimensional (3-D) architecture and interact with neighboring cells through cell-cell and cell-ECM interactions. *Ex vivo* 3-D model is mimic *in vivo* primary tumor cell environment. Now, 3-D models have been quickly developing, consisting of (A) scaffold-free, which aggregates in suspension without the use of matrix-based substances; (B) scaffold utilizing either biomaterial-based matrices or solid scaffolds in which different materials and fabrication have been employed [9].

3-D spheroid cultures are one of scaffold-free method that can be used for a wide range of primary tumor cell culture to form tumor spheroids analyzed by imaging of light, fluorescence, and confocal microscopy, and thus now the 3-D tumor spheroid culture has been used for high throughput screening tumor cells from NSCLC, SCLC and brain tumor [10].

The scaffold of biomaterial-based matrices is comprised of natural hydrogels, synthetic hydrogels, and other solid scaffolds. Hydrogels and extracellular matrices in 3-D cultures produce networks of cross-linked polymer chains or complex protein molecules of natural or synthetic origin so that the materials possess biophysical characteristics similar to natural tissue and serve as highly effective matrices for 3-D cell culture. Solid scaffolds of 3-D cell cultures are also fabricated with a broad range of materials, including metal, ceramics, glass, and polymers. The tumor cells binding to scaffolds of the surface of matrix stiffness can support tumor cell adhesion, growth, and behavior as primary tumor cells growth *in vivo*. Now scaffolds method has extensively used in primary cell culture so that the primary tumor cell cultures can play an important role in clinical application [11].

4. 3-D Bio-printing Primary Tumor Cell and Tissue Culture

The 3-D bio-printed tissues and organs could be designed to mimic the exact cellular density of target tissues and organs with a proper cellular component, extracellular matrix, and 3-D spatial components. The bio-printing is now feasible to combine the important elements to generate 3-D *in vitro* tissue/organ systems mimic cellular and extracellular functional machinery. Technological advancement in imaging and digital design can visualize print-tissues and organs by inkjet, micro-extrusion, and laser-assisted printing [12]. The 3-D bio-printed materials are comprised of natural polymers such as alginate, gelatin, collagen, chitosan, fibrin, and synthetic molecules such as polyethylene glycol. The major advantages of the natural polymers in 3-D bioprinting can be personalized and tailored to the specific application. The challenges of the technique are the loss of mechanical strength, overtime culture and immunogenicity. Although the new methods now make it reliable for regeneration constructs, clinically, bio-printing is a potential possibility for primary tumor cell cultures at tissue and organ levels.

5. Multiple D Primary Tumor Cell Culture

Because primary cells such as cancer stem cells from patients are dynamic growths with differentiation mechanism, in order to study the primary cells as *in vivo* growth, we have reported mimicking dynamic growths as *in vivo* primary cell growth with the change of time course. For example, 4-D culture systems adding time-course curves have been developed into stem cells [13] and cancer stem cells culture, which can support differential induction for CD34 cell or reverse differential induction for cancer stem cells [14].

T-CELL CLONING WITH CULTURE

According to research & development (R&D) of T-cell clonal techniques with their cultures, at least five tumor-specific T-cell cloning techniques and strategies are emerging in thirty years: (1) TIL culture with TIL polyclonal strategy and techniques; (2) specific peptides pulsed dendritic cells (DC) including co-culture CD8+cell with CTL cloning and culture; (3) shared neoantigen CAR T-cell and TCR T-cell construction with their cloning culture and engineering; (4) genomics technique (SNP and neoantigen screening) combined CAR T-cell and TCR T-cell engineering; (5) genomics technique (SNP and neoantigen screening) supporting TIL functional polyclonal culture techniques. The cloning cultures of T-cell immunotherapy obtained/induced by tumor antigen and T-cell reconstructed by tumor immunogenicity can specifically target their own tumor cells *in vivo*.

1. TIL Culture with TIL Polyclonal Strategy and Techniques

In an early adoptive TIL immunotherapy, in order to increase TIL CTL specific to autologous tumor cells, we have performed T-cells collected from TIL residing tumor tissue of patients to set up and perform CTL assay to determine and define the lymphocyte killing autologous primary tumor-cells for clinical efficacy of polyclonal TIL. After the techniques were developed from CTL assay using radioactivity (such as H^3 releasing assay) and GMM staining into MTT assay, we have routinely screen polyclonal TIL efficacy for personalized TIL immunotherapy with reports of several hundred patients suffering from solid tumors as Fig. (**2**) [15, 16]. Although patients demonstrated good response by both sensitive polyclonal TIL culture confirmed by CTL assay, combining sensitive drugs by CSA for clinical application as our early publication [17], it is not cost-effective to extend into most patients in our early periods. Moreover, TIL polyclonal culture techniques are not easy to popularize, so that we have only used these protocols for adoptive TIL immunotherapy of clinical patients with solid tumors in a decade [18].

Table 2. Tumor-specific antigen T-cell cloning with their cultures.

	TIL Culture with Polyclonal Techniques	**Specific CTL Cell Cloning and Culture**	**Shared Neoantigen CAR/TCR Cloning Culture**	**Genomic Based CAR/TCR Cloning Culture**	**Genomic Based Polyclonal TIL Culture**
First efficacy	1987	2000	2013	2018	2015
Production method	Isolation of T cells from tumors and expansion *ex vivo*	Isolation of peripheral T cells *via* apheresis and *ex vivo* transduction with a TCR against the tumor antigen	Isolation of peripheral T cells *via* apheresis and *ex vivo* transduction with a CAR against the tumor antigen	Isolation of peripheral T cells *via* apheresis and *ex vivo* transduction with a CAR against the tumor antigen	Isolation of T cells from tumors and expansion *ex vivo*
Specificity	Polyclonal	Monoclonal	Monoclonal	Monoclonal	Polyclonal
Safety	IL-2 mediated (chills, fever, edema)	"On-target, off-tumor"	"On-target, off-tumor"	Few On-target, off-tumor	IL-2 mediated (chills, fever, edema)
	Seldom autoimmune	CRS	CRS	CRS	Seldom autoimmune

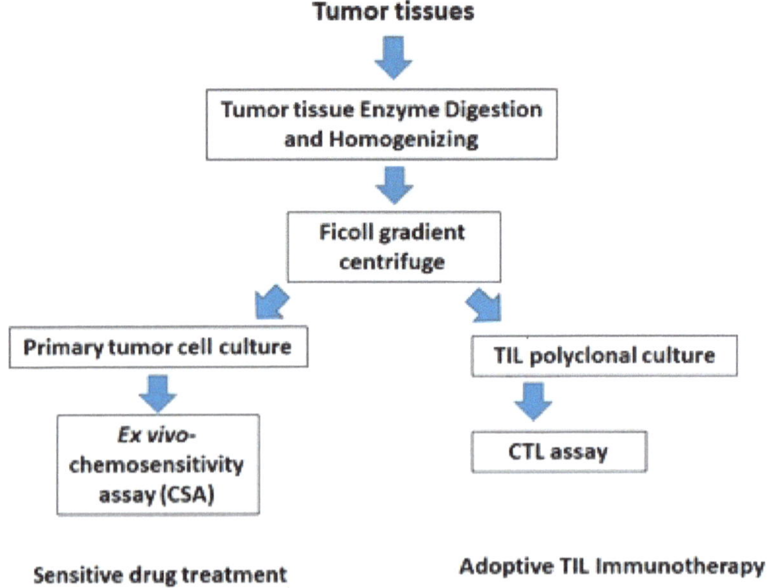

Fig. (2). Polyclonal TIL culture. In our early model, which was polyclonal T-cell by TIL culture combined with CTL assay using autologous primary tumor cells for adoptive immunotherapy.

2. Specific Peptides Pulsed Dendritic Cells (DC) Co-Culture CD8+Cell with CTL Cell Cloning and Culture

As described above, polyclonal TIL cultures are not easy to set up criteria culture, especially from solid tumor tissues, so that some methods have been developed since then. The first technique is developed by synthesized peptides or protein inducing CTLs. For example, HLA-A2-restrictive peptide PR1 could destroy leukemia cells, thus use the elimination of chronic myeloid leukemia [19]. Bernhard *et al.* demonstrated that CTLs specific for E75 peptide of the HER2/neu tumor antigen could eliminate breast cancer cells in patients after the adoptive transfer of HER2-specific CTL populations [20]. In the tumor neoantigen induction, DCs are widely used in cancer immunotherapy to stimulate specific antitumor immune responses, because they can effectively recognize and present tumor antigens to T-cells both *in vitro* and *in vivo* [21 - 23]. Moreover, because the T-cells are obtained from autologous PBMC, this advantage of adoptive transfer of autologous T-cells activated *ex vivo*, makes these easy to culture and possible to target specific cell-mediated immune responses against autologous tumor cells [24 - 26]. For example, recombinant MHC molecules are conjugated to antigen epitopes of tumor antigens so that some models (such as overexpression of HER2, human epidermal growth factor receptor 2: HER2/neu) are observed in various types of carcinomas, including breast, colon, stomach, pancreatic, and thyroid carcinomas, as well as ovarian cancer [27]. Now, the development of optimized protocol for generating populations of antitumor antigen-specific CTLs using DCs and isolating antigen-specific cells is promising for the most efficient production of T-cell eliminating tumor cells disseminated in the patient's body. Moreover, this approach can be used to generate functionally active antigen-specific T-lymphocytes from PBMC of patients for adoptive T-cell transfer to eliminate peptide-positive tumor cells, prevent metastasis, and relapse. At present, pure populations of monospecific polyclonal T cells can be sorted efficiently, their TCR repertoire can be analyzed by polymerase chain reaction (PCR) techniques, and their functional potential can be assessed without the interference of the nonspecific T-cell universe. Thus, it can rapidly change as a consequence of the information provided by recent tetramer-based quantitative analyses. In addition, one human tumor antigen from melanoma has proven to be extremely informative, the melanocyte/melanoma differentiation antigen known as Melan-A (for melanoma antigen A) or MART-1 (melanoma antigen recognized by T cells), which was among the first human tumor antigens to be cloned. Scientists have used tetramers of HLA-A2, and Melan-A/MART-1 derived peptide to carefully quantify the specific CD8 T-cell response against this antigen in both melanoma patients and healthy donors as Fig. (**3**) [28, 29].

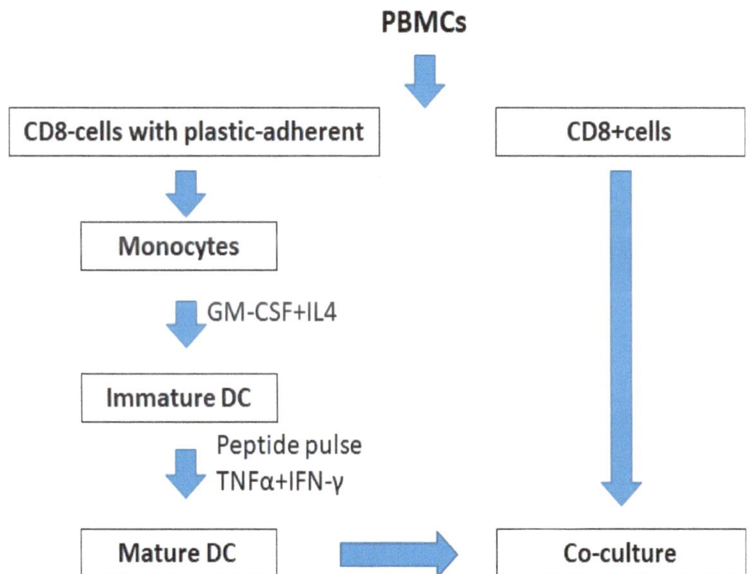

Fig. (3). Specific T-cell culture. Specific T-cell by co-culture with T-cell from PBMC and with DC by peptide pulse. Following T-cell coculture, the T-cells can be used for adoptive immunotherapy.

3. Shared Antigen CAR and TCR T-cell Construct with Cloning Culture

Human tumor antigens are classified into two main types: tumor-specific antigens

(TSA) such as HBV, EBV, CMV, and human papillomavirus (HPV) E6/E7 protein, and shared tumor-associated antigens (TAAs). Most of TCR T-cell and CAR T-cell therapy relies on shared tumor antigens expressed in tumor cells. TAA includes cancer-testis (CT) antigens, differentiation antigens, an oncofetal antigen.

i. CT antigens are protein antigens with normal expression restricted to adult testicular germ cells aberrantly activated and expressed in different types of human cancer. At least a group of antigens has been found to elicit spontaneous immune responses in cancer patients, raising the possibility that these antigens could produce TCR T-cell targets as Table **3** [30].
ii. Differentiation antigens are encoded by genes that express in a tissue-specific manner. The proteins are normally produced in very low quantities but whose production is dramatically increased in tumor cells, activating an immune response. MART-1 (melanoma antigen) and tyrosinase are recognized by T-cells which are mainly found in melanomas and normal melanocytes [31, 32].
iii. Oncofetal antigen is third important tumor antigens such as alpha fetal protein (AFP) and carcinoembryonic antigen (CEA) [33, 34]. These proteins are normally produced in the early stages of embryonic development and disappeared by the time the immune system is fully developed at adults. Thus, self-tolerance does not develop against these antigens. CEA is often highly expressed in colon cancer and other tumor diseases, including NSCLC (non-small cell lung cancer), in which CEA is identified as one biomarker of lung adenocarcinoma.

A study on T-cell specific affinity to tumor cells of T-cell adoptive immunology is over 30 years. First chimeric TCR for T-cell specific affinity by anti-TNP mRNA cloning into TCR v-chain and c-chain to targeting cell was reported in 1989 [35]. According to the evidence reported in PNAS, in 1989, we had studied a plan with DHBsAb from Duck Hepatitis B Virus (DHBV) to clone into CD3 of TIL forming DHBsAb-CD3 CAR T-cells. Although we achieved a successful result for DHBV-LSP inducting animal model of hepatic necrosis as reported in 1989 [36] and successfully set up TIL culture and clone technique as reported in 1995 [37], we failed to achieve DHBsAb-CD3 chimeric TILs to specific affinity both DHBV and HBV infected HCC cells due to knowledge limitation of CD3 and TCR structure in that early period [38].

After successfully reported synthetic immunoglobulin/TCR chimeric molecule with antibody-like specificity in 1987-1989, Irving and Weiss discovered that CD8 and the CD3ζ chain could independently mediate T-cell activation of the endogenous TCR [39], so that CAR T-cells begin to be largely studied. After at least three generations of development of CAR T-cells, now CAR T-cells have at least three signaling domain CD28- 4-1BB-CD3 ζ in CAR T-cells [40, 41]. These CAR T-cells are capable of on-target chronic lymphocytic leukemia (CLL) with clinical significance so that these designs lead to producing autologous CD19 CAR-T cells to treat B-cell lymphoma [42, 43]. Recent trials of CAR T-cells have been quickly developed in different hematological malignancies.

Although CAR T-cell therapy has shown excellent results against hematological malignancies, its effect against solid tumors is unsatisfactory by comparison of TCR T-cells. After several years' effort, TCR engineered T-cells have demonstrated better responses against solid tumors than those of CAR engineering T-cells. TCRs depend on their interaction with peptide-major histocompatibility complex (MHC), complexes formed by peptide bound to MHC [44]. The different structures of CAR and TCR are that CAR T-cells employ antibody-antigen recognition machinery that consists of a scFv derived from an antibody to bind to antigens on the target cell's surface and TCR has full-length TCR structures that have greater sensitivity than CAR T-cells, enable quicker killing solid tumor cells. As Fig. (**4**), CAR T-cells and TCR T-cells involves at least four steps: (I) cell collection from a patient, (II) T-cell enrichment with removal of other cells, (III) transgene delivery, and (IV) *ex vivo* TCR or CAR T-cell expansion [45].

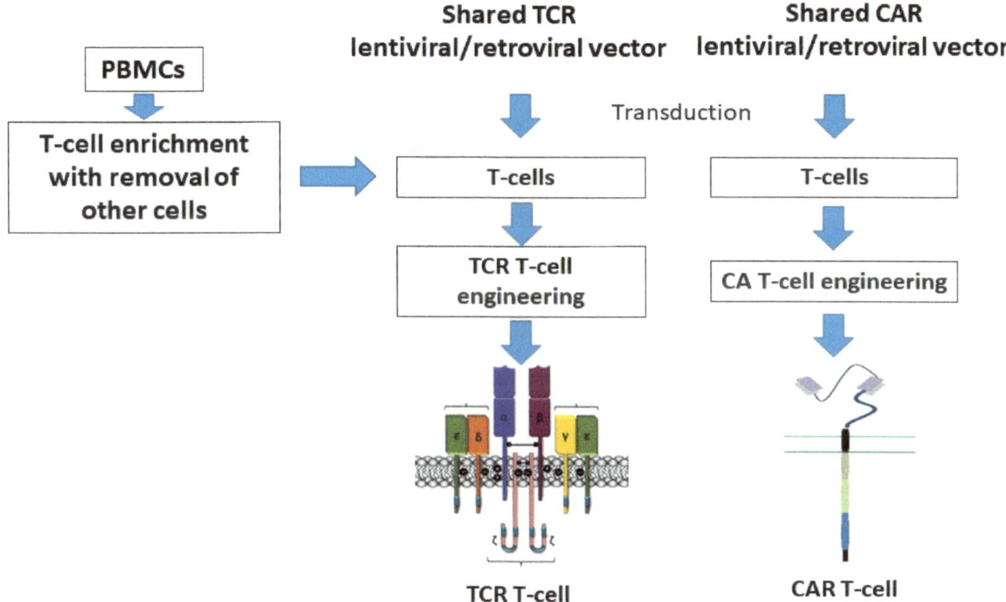

Fig. (4). TCR T-cell and CAR T-cell culture by shred antigen. T-cell clonal shared specific T-cell by shared Ag transducing into T-cell from PBMC. Following T-cell engineering, the T-cells can be used for adoptive immunotherapy.

As shown in Fig. (**4**), one of the critical manufacturing is the efficient isolation of T-cells from leukapheresis. Leukapheresis products from cancer patients consist of a heterogeneous population of cells, including T-cells, myeloid cells, natural killer cells, erythroid cells, and malignant cells. The application of positive and negative selection methods can enrich T-cells to exclude autologous peripheral blood mononuclear cells and leukemia cells. Thus, efficient T-cell purification and tumor cell purging will improve the safety and potency of cellular products for adoptive transfer therapies [46]. In order to achieve durable clinical responses to cell-based gene therapies, permanent transgene expression is often required. At present, murine gamma-retroviruses and lentiviruses are two available clinical gene therapy vector systems that afford long-term CAR and TCR transgene expression. Considerable clinical evidence shows that retroviral vectors are safe when expressed in human T-cells [47]. In contrast, lentiviral vectors, especially third-generation self-inactivating vectors, have a lower risk of insertional mutagenesis, which may be attributed to the absence of strong enhancer elements present in oncogenic murine gamma-retroviruses. Lentiviral vectors also have substantially higher efficiency for genetically engineering human T-cells [48, 49]. Clinical studies are currently being conducted to evaluate the safety and efficacy of CAR T-cells and TCR T-cells, including leukapheresis, T-cell enrichment with purity and quantity, transgene delivery with vector selection, and *ex vivo* expansion under GMP condition [50].

4. Genomic Supporting Patient's Neoantigen-Specific CAR T-cell and TCR T-cell Construction with their Cloning Culture

Some scientists have established the rapid identification of antigen-specific T cells from PBMCs to meet clinical application using TCR engineered T cells as Fig. (**5**) [51, 52]. During the procedure, there are two steps by using genomic analysis: (I) comparison between healthy cells and patient tumor cells to discover mutant proteins and genomic expression profile; (II) TCR sequencing to define specific TCR to downstream specific T-cell engineering.

After screening candidate neoantigens by genomic analysis such as whole-exome and RNA sequencing, scientists used dendritic cells (DCs) loaded with neoantigen peptides from genomic analysis to process MHC-antigen presenting a process with co-culture autologous CD8+cell. The personalized TCR T-cell cloning culture includes priming of autologous CD8+T cells after incubation with peptide-pulsed DC; antigen-depending T-cells are stimulated by supplementing the culture with of IL-7 and IL-15 [53]; sorting neoantigen-specific CD8+T-cells were stained using peptide-HLA dextramers by fluorescence-activated cell sorting (FACS); TCR sequencing identify TCR alpha (TCRA) and beta (TCRB) chains. After determining TCRA and TCRB genes with neoantigen-specific TCRs, autologous T-cells are performed by TCR T-cell engineering including four steps as shared Ag TCR engineering: (I) PBMC collection from a patient, (II) T-cell enrichment with removal of other cells, (III) transgene delivery from identified specific neoantigen-TCRs, and (IV) *ex vivo* specific TCR T-cell expansion after initiating the priming of CD8+ T cells.

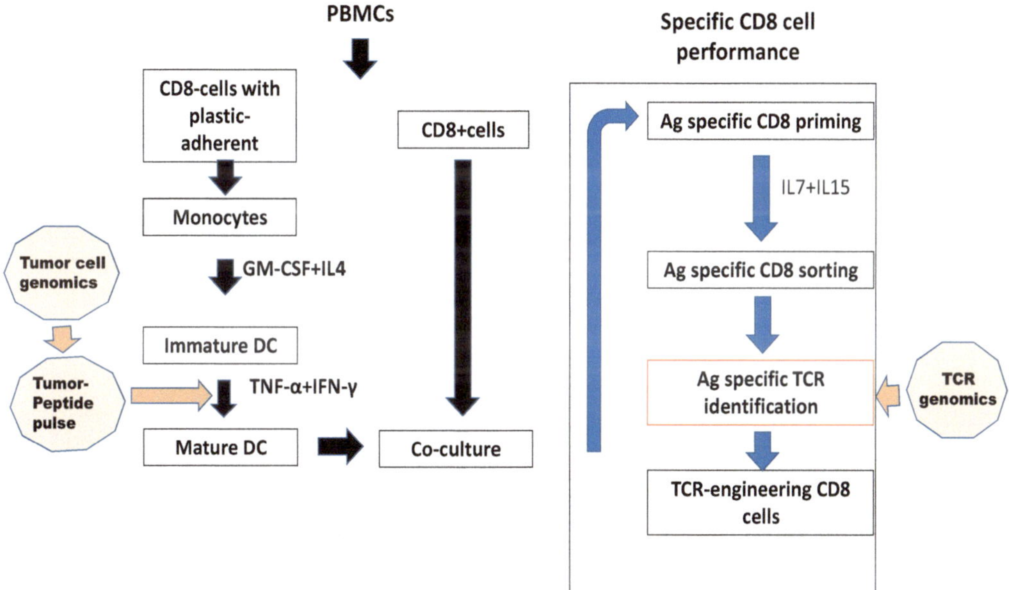

Fig. (5). Personalized TCR T-cell and cloning culture. During the procedure, there are two steps regarding cell biology as PBMC culture and specific T-cell culture. Additionally, pink color for genomic analysis: (I) comparison between healthy cells and patient tumor cells to assay SNP and genomic expression profile to produce tumor-specific peptide; (II) TCR sequencing to define specific TCR to downstream specific T-cell engineering.

5. Genomic Supporting Functional TIL with their Polyclonal Cultures

As our TIL isolation and culture model for adoptive TIL immunotherapy, we have resolved TIL efficacy to tumor cells from solid tumors. After thirty years R&D, a lot of clinical laboratories have supported our early work and further confirmed that TILs could be used for adoptive T-cell immunotherapy for solid tumors, including H&N tumor, brain tumor, lung cancer, liver cancer and ovarian tumors [54]. TILs have at least four advantages while those without TCR and CAR T-cells: (I) TIL has polyclonal T-cells to *in vivo* recognize a few tumor antigens of tumor cells from tumor site; (II) autologous TILs have MHC system to recognize tumor cells MHC system so that TILs do not need to reconstruct as TCR T-cells; (III) TIL immunotherapy are much safer than TCR and CAR T-cells because TILs have not cytokine release syndrome (CRS); (IV) TIL more than 100-fold to kill tumor cells to compare T-cell from peripheral blood [55]. Because TIL isolation and effective cultures are not easy for some research laboratories, TILs are reported to only efficacy to treat melanoma in some early evidence. After long-term arguments, now most TIL culture laboratories have confirmed that TILs can be used for adoptive T-cell immunotherapy of solid tumors.

After we addressed TIL to effectively treat tumor cells from solid tumors, in order to increase TIL efficacy, we begin to study functional TIL immunotherapy since 1998, including (I) TIL CD8+cells are an actively maintained quiescent status in TME by single-cell genomics technique; (II) TIL quiescent pathways with their topology study; (III) TIL quantitative networks with their drug-bank linker to activate related factors to kill tumor cells and to inhibit related factors from blocking TME inhibiting factors.

Following more than twenty's year study, the personalized TIL functional poly-cloning culture as Fig. (6) includes (I) genomic analysis for both TIL and tumor cells; (II) functional inhibiting tumor cells after genomic results from tumor cells and (III) functional inducing CTL and (IV) functional inhibiting TME when TIL culture.

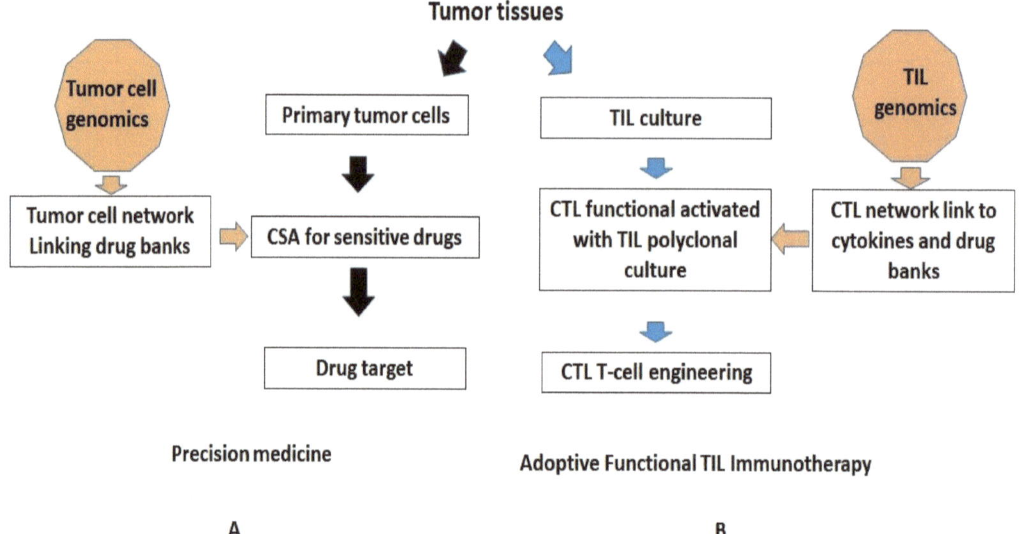

Fig. (6). Personalized polyclonal TIL culture combined with CSA for personalized chemotherapy for tumor cells.

During the procedure, there are two steps to support polyclonal TIL culture by genomic analysis as a pink color for (I) TIL genomics to define increase CTL function and decrease TME function for personalized functional TIL therapy and

(II) genomic comparison between healthy cells and patient tumor cells to define targets to personalized chemotherapy for antitumor cells.

Through more than twenty years' effort, now we have successfully set the functional and polyclonal TIL culture to treat clinical cancer as Fig. (**7**). The personalized polyclonal T-cell immunotherapy is based on individual genomics,

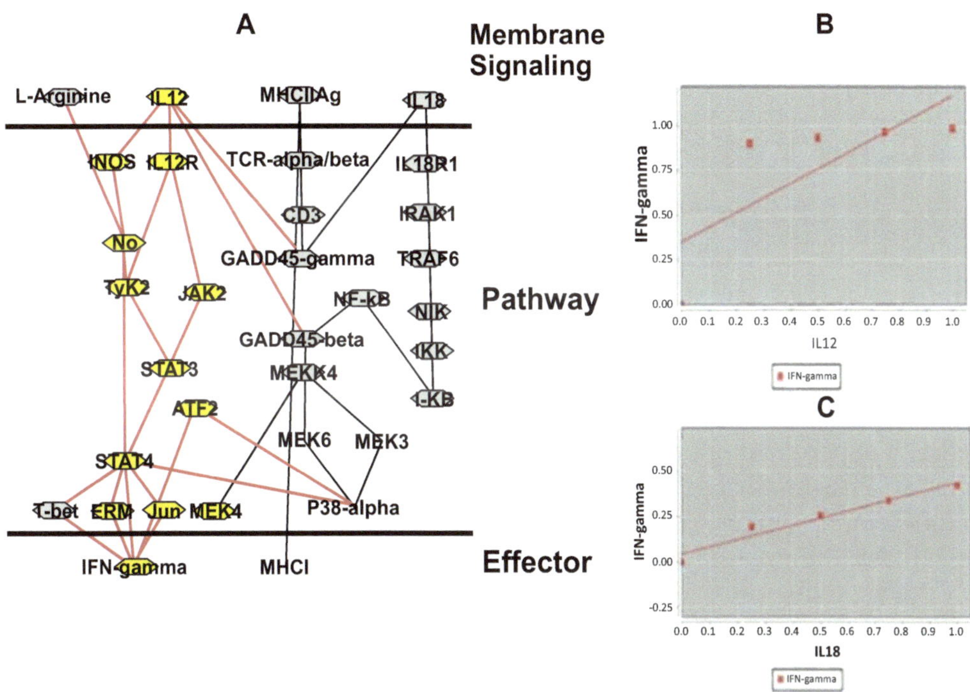

Fig. (7). Bioinformatics supporting T-cell culture for functional cell immunotherapy.

which will be discussed in Chapter 12. Personalized T-cell immunotherapy based on system modeling and/or GWAS has at least four advantages to contrast genetically- modified adoptive immunotherapy: (a) induced T-cells are based on system biology rather than any genetic modification performance so that personalized immunotherapy can keep T-cells good proliferation during culture; (b) CD8+cell culture based on personalized genomic profiles with their network also can release some special substances (such as TNF-α and IFN-γ) or inhibiting some genes expression (such as inhibiting TGF-β) after the functional T-cell *in vivo* infusion; (c) Functional inducing or inhibiting T-cells could be much safer than genetically-modified T-cell immunotherapy with a good efficacy as Fig. (**7c** and **7d**); (d) Once new antibodies, antigens, cytokines, growth factors and receptors are discovered such as antibody to anti-PD-1 and anti-cytotoxic T-lymphocyte antigen-4 (CTLA-4), individual T-cell genomic profiles related to network to link the new compounds can be quickly applied to personalized immunotherapy for different patients.

CYTOKINES OF SPECIFIC T-CELL THERAPY

Since the discovery of IL-1 in 1977, approximately 360,000 published scientific articles have referred to interleukins [57 - 59]. Secreted proteins that bind to their specific receptors and play a role in intercellular communication among T-cells, macrophages, and NK cells are called interleukins. Almost all immune cells display functions characterized by distinct surface receptors and cytokine profiles, such as CD4 and CD8 T-cells, B-cells, NK cells, and dendritic cells (DCs).

Investigations of adoptive immunotherapy have identified a growing list of interleukins [60] or published linker (https://www.jacionline.org/)). Their functions contribute different cell types for adoptive immunotherapy such as T-cells, TIL, CAR T-cells, and TCR T-cells, specific T-cells, and dendritic cells (DCs) are shown in Table **4**, which will be discussed in chapters of adoptive T-cell therapy.

In order to support functional personalized T-cell immunotherapy, after genomic profiles of TILs are discovered for patients, we have set up and use the webpage immunotherapies-linker (http://www.dgidb.org/search_interactions) to support personalized immunotherapy and webpage FDA approval-drug-linker (http://www.dgidb.org/search_interactions) to reprogram TIL functions which we also discuss in chapter 12. The combinations of immunotherapies will play an important role in activating TIL with FDA approval-drug reprograming TIL function to block mechanism to TME factors and cells.

Table **4** . **Growth factors for a culture of immunotherapy.**

Class	Times	Some Modification
TIL	whole periods	IL2 and/or CD3 Ab
Specific T-cells	Monocyte	GM-CSF, IL4
	DC	IFN-Υ, LPS
	Co-culture	IL7, IL15
	T-cells	IL2
TCR T-cells	T-cell engineering	IL2
CAR T-cells	T-cell engineering	IL2

(Table 4) cont.....

	Monocyte	GM-CSF, IL4
Personalized TCR T-cells	DC	IFN-Υ, LPS
	Co-culture	IL7, IL15
	T-cells	IL2
Personalized Functional TIL	Whole periods	IL2 and/or CD3 Ab
	Functional inducing	Inducing and blocking

CONCLUSION

Tumor antigen is essential to a target of tumor-specific T-cells such as TIL, TCR T-cells, and CAR-T-cells for adoptive T-cell immunotherapy. Because tumor cells often accumulate hundreds of mutations with several immunogenic neoantigens, two strategies are going to be used to immunogenetic adoptive immunotherapy: polyclonal tumor antigen recognized by TIL (1) directly isolated from tumor tissue with *ex vivo* culture and (2) functional TIL culture based on genomic profiles from TIL, both of TIL and functional TIL can be used for polyclonal culture for personalized adoptive immunotherapy; shared tumor antigen, recognized by (1) specific T-cell, (2) CAR T-cell and (3) TCR T-cell, can be used for shared antigen immunogenicity for T-cell adoptive immunotherapy. Now the tumor antigen with mutants and neoantigen from patient tumor cells can be mined by a genomic performance with screening techniques to uncover for engineering TCR T-cells. These new methodologies are increasingly supporting clinical oncologists to apply for a new generation of T-cell adoptive immunotherapy for patients.

CONSENT FOR PUBLICATION

The authors declare no financial interests.

CONFLICT OF INTEREST

The authors declare no financial interests.

ACKNOWLEDGEMENTS

During the early period, BL with his colleagues, including HLH set up the first TIL polyclonal culture in China, as described in the chapter. BL further study more than 25 years for TIL immunotherapy, including setting up single-cell cloning culture to analyze genomic profiles including CD3+, CD3+CD8+ during 1996-2000 in Rush Medical Center. The research was previously supported by National Cancer Institute IRG-91-022-09, USA (to BL). The mention of trade names or commercial products in this article is solely to provide specific information and does not imply recommendation.

REFERENCES

[1]   Berggren JR, Tanner CJ, Houmard JA. Primary cell cultures in the study of human muscle metabolism. Exerc Sport Sci Rev 2007; 35(2): 56-61.
[http://dx.doi.org/10.1249/JES.0b013e31803eae63] [PMID: 17417051]

[2]   Moridani M, Harirforoosh S. Drug development and discovery: challenges and opportunities. Drug Discov Today 2014; 19(11): 1679-81.
[http://dx.doi.org/10.1016/j.drudis.2014.06.003] [PMID: 24928030]

[3]   Mak IW, Evaniew N, Ghert M. Lost in translation: animal models and clinical trials in cancer treatment. Am J Transl Res 2014; 6(2): 114-8.
[PMID: 24489990]

[4]   Perel P, Roberts I, Sena E, *et al*. Comparison of treatment effects between animal experiments and clinical trials: systematic review. BMJ 2007; 334(7586): 197.
[http://dx.doi.org/10.1136/bmj.39048.407928.BE] [PMID: 17175568]

[5]   DiMasi JA, Hansen RW, Grabowski HG. The price of innovation: new estimates of drug development costs. J Health Econ 2003; 22(2): 151-85.
[http://dx.doi.org/10.1016/S0167-6296(02)00126-1] [PMID: 12606142]

[6]   Li BR, Tong SQ, Zhang XH, Lu J, Gu QL, Lu DY. A new experimental and clinical approach of combining usage of highly active tumor-infiltrating lymphocytes and highly sensitive antitumor drugs for the advanced malignant tumor. Chin Med J (Engl) 1994; 107(11): 803-7.
[PMID: 7867384]

[7]   Huang XK, Meyer P, Li B, Raza A, Preisler HD. The effects of the farnesyl transferase inhibitor FTI L-778,123 on normal, myelodysplastic, and myeloid leukemia bone marrow progenitor proliferation *in vitro*. Leuk Lymphoma 2003; 44(1): 157-64.
[http://dx.doi.org/10.1080/1042819021000040387] [PMID: 12691158]

[8]   Morton CL, Houghton PJ. Establishment of human tumor xenografts in immunodeficient mice. Nat Protoc 2007; 2(2): 247-50.
[http://dx.doi.org/10.1038/nprot.2007.25] [PMID: 17406581]

[9]   Haycock JW. 3D cell culture: a review of current approaches and techniques. Methods Mol Biol 2011; 695: 1-15.
[http://dx.doi.org/10.1007/978-1-60761-984-0_1] [PMID: 21042962]

[10]   Si Plain-Laid, Live Lu, Zhou Wen-Hui, Hu Wei-Dong. Establishment and Identification of human primary lung cancer cell culture in vitro Nit J Clan Expr Patrol 2015; 8(6): 6540-6.

[11]   Klebe RJ. Cytoscribing: a method for micropositioning cells and the construction of two- and three-dimensional synthetic tissues. Exp Cell Res 1988; 179(2): 362-73.
[http://dx.doi.org/10.1016/0014-4827(88)90275-3] [PMID: 3191947]

[12]   Xu T, Zhao W, Zhu JM, Albanna MZ, Yoo JJ, Atala A. Complex heterogeneous tissue constructs containing multiple cell types prepared by inkjet printing technology. Biomaterials 2013; 34(1): 130-9.
[http://dx.doi.org/10.1016/j.biomaterials.2012.09.035] [PMID: 23063369]

[13]   Li B, Ding L, Yang C, *et al*. Characterization of transcription factor networks involved in umbilical cord blood CD34+ stem cells-derived erythropoiesis. PLoS One 2014; 9(9)e107133
[http://dx.doi.org/10.1371/journal.pone.0107133] [PMID: 25211130]

[14]   Li B, Ding J, Larson A, Song S. Tumor tissue recycling--a new combination treatment for solid tumors: experimental and preliminary clinical research. *In Vivo* 1999; 13(5): 433-8.
[PMID: 10654199]

[15]   Deng YD, Gu QL, Li B, *et al*. MTT colorimetric assay for LAK and TIL cell activity in cord blood

Journal of Shanghai Jiaotong University (Medical Science Edition, Chinese) 1995. 02.

[16]   Hu BC, Li GW, Cheng W, Shen JK, *et al.* Clinical application of infiltrating lymphocytes in malignant brain tumors. Journal of Immunology (Chinese): 1997; 02.

[17]   Hua ZD, Lu J, Li HF, Li B, *et al.* Clinical study of tumor-infiltrating lymphocytes in ovarian cancer Chinese Journal of Obstetrics and Gynecology. Chinese 1996; p. 09.

[18]   Lu J, Hu LW, Hua ZD, Li B, *et al.* analysis of the therapeutic effects of different therapeutic approaches for TIL. Journal of Chinese Tumor Biological Treatment (Chinese): 1996; 02.

[19]   Molldrem JJ, Lee PP, Wang C, *et al.* Evidence that specific T lymphocytes may participate in the elimination of chronic myelogenous leukemia. Nat Med 2000; 6(9): 1018-23.
         [http://dx.doi.org/10.1038/79526] [PMID: 10973322]

[20]   Bernhard H, Neudorfer J, Gebhard K, *et al.* Adoptive transfer of autologous, HER2-specific, cytotoxic T lymphocytes for the treatment of HER2-overexpressing breast cancer. Cancer Immunol Immunother 2008; 57(2): 271-80.
         [http://dx.doi.org/10.1007/s00262-007-0355-7] [PMID: 17646988]

[21]   Boudreau JE, Bonehill A, Thielemans K, Wan Y. Engineering dendritic cells to enhance cancer immunotherapy. Mol Ther 2011; 19(5): 841-53.
         [http://dx.doi.org/10.1038/mt.2011.57] [PMID: 21468005]

[22]   Jeras M, Bergant M, Repnik U. *In vitro* preparation and functional assessment of human monocyte-derived dendritic cells-potential antigen-specific modulators of *in vivo* immune responses. Transpl Immunol 2005; 14(3-4): 231-44.
         [http://dx.doi.org/10.1016/j.trim.2005.03.012] [PMID: 15982568]

[23]   Sennikov SV, Shevchenko JA, Kurilin VV, *et al.* Induction of an antitumor response using dendritic cells transfected with DNA constructs encoding the HLA-A*02:01-restricted epitopes of tumor-associated antigens in culture of mononuclear cells of breast cancer patients. Immunol Res 2016; 64(1): 171-80.
         [http://dx.doi.org/10.1007/s12026-015-8735-0] [PMID: 26590947]

[24]   Gelao L, Criscitiello C, Esposito A, *et al.* Dendritic cell-based vaccines: clinical applications in breast cancer
         [http://dx.doi.org/10.2217/imt.13.169]

[25]   Frankenberger B, Schendel DJ. Third generation dendritic cell vaccines for tumor immunotherapy. Eur J Cell Biol 2012; 91(1): 53-8.
         [http://dx.doi.org/10.1016/j.ejcb.2011.01.012] [PMID: 21439674]

[26]   Schürch CM, Riether C, Ochsenbein AF. Dendritic cell-based immunotherapy for myeloid leukemias. Front Immunol 2013; 4: 496.
         [http://dx.doi.org/10.3389/fimmu.2013.00496] [PMID: 24427158]

[27]   Goebel SU, Iwamoto M, Raffeld M, *et al.* Her-2/neu expression and gene amplification in gastrinomas: correlations with tumor biology, growth, and aggressiveness. Cancer Res 2002; 62(13): 3702-10.
         [PMID: 12097278]

[28]   Tran E, Robbins PF, Lu YC, *et al.* T-Cell Transfer Therapy Targeting Mutant KRAS in Cancer. N Engl J Med 2016; 375: 62-2255. 13.

[29]   Ott PA, Hu Z, Keskin DB, *et al.* An immunogenic personal neoantigen vaccine for patients with melanoma Nature 2017; 547: 21-217. 14.
         [http://dx.doi.org/10.1038/nature22991]

[30]   De Smet C, Lurquin C, van der Bruggen P, De Plaen E, Brasseur F, Boon T. Sequence and expression pattern of the human MAGE2 gene. Immunogenetics 1994; 39(2): 121-9.
         [http://dx.doi.org/10.1007/BF00188615] [PMID: 8276455]

[31]   Bakker AB, Schreurs MWJ, de Boer AJ, *et al.* Melanocyte lineage-specific antigen gp100 is recognized by melanoma-derived tumor-infiltrating lymphocytes. J Exp Med 1994; 179(3): 1005-9. [http://dx.doi.org/10.1084/jem.179.3.1005] [PMID: 8113668]

[32]   Kawakami Y, Eliyahu S, Sakaguchi K, *et al.* Identification of the immunodominant peptides of the MART-1 human melanoma antigen recognized by the majority of HLA-A2-restricted tumor infiltrating lymphocytes. J Exp Med 1994; 180(1): 347-52. [http://dx.doi.org/10.1084/jem.180.1.347] [PMID: 7516411]

[33]   Tsang KY, Zaremba S, Nieroda CA, Zhu MZ, Hamilton JM, Schlom J. Generation of human cytotoxic T cells specific for human carcinoembryonic antigen epitopes from patients immunized with recombinant vaccinia-CEA vaccine. J Natl Cancer Inst 1995; 87(13): 982-90. [http://dx.doi.org/10.1093/jnci/87.13.982] [PMID: 7629885]

[34]   Wang X, Wang Q. Alpha-fetoprotein and hepatocellular carcinoma immunity. Can J Gastroenterol Hepatol 2018; 20189049252 [http://dx.doi.org/10.1155/2018/9049252] [PMID: 29805966]

[35]   Gross G, Waks T, Eshhar Z. Expression of immunoglobulin-T-cell receptor chimeric molecules as functional receptors with antibody-type specificity. Proc Natl Acad Sci USA 1989; 86(24): 10024-8. [http://dx.doi.org/10.1073/pnas.86.24.10024] [PMID: 2513569]

[36]   Li B, Tong SQ, Lu DY, *et al.* DHBV induced acute hepatic cell necrosis in a duck-An experimental model for fulminant hepatitis. Acta Shanghai Second Medical University 1990; 10(3): 189-93.

[37]   Li B, Xu W, Qian GX, Zhang XH, Dong SQ, Chen SS. Methodology of TNF gene transduction of tumor infiltrating lymphocytes. Journal of Shanghai Second Medical University 1995; 15(3): 3-6.

[38]   Cai X, Zheng W, Pan S, *et al.* A virus-like particle of the hepatitis B virus preS antigen elicits robust neutralizing antibodies and T cell responses in mice. Antiviral Res 2018; 149: 48-57. [http://dx.doi.org/10.1016/j.antiviral.2017.11.007] [PMID: 29129705]

[39]   Irving BA, Weiss A. The cytoplasmic domain of the T cell receptor zeta chain is sufficient to couple to receptor-associated signal transduction pathways. Cell 1991; 64(5): 891-901. [http://dx.doi.org/10.1016/0092-8674(91)90314-O] [PMID: 1705867]

[40]   Park JR, Digiusto DL, Slovak M, *et al.* Adoptive transfer of chimeric antigen receptor re-directed cytolytic T lymphocyte clones in patients with neuroblastoma. Mol Ther 2007; 15(4): 825-33. [http://dx.doi.org/10.1038/sj.mt.6300104] [PMID: 17299405]

[41]   Lamers CH, Sleijfer S, Vulto AG, *et al.* Treatment of metastatic renal cell carcinoma with autologous T-lymphocytes genetically retargeted against carbonic anhydrase IX: first clinical experience. J Clin Oncol 2006; 24(13): e20-2. [http://dx.doi.org/10.1200/JCO.2006.05.9964] [PMID: 16648493]

[42]   Till BG, Jensen MC, Wang J, *et al.* Adoptive immunotherapy for indolent non-Hodgkin lymphoma and mantle cell lymphoma using genetically modified autologous CD20-specific T cells. Blood 2008; 112(6): 2261-71. [http://dx.doi.org/10.1182/blood-2007-12-128843] [PMID: 18509084]

[43]   Finney HM, Lawson AD, Bebbington CR, Weir AN. Chimeric receptors providing both primary and costimulatory signaling in T cells from a single gene product. J Immunol 1998; 161(6): 2791-7. [PMID: 9743337]

[44]   Friedmann-Morvinski D, Bendavid A, Waks T, Schindler D, Eshhar Z. Redirected primary T cells harboring a chimeric receptor require costimulation for their antigen-specific activation. Blood 2005; 105(8): 3087-93. [http://dx.doi.org/10.1182/blood-2004-09-3737] [PMID: 15626734]

[45]   Ruella M, Xu J, Barrett DM, *et al.* Induction of resistance to chimeric antigen receptor T cell therapy by transduction of a single leukemic B cell. Nat Med 2018; 24(10): 1499-503. [http://dx.doi.org/10.1038/s41591-018-0201-9] [PMID: 30275568]

[46]   Scholler J, Brady TL, Binder-Scholl G, *et al.* Decade-long safety and function of retroviral-modified chimeric antigen receptor T cells. Sci Transl Med 2012; 4(132)132ra53
[http://dx.doi.org/10.1126/scitranslmed.3003761] [PMID: 22553251]

[47]   Hacein-Bey-Abina S, Garrigue A, Wang GP, *et al.* Insertional oncogenesis in 4 patients after retrovirus-mediated gene therapy of SCID-X1. J Clin Invest 2008; 118(9): 3132-42.
[http://dx.doi.org/10.1172/JCI35700] [PMID: 18688285]

[48]   Montini E, Cesana D, Schmidt M, *et al.* The genotoxic potential of retroviral vectors is strongly modulated by vector design and integration site selection in a mouse model of HSC gene therapy. J Clin Invest 2009; 119(4): 964-75.
[http://dx.doi.org/10.1172/JCI37630] [PMID: 19307726]

[49]   Naldini L, Blömer U, Gallay P, *et al. In vivo* gene delivery and stable transduction of nondividing cells by a lentiviral vector. Science 1996; 272(5259): 263-7.
[http://dx.doi.org/10.1126/science.272.5259.263] [PMID: 8602510]

[50]   Stroncek DF, Ren J, Lee DW, *et al.* Myeloid cells in peripheral blood mononuclear cell concentrates inhibit the expansion of chimeric antigen receptor T cells. Cytotherapy 2016; 18(7): 893-901.
[http://dx.doi.org/10.1016/j.jcyt.2016.04.003] [PMID: 27210719]

[51]   Oncotarget 2018; 9(13): 11009-11019. eCollection 2018 Feb 16.
[http://dx.doi.org/10.18632/oncotarget.24232]

[52]   Effective screening of T cells recognizing neoantigens and construction of T-cell receptor-engineered T cells.

[53]   Kato T, Matsuda T, Ikeda Y, *et al.* Effective screening of T cells recognizing neoantigens and construction of T-cell receptor-engineered T cells. Oncotarget 2018; 9(13): 11009-19.
[http://dx.doi.org/10.18632/oncotarget.24232] [PMID: 29541393]

[54]   Ben-Avi R, Farhi R, Ben-Nun A, *et al.* Establishment of adoptive cell therapy with tumor infiltrating lymphocytes for non-small cell lung cancer patients. Cancer Immunol Immunother 2018; 67(8): 1221-30.
[http://dx.doi.org/10.1007/s00262-018-2174-4] [PMID: 29845338]

[55]   Topalian SL, Muul LM, Solomon D, Rosenberg SA. Expansion of human tumor infiltrating lymphocytes for use in immunotherapy trials. J Immunol Methods 1987; 102(1): 127-41.
[http://dx.doi.org/10.1016/S0022-1759(87)80018-2] [PMID: 3305708]

[56]   Li B. Breakthroughs of 2015-Personalized Immunotherapy Based on Individual GWAS and Biomarkers. Biom J 2015; 1: 1-2.

[57]   Dinarello C, Arend W, Sims J, *et al.* IL-1 family nomenclature. Nat Immunol 2010; 11(11): 973.
[http://dx.doi.org/10.1038/ni1110-973] [PMID: 20959797]

[58]   Lloyd CM, Saglani S. T cells in asthma: influences of genetics, environment, and T-cell plasticity. J Allergy Clin Immunol 2013; 131(5): 1267-74.
[http://dx.doi.org/10.1016/j.jaci.2013.02.016] [PMID: 23541326]

[59]   Akdis M, Burgler S, Crameri R, Eiwegger T, Fujita H, Gomez E, *et al.* Interleu-kins, from 1 to 37, and interferon-gamma: receptors, functions, and roles in diseases J Allergy Clin Immunol 2011; 127:701-21, e1-70

[60]   Akdis M, Aab A, Altunbulakli C, Azkur K, Costa RA, Crameri R, *et al.* Interleukins (from IL-1 to IL-38), interferons, transforming growth factor, and TNF-a: Receptors, functions, and roles in diseases. Fundamentals of allergy and immunology 2016; 13(4): 986- 1004.

CHAPTER 8

Bioinformatics of T-cell and Primary Tumor Cells-Fundamental of Adoptive T-cell Immunotherapy

George Liu[1,2], Jie Zheng[3] and Biaoru Li[1,4,*]

[1] *Department of Biochemistry, Case Western Reserve University School of Medicine , Cleveland OH , USA*

[2] *USDA, ARS, ANRI, Bovine Functional Genomics Laboratory, Beltsville Agricultural Research Center (BARC) – East , Beltsville, MD, USA*

[3] *School of Computer Engineering, Nanyang Technological University, 639798, Singapore*

[4] *Georgia Cancer Center and Department of Pediatrics, Medical College at GA, Augusta, GA 30912, USA*

Abstract: Epitope discovery of tumor antigen and mutant proteins has enabled a better application of T-cell immunotherapy. Genomic profiles analyzed by genomic expression and single nucleotide polymorphisms (SNP) by genome-wide association studies (GWAS) are an essential fundamental to screen and define T-cell therapeutic targets. To determine tumor antigens or mutant proteins related to T-cell targets with their TCR or CAR reconstruction, we will introduce the SNP technique related to primary tumor cells for personalized T-cell immunotherapy, including global and local SNP detection of the therapeutic targets. Moreover, the use of mRNA genomic expression can discover gene expression signature and further uncover tumor-associated antigen (TAA) or tumor-specific antigen (TSA) for T-cell immunotherapy. Accompany with the ongoing development of next-generation sequencing, epitope discovery of tumor neoantigen and mutant proteins will be irreplaceable for a novel generation of T-cell adoptive immunotherapy. System biology, which is a mathematical modeling of complex biological systems,can integrate data of SNP signature and genomic expression signature. Thus, a new bioinformatics platform with the analysis of GWAS and genomic expression profile along with system modeling is an essential fundamental for T-cell adoptive immunotherapy.

Keywords: And system modeling, Genome-wide association studies (GWAS), gene expression signature (GES), Networks, Proteomics, Single nucleotide polymorphisms (SNP), System biology, T-cell adoptive immunotherapy, Therapeutic targeting, Transcriptome.

---

* **Corresponding author Biaoru Li**: Georgia Cancer Center and Department of Pediatrics, Medical College at GA, Augusta, GA 30912, USA; Tel: 440-317-1443; E-mail: bli@augusta.edu

INTRODUCTION

Detecting single nucleotide polymorphisms (SNP) and genomics expression profiles from tumor cells is an important foundation in the new generation of personalized immunotherapy or adoptive T-cell immunotherapy. The genomic profile can define mutant proteins uncovered by specific SNPs and tumor neoantigen discovered by genomic expression files [1 - 4]. Moreover, it is essential to integrate SNPs profiles with other genomic profiles among them (GWAS-transcriptome, GWAS-microRNA, GWAS-transcriptome-epigenetics) to study therapeutic targets [5, 6]. To introduce rational screening SNPs and neoantigens, according to workflow of clinical genomics workflow (Fig. **1**), in the chapter, we will first introduce necessary screening procedures: (A) tumor sampling and techniques for SNPs and genomic profile; (B) tumor cell SNP and genomic profiles detection related analysis and discovery; (C) SNP and genomic signature related system model; (D) different validation methods for the targets.

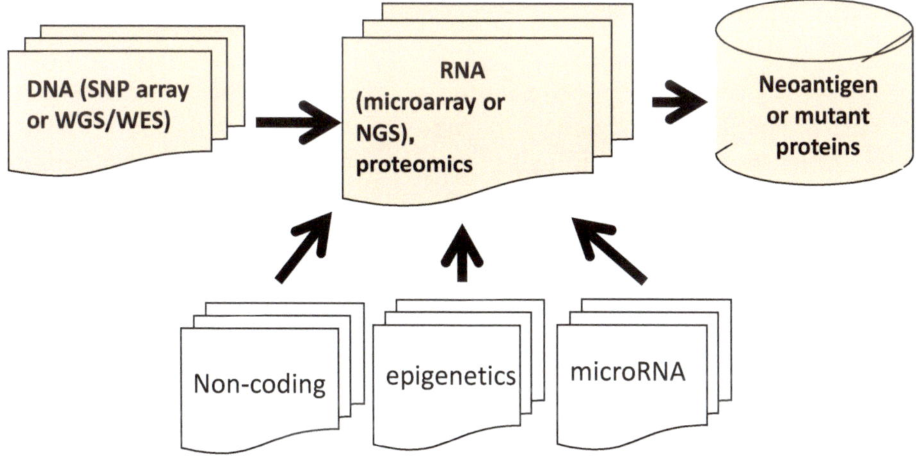

Fig. (1). Clinical genomics workflow. Three levels of analyses include genomic archives (GWAS), genomics expression analysis, including transcriptomes and proteomics, clinical phenotype changes of tumor cells. Dark-color is the central part of the manual.

Moreover, after the discovery of tumor neoantigen including mutant protein, scientists and physicians are going to study TCR sequencing to define specific TCR to downstream specific T-cell engineering and TCR T-cell engineering including peptide-pulsed DC with T-cell activity for specific T-cell engineering; or TCR T-cell workstream including peptide-pulsed DC with T-cell antigen-depending T-cells culture by IL-7 and IL-15, sorting neoantigen-specific CD8+T-cells stained by peptide-HLA dextramers and isolated by fluorescence-activated cell sorting (FACS), TCR sequencing identifying TCR alpha (TCRA) and beta (TCRB) chains. If the genomic process is combined to TCR T-cell engineering, after determining TCR sequence with neoantigen-specific TCRs, autologous PBMN T-cells are performed by TCR T-cell engineering including four steps: (I) PBMN collection from a patient, (II) T-cell enrichment with removal of other cells, (III) transgene delivery from identified specific neoantigen-TCRs, and (IV) *ex vivo* specific TCR T-cell expansion after initiating the priming of CD8+ T cells.

Genomic expression profiles or integration of genomic expression of tumor cells can uncover candidates of gene expression level by system modeling to discover tumor biomarkers (TAA) and therapeutics targets. To set up a rational network to determine neoantigen for personalized immunotherapy, at present, system biology-based on transcriptomes such as microarray and RNA-sequencing has been largely reported. According to some successful workflow, we also present one successful module detecting SNP based TCR T-cells with their reconstruction under bioinformatics support.

Finally, we also present the second bioinformatics module, which we have worked for more than 15 years, to study functional polyclonal TIL for personalized therapy. In the conclusion section, I will discuss the challenges of personalized immunotherapy based on bioinformatics and system modeling.

WORKFLOW OF TUMOR SAMPLING WITH SNP AND GENOMIC ANALYSIS

1. Clinical Tumor Sampling to the Isolation of Tumor Cells and TIL

Mixed-cells from tumor samples are great challenges for genetic analysis and genomic data analysis. To achieve objective results of genetic analysis and genomics data analysis for personalized targets, we will first introduce SNP and genomic analysis from clinical tumor samples. In the clinical workflow of tumor genomic analysis from reported evidence, several sampling techniques have been applied for tumor SNP and genomic analysis [7, 8]: tumor sampling *in vitro* (single-cell sampling for SNP and genomic analysis), tumor sampling *ex vivo* (purifying/expanding primary cells *ex vivo* from clinical tumor samples for SNP and genomic analysis) and direct tumor tissue SNP and genomic analysis *in silico*.

1. Clinical Tumor Sampling In Vitro

Clinical sampling *in vitro* includes isolation of primary tumor cells consisting of flow-cytometric cell sorting (FACS) [9], magnetic cell separation (MACS) [10, 11], and laser-captured micro-dis-section (LCM) [12] with downstream SNP and genomic analysis. FACS can isolate tumor cells by a specific biomarker on the cell surface and intracellular parts such as CD133/CD34 for cancer stem cells (CSCs) [13] and EpCAM for circulating tumor cells (CTCs) [14]. At present, multi-colored FACS can specifically harvest identified cells in a vial by combined biomarkers so that FACS can enhance its ability to mine SNP and genomic profile. MACS technique. The second cell harvesting technique *in vitro* for clinical genomics analysis is to use the MACS technique to sort primary cells by cell-surface biomarkers. At present, MACS can use multi-labeling Abs to negative or positive select identified cells with surface biomarkers; therefore, it also can increase its ability to uncover SNP and gene profile in a given cell at the tissue level. Among LCM techniques, LCM can achieve tumor cells based on morphology change on glass slides or rely on specific mRNA/protein biomarkers. LCMs can specifically harvest clinical cells *in vivo* environment [15]. LCMs also can combine Ab-based stains and DNA/RNA FISH stains to increase the cell specificity from their biomarkers. In these several years, along with R&D of LCM techniques and biomarker identification for primary tumor cells and TIL, LCM has been quickly developed (A) from fixed cells into living cells which can be further cultured for primary cells due to downstream genomic analysis [16]; (B) LCM can be used for an automation system for high-throughput screening [17].

2. Clinical Tumor Sampling Ex Vivo

Clinical sampling *ex vivo* includes primary tumor-cell culture with downstream SNP and genomic analysis. In 1977, Drs. Hamburger and Salmon first set up primary tumor-cell culture to assay drug sensitivity for tumor patients [18]. In 1994, we reported 50 cases of primary tumor-cell culture for chemosensitivity assay (CSA) [19]. Along with R&D of the culture of primary tumor cells, genomic analyses are going to play an important role in personalized immunotherapy. Furthermore, the *ex vivo* CSA system can verify suggested targeted molecules for personalized therapy.

3. Tumor Tissue SNP with Genomic Analysis In Silico

In clinics, most clinical specimens are directly frozen at tissue level after surgical removal. If the specimens are performed by SNP microarray and NGS at the tissue level, genomic analysis *in silico* is a very important strategy for tumor tissue SNP and genomic analysis because the SNPs and genomic data are mixed with different those from the mixed cells. According to published data [20], two combined groups of bioinformatics techniques can increase the purity of clinical genomic analysis from the mixed cells: (A) tissue-level by hierarchical cluster, principal component analysis (PCA), and self-organizing map (SOM) and (B) molecular-level by supervised learning based on cell-biomarkers and time-courses relied on time-course of biomarker change.

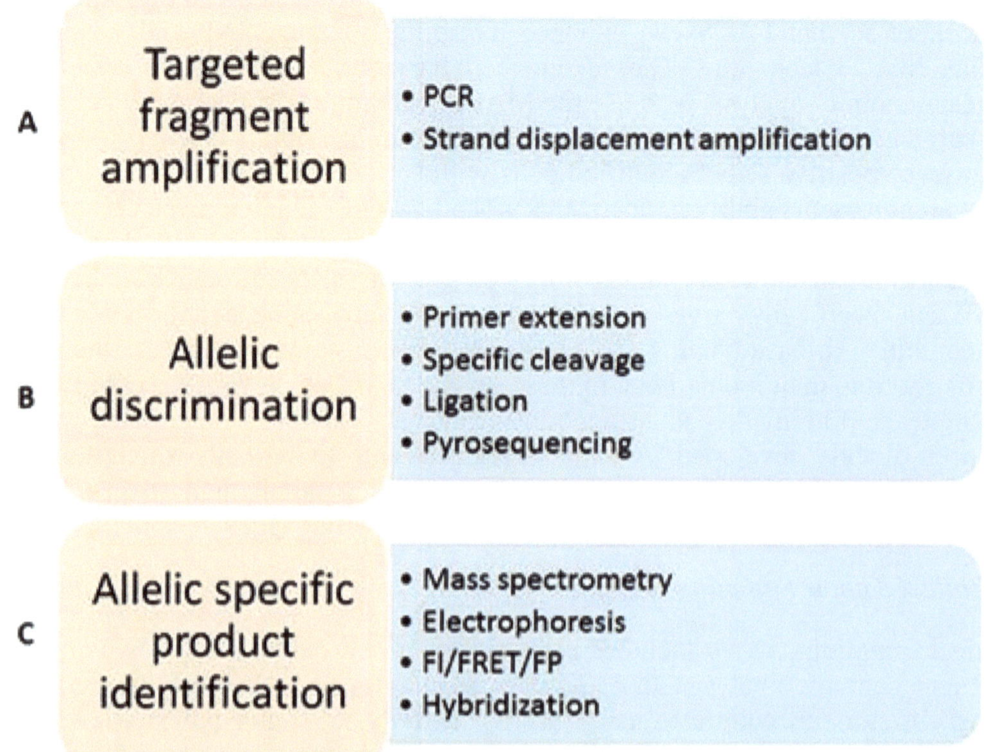

Fig. (2). The diagram of the procedure of designed SNP detection. **A.** Targeted Fragment amplification by PCR; **B.** Allelic discrimination reaction by ligase, cleavage, and extension; **C.** Allele-specific product identification by mass spectrometry, electrophoresis, fluorescence, and hybridization.

TUMOR GWAS AND GENOMIC PROFILE WITH ANALYSIS

1. SNP Detection and Analysis

SNP is a single base-pair mutation at a specific locus, usually consisting of two alleles (where the rare allele frequency is >1%). SNPs can provide information on mutant protein for immunotherapy. To discover mutant proteins, detecting assays include global approaches and local approaches. Global SNP analysis is to use SNP microarray and next-generation sequencing (NGS) to uncover mutant proteins [21, 22]. At present, Affymetrix is available for these kinds of products, such as Human SNP 5.0 Gene Chip. NGS is the second universal SNP detection quickly developed due to more throughput than SNP microarray. As our several publications, SNP detection of NGS can utilize whole genomic DNA-Seq (WGS), whole-exome-Seq (WES), and RNA-Seq to detect SNPs [23 - 25]. On the other hand, designed-local SNP detection is also quickly developed. Designed SNPs genotyping protocols include three steps as Fig. (**2**) [26]: target amplification, allelic discrimination, and product detection/identification. Target DNA Amplifications use almost all the polymerase chain reaction (PCR) techniques. Allelic discriminations are a key of SNP genotyping. The discriminating power generating from DNA polymerases and DNA ligases can differ matched and mismatched DNA duplexes with high specificity and accuracy. Allele discrimination can be used by hybridization, ligation, and the 5' nuclease activity of DNA polymerases. The final step is the identification of allele-specific products. Now amplified local DNA or RNA can combine NGS to detect a pair of tumor cells or T-cells.

Most detection systems have built-in mechanisms to perform repetitive work for many samples, such as 96- and 384-well plates or hybridization on a solid membrane [27 - 30]. Because so many products are available on the markets that clinical scientists are difficult to select an appropriate one for their applications. In this manual, we conclude some SNPs techniques and kits with their strengths/weaknesses, ranking/throughputs, and cost range of these technologies for clinical application as a Table **1**.

2. Detection of Genomic Expression

In order to detect genomics expression level, we have evaluated three groups of transcriptome profiles as our reports: tumor-normal cell pairing from cardiac sarcoma by LCM sampling to study 15 genes for sensitivity test and 14 genes for specificity test indicated 87% sensitivity and 60% specificity. In contrast, genomic expression level from non-pairing tumor-cells (NSCLC from biopsy and SCLC from surgical specimens) using 10 and 20 genes for sensitivity test, as well as 13 and 20 genes for specificity test indicated sensitivity 70% and 91% and specificity 47% and 31%, respectively [31]. At present, mRNA microarray and RNA-seq are routinely employed to uncover abnormal expressive proteins. Finally, sensitivity and specificity of matched tumor-normal genomics profiles should be validated by quantitative RT-PCR.

Table 1. Comparison of routine SNPs detection kits for PTT.

Types	Methods	Scales (SNP)	Samples	Strength	Weakness	Cost
Local	Taq Man assay	about 10	96-384	Simple and easy to automate	lower throughput	0.6 per SNP/genotype
	Sequenom	10-300	50-1000	Medium throughput	Higher cost for equipment	0.2 per SNP/genotype
	Illumina Golden Gate	384-3072	96-1000	Medium throughput	Higher cost for equipment	0.2 per SNP/genotype
	Captured-seq	targeted all SNPs disease	depending	Higher throughput for a given	Higher cost equipment	depending on the sample size
Global	SNP Microarray	Universal	12	higher throughput	Costly equipment and bioinformatics	expensive
	WGS	Universal	1	coding and noncoding	Costly equipment and bioinformatics	expensive
	WES	Universal	1	exome	Costly equipment and bioinformatics	expensive
	RNA- Seq	Universal	1	SNVs and transcriptome	Costly equipment and bioinformatics	expensive

SYSTEM MODELING FOR TUMOR CELLS AND TILS

When we achieve both files of SNP and genomics expression, we require to integrate those to discover mutant proteins or biomarkers. Here we will discuss system biology, including network with topology analysis for personalized biomarkers with their targets.

1. System Modeling of a Network to Discover GES

Networks are intracellular biological and molecular components and their direct or indirect interactions as links within a system modeling [32]. There are many different approaches of a network to apply for system models such as directed or undirected, Boolean networks, and Steiner trees [33]. For in-depth coverage of these data structures and algorithms, bioinformatics science enables the integration of data from many different studies into a single framework. For example, networks can be generated directly from time-series data or from perturbation data. The topology of networks can be "simulating-engineer" directly from data tables to changing quantities of mRNA expression/mutant protein so that they can define gene expression signature (GES) with validated specificity in system modeling for therapeutic targets [34]. Currently, the Cytoscape platform can be used to integrate different bioinformatic information by algorithms [35 - 37].

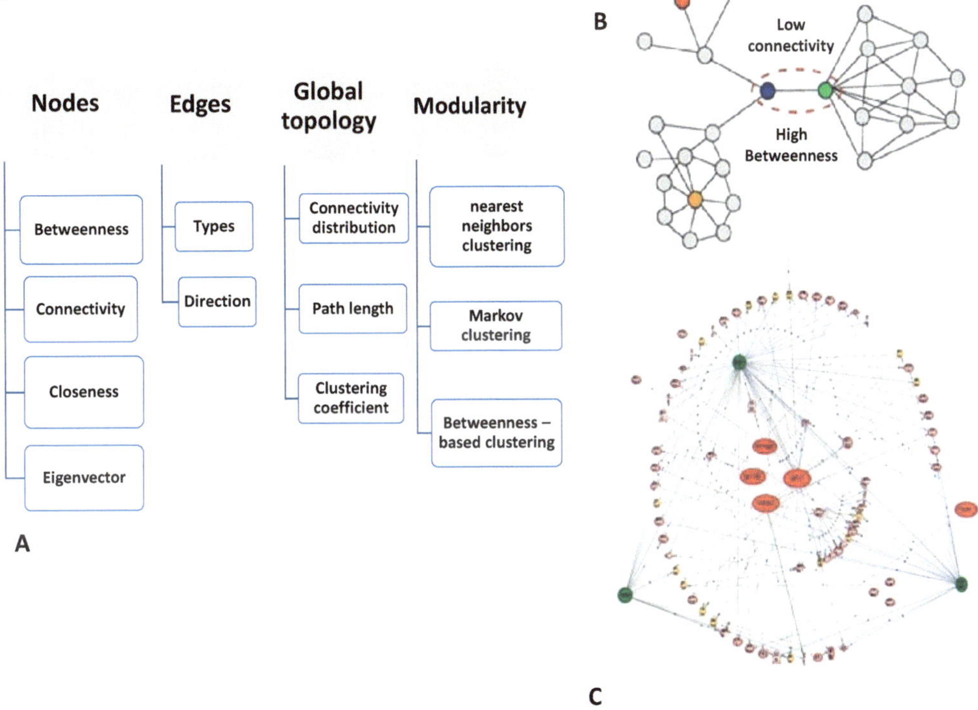

Fig. (3). The diagram of a quantitative network for GES. **A.** entire quantitative network analysis; **B.** GES with higher "Betweenness" and lower "connectivity"; **C.** example of GES with higher "Betweenness" and lower "connectivity." The red color is type-I targeting with higher "Betweenness," and lower "connectivity" and Green color is type-II with lower "Betweenness" and higher "connectivity." Targeted Fragment amplification by PCR; B. Allelic discrimination reaction by ligase, cleavage, and extension; C. Allele-specific product identification by mass spectrometry, electrophoresis, fluorescence, and hybridization.

2. GES Determining Targets

A network's topology enables providing GES insight into the key targets from tumor cells and TILs. Network topology consists of general and specific properties of nodes, properties of edges, properties of the entire network (global topological properties) and modules within the network (Fig. **3**) [38, 39]: (A) Properties of nodes include connectivity degree (number of links for each node), betweenness centrality (number of shortest paths that go through a node among all shortest paths between all possible pairs of nodes), closeness centrality (average shortest path from one node to all other nodes) and eigenvector centrality (a more sophisticated centrality measure that assesses the closeness to highly connected nodes); (B) Properties of edges include the types of relationship (activating or inhibiting by phosphorylation, binding, gene regulation between a pair of nodes) and edge directionality (upstream and downstream); (C) Global topological characteristics of networks include connectivity distribution (a histogram showing nodes with their links), path length (Floyd-Warshall's or Dijkstra's algorithms) and clustering coefficient (local density of interactions by measuring the connectivity of neighbors for each node averaged over the entire network); (D) Modularity or network clusters includes unsupervised clustering algorithms, such as nearest neighbors clustering, Markov clustering, and betweenness centrality–based clustering with high betweenness centrality and low Connectivity to separate clusters. After understanding the structure of networks and topology analysis as above, the results of measurement should select GES with the best target effect of tumor cells and TILs in the biological networks. Although many measures can be used as the importance of nodes in a network, we often select high values of Betweenness Centrality (BC), and Connectivity Degree (CD) with their mutants are to use for their immune-targets [40].

NEOANTIGEN ANALYSIS AND DETERMINATION

Once target proteins are discovered, as shown above, predicted proteins should be validated for personalized or immune targets [41]. According to published evidence, here I concluded most of approving ways as below as Fig. (4) and Table 2.

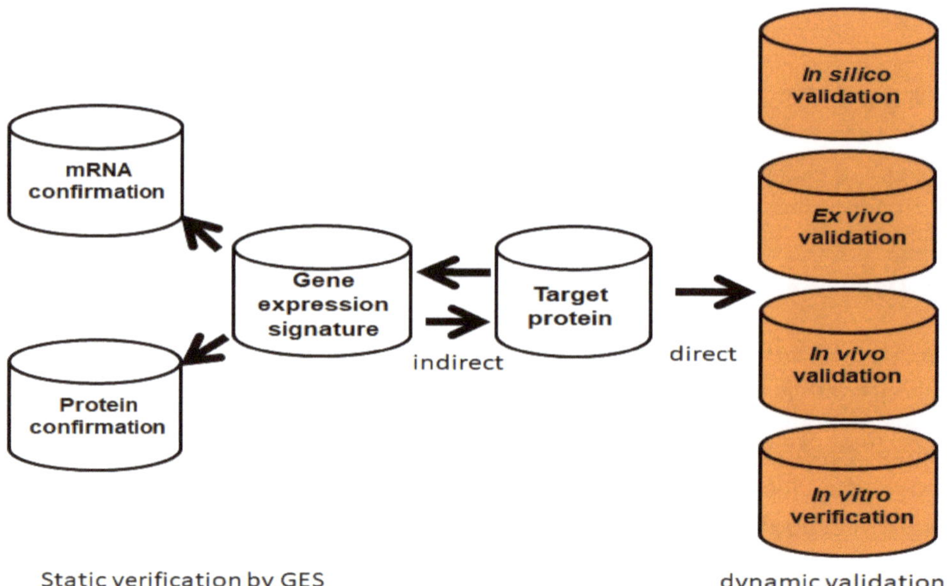

Fig. (4). The diagram of neoantigen analysis and determination. **A.** indirect methods regarding GES confirmation by Qrt-PCR and protein levels; **B.** direct methods regarding in silico validation, *ex vivo* validation, *in vivo* validation, and *in Vitro* verification. The pink color is mainly used in laboratories.

Indirect confirmation: It is essential to identify gene-expression signatures on targeting such as polymerase chain reaction (PCR), immunohistochemistry, and proteomics [42]. Based on the results of sensitivity and specificity, as discussed above, we have routinely used quantitative RT-PCR measurement as essential verification steps after GES and target discovery.

Direct validation: Direct validation-assay has been successfully reported to predict outcomes of target efficacy, including *in silico* module, *ex vivo* module, *in vivo* module and *in vitro* module.

Table 2 . Verification of therapeutic targets.

Methods	Technology	Advantages	Disadvantages
Indirect-confirmation	Qrt-PCR or ICC/IHC staining	Simple and cheap	Indirect data
***In silico* validation**	Bioinformatics modules	Bioinformatics supports	Mimic data
***Ex vivo* validation**	Primary tumor cell or CSC culture	Objective response for different targets	Difficult techniques
***In vivo* validation**	Xenografts of human cancer cells	Objective response for different targets	Very cost and limiting time
***In vitro* confirmation**	Tumor cell lines cultures	Simple and easy for different drugs	Non- individual responses

a. *in silico* **module**: Network related to target discovery has been largely reported. Dr. Zheng first set up a python-based network to study tumor cell-line proliferation using scoring analysis, and then they used the model to score agents in the network [43]. In 2015, we further reported the model for a patient genomic analysis who suffered from triple-negative breast cancer (TNBC). Excitingly, after prediction and validation-mimic-assay by the python model, two groups' drugs were uncovered and confirmed for the patient, the patient achieved complete response [44]. Some laboratories performed similar mimic-mining and confirmation. For example, in 2013, *in silico* screening combined with CSCs from glioblastoma are used for predictive models of drug response. They reported that 185 compounds by *in silico* screening, and seven were confirmed in glioma cell lines, and 21 compounds were done in three glioblastoma stem cells [45]. The verification steps also can be used for the target discovery of tumor cell immunotherapy.

b. *ex vivo* **module**: As discussed above, the culture of primary tumor-cell is an assay drug sensitivity by Drs. Hamburger and Salmon and is long-term developed in our laboratories for more than 20 years. Now several culture protocols of a primary tumor cell with their techniques are going to apply for a validation system of personalized therapy [46]. Thus, the *ex vivo* module also can be used for target discovery of tumor cell immunotherapy.

c. ***in vivo* module**: xenografts of human cancer cells also are a very good model to verify the drugs. Some scientists developed xenografts of human cancer cells *in vivo* to validate drugs. For example, scientists selectively isolated the migratory cell subpopulation of the primary tumor for gene expression profiling. In that way, they discovered a gene signature specific to breast cancer migration and invasion called Human Invasion Signature (HIS). They confirmed that genes involved in these functions are upregulated in the migratory tumor cells with independent biological repeats. They also demonstrate that specific genes are functionally required for *in vivo* invasion from patient-derived breast tumors. Finally, they used statistical analysis to show that the signature can significantly predict the risk of breast cancer metastasis [47]. Accordingly, *in vivo* xenografts module also can be used for target discovery of tumor cell immunotherapy

d. ***in vitro* module**: Some scientists developed tumor cell-lines as a model to verify neoantigen as reports [48].

BIOIFNROAMTICS INTEGRATION FOR T-CELL TARGETS

A group of scientists has successfully set up a bioinformatics module to identify neoantigen-specific T-cells from epithelial ovarian cancer (EOC) as Fig. (5) [49]. They perform whole-exome sequence (WES) and transcriptome sequencing to 20 EOC patients. After both data were analyzed, they first used immunogenicity prediction (NetMHC) combined with transcriptome from RNA-seq to set up candidates of profiles and then prioritize the tumor neoantigens. They also evaluated the capacity of autologous ovarian tumor recognition. For example, a genetic transfer of T-cell receptor (TCR) from these neoantigen-specific T-cell clones into peripheral blood T-cells was conducted to generate neoepitope-specific T-cells. Their results demonstrated a small subset of prioritized neoantigen candidates were able to detect spontaneous CD4+ and/ or CD8+ T-cell responses against neoepitopes from autologous lymphocytes with a significantly improved validation rate of 19%. They discovered that T-cells specific against two mutated cancer-associated genes, NUP214 and JAK1 to recognize autologous tumors. Also, gene-engineering with TCR from these neoantigen-specific T-cell clones conferred neoantigen-reactivity to peripheral T-cells. They concluded that their method is feasible to efficiently identify both CD4+ and CD8+ neoantigen-specific T-cells in EOC. Although they have not used their strategies for clinical application, they think that the autologous lymphocytes genetically engineered with tumor antigen-specific TCR can be used to generate cells for personalized adoptive T-cell transfer immunotherapy.

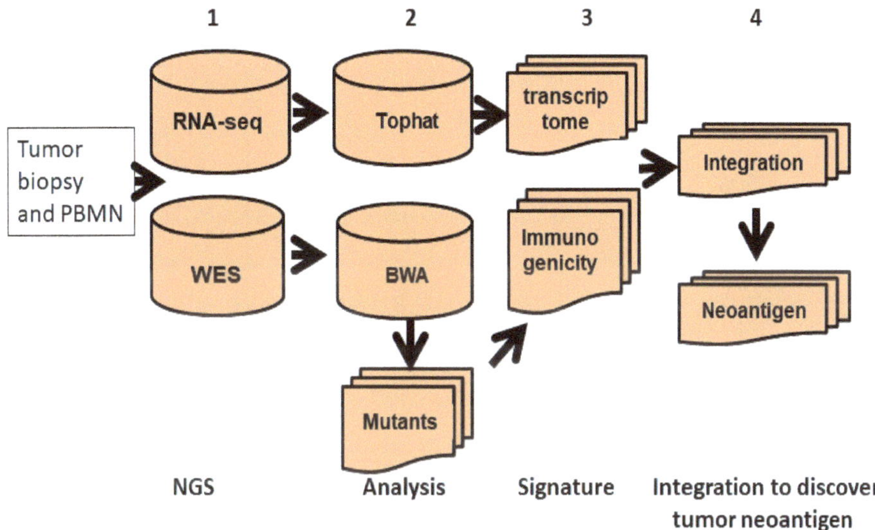

Fig. (5). The diagram of SNP based neoantigen analysis and determination. **(1)**. NGS including GES and RNA-seq; **(2)**. analysis with their methods; **(3)**. discovery signature by NetMHC combined transcriptome; **(4)**. an integration and prioritization to uncover neoantigens with immunogenicity.

SUCCESSFUL SYSTEM BIOLOGY INTEGRATION FOR FUNCTIONAL POLYCLONAL TIL TARGETS

As our modification of TIL isolation and culture for adoptive TIL immunotherapy, we have resolved TIL efficacy to tumor cells from solid tumors as published since 1995 [50]. After thirty years of R&D, a lot of clinical laboratories have confirmed that TILs can be used for adoptive T-cell immunotherapy of solid tumors, including H&N tumor, brain tumor, lung cancer, liver cancer, and ovarian tumors [51]. TILs have at least four advantages: (I) TIL has polyclonal T-cells to *in vivo* recognize tumor antigens of tumor cells from tumor site; (II) autologous TILs have similar MHC-Antigen so that TILs do not need reconstruct as TCR T-cells; (III) TIL immunotherapy have not cytokine release syndrome (CRS) which are much safer than TCR and CAR T-cells; (IV) TIL has more than 100-fold to kill tumor cells to compare T-cell from peripheral blood [52]. TILs have at least two disadvantages: (I) criteria of TIL isolation is different so that TILs are reported different efficacy; (II) effective TIL cultures are difficult for some research laboratories. In the early period, TILs are only reported to efficacy to treat melanoma in some early evidence. After long-term arguments, now most TIL culture laboratories have confirmed that TILs can be used for adoptive T-cell immunotherapy of solid tumors.

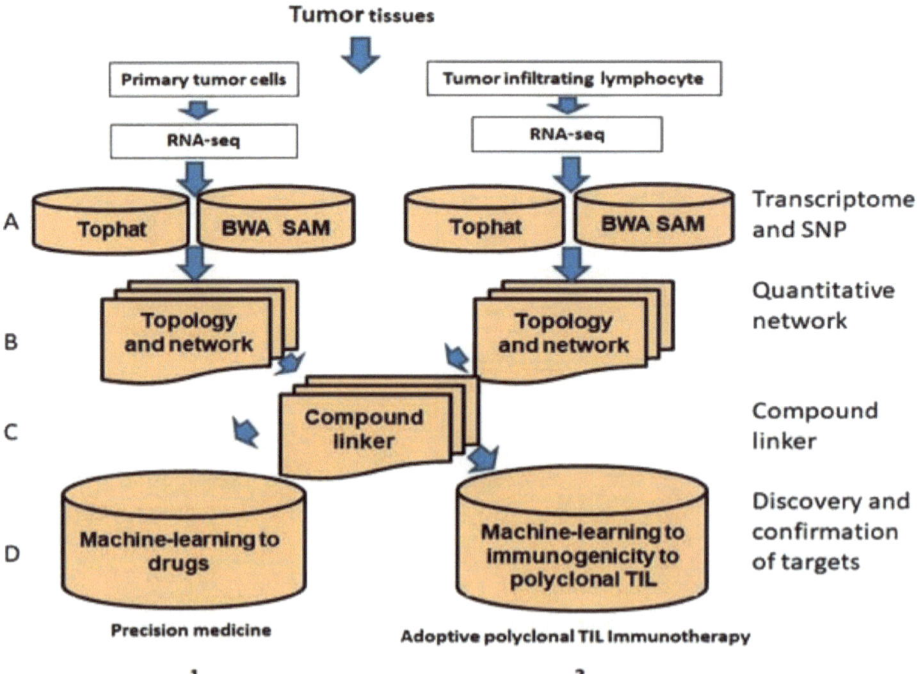

Fig. (6). The diagram of polyclonal functional TIL and precision medicine. **A.** Discovery of transcriptome and SNP; from RNA-seq; **B.** network analyses by topology; **C.** compound linker to discover targets; **D.** Machine-learning to confirm targets and drugs under primary cell culture.

Table 3. Functional polyclonal TIL and personalized TCR T-cells.

	Functional TIL	**Personalized TCR T-cells**
First efficacy	2009-2015	2019
First clinical trial	2015	Not yet
Target	MHC-peptide complex	MHC-peptide complex
Supportive IL-2	Yes	Varying
Specificity	Polyclonal	Monoclonal
Main toxicity	Lymphodepleting regimen	Lymphodepleting regimen
	IL-2 mediated (chills, fever, edema)	"On-target, off-tumor."
	Seldom autoimmune	CRS
Restrictions	Heterogeneous infusion product	MHC-restricted

After we addressed TIL to effectively treat tumor cells from solid tumors in our publication, in order to increase TIL efficacy, we begin to study functional TIL immunotherapy since 1998 [53], including (I) TIL CD8+cells are an actively maintained quiescent status in TME by single-cell genomics technique; (II) TIL quiescent pathways with their study of topology; (III) TIL quantitative networks with their drug-bank linker to activate related factors to kill tumor cells and to inhibit related factors to block TME inhibiting factors. After more than twenty's year efforts, the personalized TIL functional poly-cloning culture with their clinical application includes (I) genomic analysis for both TIL and tumor cells; (II) functional inhibiting tumor cells after genomic results from tumor cells and (III) functional inducing TIL CTL and (IV) functional inhibiting TME when TIL culture.

After study, as shown above, we have successfully set up a bioinformatics module to identify functional polyclonal TIL as Fig. (**6**) [54] including (A) RNA-seq or mRNA microarray with their mining a transcriptome profile from both tumor cells and TILs; (B) set up network under topology; (C) compound linker to uncover targets; (D) Machine-learning to confirm targets and drugs under primary cell culture.

After more than twenty years of study, now we have successfully used the functional TIL to treat a case with primary hepatocellular cancer [55]. The polyclonal functional TIL at least has four advantages to contrast genetically-modified adoptive immunotherapy as Table **3**: (a) induced T-cells are based on system biology rather than any genetic modification so that personalized immunotherapy can keep T-cells good proliferation during culture; (b) CD8+cell culture based on personalized genomic profiles with their network also can release some special substances (such as TNF-α and IFN-γ) or inhibiting some genes expression (such as inhibiting TGF-β) after the functional T-cell *in vivo* infusion; (c) functional inducing or inhibiting T-cells could be much safer than genetically-modified T-cell immunotherapy; (d) once new antibodies, antigens, cytokines, growth factors and receptors are discovered such as antibody to anti-PD-1 and anti-cytotoxic T-lymphocyte antigen-4 (CTLA-4), individual T-cell genomic profiles related to network to link the new compounds can be quickly applied to personalized immunotherapy for different patients.

CONCLUSION

Genomic profiles analyzed by bioinformatics to mine genomic expression level and SNP are an essential fundamental to global screen T-cell targets for tumor neoantigen or mutant peptides/proteins. Following the development of next-generation sequencing, epitope discovery of tumor neoantigen and mutant proteins will be increasingly applied for a novel generation of T-cell adoptive immunotherapy. New bioinformatics platform with system biology can integrate data of SNP and genomic expression signature, and therefore, system modeling is an important fundamental for T-cell adoptive immunotherapy. For example, personalized TCR T-cells and functional TIL is required to search and define tumor-specific T-cells such as TIL, TCR T-cells under the support of bioinformatics and system biology for adoptive T-cell immunotherapy.

The advent of a new generation of personalized immunotherapy allows for the treatment of individual patients based on their own genomic data. Although a comprehensive bioinformatic analysis has successfully applied for personalized immunotherapy, several questions still need to be addressed so that here we list several challenges which I want to further be resolving:

1. Tumor sampling for genomic analysis: (A) tumor sampling *in vitro* with genomic expression analyses needs more specific biomarkers on the cell surface, cytoplasmic proteins, mRNA or DNA. (B) Tumor sampling *ex vivo* with genomic expression analyses requires developing a criterial culture technique and culture system for a primary tumor cell. We have largely reported culture techniques from a primary tumor cell and TIL. Because different samples have different culture conditions such as primary-cells harvested from before-chemotherapy and after-chemotherapy, "one size fits all" culture system cannot adapt targets for a personalized application so that it needs a more experienced expert to perform the clinical sampling.

2. Tumor and TIL genomic profiles require a quantity of data so that we always use specificity and sensitivity tests while other groups utilized prioritization to conclude a genomic profile. According to current data, criteria should be set up for quantitation or prioritization for each sample.

3. System modeling for genomics (GES and SNP signature): In order to set up rational network for personalized immunotherapy, in future, transcriptome-based system biology should also include genomic archives such as epigenetics or microRNA. A quantitative scoring network should cover all genomic profiles, including transcriptome, GWAS, epigenetics, and microRNA.

4. Bioinformatics of personalized targets demands to develop other options with their techniques. For example, after neoantigens or mutant peptides are discovered by bioinformatics, DC pulsed-peptides can be replaced by easy ways such as transaction by RNA level or DNA level into DC, which can be extensively used for most of the laboratories.

CONSENT FOR PUBLICATION

The authors declare no financial interests.

CONFLICT OF INTEREST

The authors declare no financial interests.

ACKNOWLEDGEMENTS

During the period of Case Western Reserve University 2000-2007, BL and GL set up single-cell genomics analysis for TIL. BL and JC further study bioinformatics modules for functional TIL immunotherapy after 2007. The research was previously supported by National Cancer Institute IRG-91-022-09, USA (to BL).

Mention of trade names or commercial products in this article is solely to provide specific information and does not imply recommendation.

REFERENCES

[1]   Rodríguez-Antona C, Taron M. Pharmacogenomic biomarkers for personalized cancer treatment. J Intern Med 2015; 277(2): 201-17.
[http://dx.doi.org/10.1111/joim.12321] [PMID: 25338550]

[2]   Schilsky RL. Personalized medicine in oncology: the future is now. Nat Rev Drug Discov 2010; 9(5): 363-6.
[http://dx.doi.org/10.1038/nrd3181] [PMID: 20431568]

[3]   Yap TA, Bjerke L, Clarke PA, Workman P. Drugging PI3K in cancer: refining targets and therapeutic strategies. Curr Opin Pharmacol 2015; 23: 98-107.
[http://dx.doi.org/10.1016/j.coph.2015.05.016] [PMID: 26117819]

[4]   Hudson TJ. Genome variation and personalized cancer medicine. J Intern Med 2013; 274(5): 440-50.
[http://dx.doi.org/10.1111/joim.12097] [PMID: 23751076]

[5]   Yoshida T, Ono H, Kuchiba A, Saeki N, Sakamoto H. Genome-wide germline analyses on cancer susceptibility and GeMDBJ database: Gastric cancer as an example. Cancer Sci 2010; 101(7): 1582-9.
[http://dx.doi.org/10.1111/j.1349-7006.2010.01590.x] [PMID: 20507324]

[6]   Pazin MJ. Using the ENCODE Resource for Functional Annotation of Genetic Variants. Cold Spring Harb Protoc 2015; 2015(6): 522-36.
[http://dx.doi.org/10.1101/pdb.top084988] [PMID: 25762420]

[7]   Li BA. strategy to identify genomic expression at single-cell level or a small number of cells. J Biotechnol 2005; 8(1): 71-81.
[PMID: 16290242]

[8]   Li B. Clinical Genomic Analysis and Diagnosis --Genomic Analysis *Ex Vivo*, *in Vitro* and in Silico. Clinical Medicine and Diagnostics 2012; 2(4): 37-44.
[http://dx.doi.org/10.5923/j.cmd.20120204.04]

[9]   Ormerod GM. Flow Cytometry: A Practical Approach. Ox-ford University Press 2000.

[10]   Zhang Q, Zhang P, Gou H, *et al.* Towards high-throughput microfluidic Raman-activated cell sorting. Analyst (Lond) 2015; 140(18): 6163-74.
[http://dx.doi.org/10.1039/C5AN01074H] [PMID: 26225617]

[11]   Zhang DG, Jiang AG, Lu HY, Zhang LX, Gao XY. Isolation, cultivation and identification of human lung adenocarcinoma stem cells. Oncol Lett 2015; 9(1): 47-54.
[http://dx.doi.org/10.3892/ol.2014.2639] [PMID: 25435932]

[12]   Emmert-Buck MR, Bonner RF, Smith PD, *et al.* Laser capture microdissection. Science 1996; 274(5289): 998-1001.
[http://dx.doi.org/10.1126/science.274.5289.998] [PMID: 8875945]

[13]   Skvortsov S, Debbage P, Skvortsova I. Proteomics of cancer stem cells. Int J Radiat Biol 2014; 90(8): 653-8.
[http://dx.doi.org/10.3109/09553002.2013.873559] [PMID: 24350919]

[14]   Magbanua MJ, Park JW. Isolation of circulating tumor cells by immunomagnetic enrichment and fluorescence-activated cell sorting (IE/FACS) for molecular profiling. Methods 2013; 64(2): 114-8.
[http://dx.doi.org/10.1016/j.ymeth.2013.07.029] [PMID: 23896286]

[15]   Niyaz Y, Stich M, Sägmüller B, *et al.* Noncontact laser microdissection and pressure catapulting: sample preparation for genomic, transcriptomic, and proteomic analysis. Methods Mol Med 2005; 114: 1-24.
[PMID: 16156095]

[16]   Steen J, Morrison JA, Kulesa PM. Multi-position photoactivation and multi-time acquisition for large-scale cell tracing in avian embryos. Cold Spring Harb Protoc 2010; 2010(6)prot5447
[http://dx.doi.org/10.1101/pdb.prot5447] [PMID: 20516185]

[17]   Vandewoestyne M, Van Hoofstat D, Van Nieuwerburgh F, Deforce D. Automatic detection of spermatozoa for laser capture microdissection. Int J Legal Med 2009; 123(2): 169-75.
[http://dx.doi.org/10.1007/s00414-008-0271-1] [PMID: 18661142]

[18]   Hamburger AW, Salmon SE. Primary bioassay of human tumor stem cells. Science 1977; 197(4302): 461-3.
[http://dx.doi.org/10.1126/science.560061] [PMID: 560061]

[19]   Li BR, Tong SQ, Zhang XH, Lu J, Gu QL, Lu DY. A new experimental and clinical approach of combining usage of highly active tumor-infiltrating lymphocytes and highly sensitive antitumor drugs for the advanced malignant tumor. Chin Med J (Engl) 1994; 107(11): 803-7.
[PMID: 7867384]

[20]   Lähdesmäki H, Shmulevich L, Dunmire V, Yli-Harja O, Zhang W. In silico microdissection of microarray data from heterogeneous cell populations. BMC Bioinformatics 2005; 6: 54-8.
[http://dx.doi.org/10.1186/1471-2105-6-54] [PMID: 15766384]

[21]   McBean RS, Hyland CA, Flower RL. Approaches to determination of a full profile of blood group genotypes: single nucleotide variant mapping and massively parallel sequencing. Comput Struct Biotechnol J 2014; 11(19): 147-51.
[http://dx.doi.org/10.1016/j.csbj.2014.09.009] [PMID: 25408849]

[22]   Cui H, Dhroso A, Johnson N, Korkin D. The variation game: Cracking complex genetic disorders with NGS and omics data. Methods 2015; 79-80: 18-31.
[http://dx.doi.org/10.1016/j.ymeth.2015.04.018] [PMID: 25944472]

[23]   Hollegaard MV, Grauholm J, Nielsen R, Grove J, Mandrup S, Hougaard DM. Archived neonatal dried blood spot samples can be used for accurate whole genome and exome-targeted next-generation sequencing. Mol Genet Metab 2013; 110(1-2): 65-72.
[http://dx.doi.org/10.1016/j.ymgme.2013.06.004] [PMID: 23830478]

[24]   Koparir A, Karatas OF, Atayoglu AT, *et al.* Whole-exome sequencing revealed two novel mutations in Usher syndrome. Gene 2015; 563(2): 215-8.
[http://dx.doi.org/10.1016/j.gene.2015.03.060] [PMID: 25834954]

[25]   Li W, Calder RB, Mar JC, Vijg J. Single-cell transcriptogenomics reveals transcriptional exclusion of ENU-mutated alleles. Mutat Res 2015; 772: 55-62.

[http://dx.doi.org/10.1016/j.mrfmmm.2015.01.002] [PMID: 25733965]

[26]   Pras E, Kristal D, Shoshany N, *et al.* Rare genetic variants in Tunisian Jewish patients suffering from age-related macular degeneration. J Med Genet 2015; 52(7): 484-92.
[http://dx.doi.org/10.1136/jmedgenet-2015-103130] [PMID: 25986072]

[27]   Kwok PY, Chen X. Detection of single nucleotide polymorphisms. Curr Issues Mol Biol 2003; 5(2): 43-60.
[PMID: 12793528]

[28]   Bjørheim J, Ekstrøm PO. Review of denaturant capillary electrophoresis in DNA variation analysis. Electrophoresis 2005; 26(13): 2520-30.
[http://dx.doi.org/10.1002/elps.200410403] [PMID: 15934053]

[29]   Winchester L, Yau C, Ragoussis J. Comparing CNV detection methods for SNP arrays. Brief Funct Genomics Proteomics 2009; 8(5): 353-66.
[http://dx.doi.org/10.1093/bfgp/elp017] [PMID: 19737800]

[30]   Witherden EA, Kunde D, Tristram SG. An evaluation of SNP-based PCR methods for the detection of β-lactamase-negative ampicillin-resistant Haemophilus influenzae. J Infect Chemother 2012; 18(4): 451-5.
[http://dx.doi.org/10.1007/s10156-011-0356-5] [PMID: 22203122]

[31]   Li B. Personalized Therapy of Tumor Disease Based on System Modeling. Personalized Chemotherapy of Tumor Disease 2017; 2: 21-35.

[32]   Proulx SR, Promislow DEL, Phillips PC. Network thinking in ecology and evolution. Trends Ecol Evol (Amst) 2005; 20(6): 345-53.
[http://dx.doi.org/10.1016/j.tree.2005.04.004] [PMID: 16701391]

[33]   Ballerstein K, Haus UU, Lindquist JA, Beyer T, Schraven B, Weismantel R. Discrete, qualitative models of interaction networks. Front Biosci (Schol Ed) 2013; 5: 149-66.
[http://dx.doi.org/10.2741/S363] [PMID: 23277042]

[34]   Janjić V, Pržulj N. The topology of the growing human interactome data. J Integr Bioinform 2014; 11(2): 238.
[http://dx.doi.org/10.1515/jib-2014-238] [PMID: 24953453]

[35]   Sanders E, Diehl S. Analysis and interpretation of transcriptomic data obtained from extended Warburg effect genes in patients with clear cell renal cell carcinoma. Oncoscience 2015; 2(2): 151-86.
[http://dx.doi.org/10.18632/oncoscience.128] [PMID: 25859558]

[36]   Zhao JH. Pedigree-drawing with R and graph *viz*. Bioinformatics 2006; 22(8): 1013-4.
[http://dx.doi.org/10.1093/bioinformatics/btl058] [PMID: 16488908]

[37]   Helaers R, Bareke E, De Meulder B, *et al.* g*Viz*, a novel tool for the visualization of co-expression networks. BMC Res Notes 2011; 4: 452.
[http://dx.doi.org/10.1186/1756-0500-4-452] [PMID: 22032859]

[38]   Olesen JM, Bascompte J, Dupont YL, Jordano P. The modularity of pollination networks. Proc Natl Acad Sci USA 2007; 104(50): 19891-6.
[http://dx.doi.org/10.1073/pnas.0706375104] [PMID: 18056808]

[39]   Telesford QK, Simpson SL, Burdette JH, Hayasaka S, Laurienti PJ. The brain as a complex system: using network science as a tool for understanding the brain. Brain Connect 2011; 1(4): 295-308.
[http://dx.doi.org/10.1089/brain.2011.0055] [PMID: 22432419]

[40]   Li B, Senzer N, Rao DD, *et al.* Bioinformatics Approach to Individual Cancer Target Identification 11th Annual Meeting of the American Society of Gene Therapy.

[41]   Vari S, Pilotto S, Maugeri-Saccà M, *et al.* Advances towards the design and development of personalized non-small-cell lung cancer drug therapy. Expert Opin Drug Discov 2013; 8(11): 1381-97.
[http://dx.doi.org/10.1517/17460441.2013.843523] [PMID: 24088065]

[42]   Lossos IS, Czerwinski DK, Alizadeh AA, *et al.* Prediction of survival in diffuse large-B-cell lymphoma based on the expression of six genes. N Engl J Med 2004; 350(18): 1828-37.
[http://dx.doi.org/10.1056/NEJMoa032520] [PMID: 15115829]

[43]   Tan DS, Thomas GV, Garrett MD, *et al.* Biomarker-driven early clinical trials in oncology: a paradigm shift in drug development. Cancer J 2009; 15(5): 406-20.
[http://dx.doi.org/10.1097/PPO.0b013e3181bd0445] [PMID: 19826361]

[44]   Zheng J, Zhang D, Przytycki PF, Zielinski R, Capala J, Przytycka TM. SimBoolNet--a Cytoscape plugin for dynamic simulation of signaling networks. Bioinformatics 2010; 26(1): 141-2.
[http://dx.doi.org/10.1093/bioinformatics/btp617] [PMID: 19887508]

[45]   Hu HL, Zhang QH, Li S, *et al.* A Therapeutic Targeting Identification from Microarray Data and Quantitative Network Analysis. Open Access Journal of Science and Technology 2015; 3: 1-10.
[http://dx.doi.org/10.11131/2015/101114]

[46]   Riddick G, Song H, Holbeck SL, *et al.* An in silico screen links gene expression signatures to drug response in glioblastoma stem cells. Pharmacogenomics J 2014; 61: 10.
[PMID: 25446780]

[47]   Dairkee SH, Ji Y, Ben Y, Moore DH, Meng Z, Jeffrey SS. A molecular 'signature' of primary breast cancer cultures; patterns resembling tumor tissue. BMC Genomics 2004; 5(1): 47.
[http://dx.doi.org/10.1186/1471-2164-5-47] [PMID: 15260889]

[48]   Patsialou A, Wang Y, Lin J, *et al.* Selective gene-expression profiling of migratory tumor cells *in vivo* predicts clinical outcome in breast cancer patients. Breast Cancer Res 2012; 14(5): R139.
[http://dx.doi.org/10.1186/bcr3344] [PMID: 23113900]

[49]   Liu S, Matsuzaki J, Wei L, *et al.* Efficient identification of neoantigen-specific T-cell responses in advanced human ovarian cancer. J Immunother Cancer 2019; 7(1): 156.
[http://dx.doi.org/10.1186/s40425-019-0629-6] [PMID: 31221207]

[50]   Li B, Shen DH. Preliminary Study on the Resting Status of Tumor-infiltrating Lymphocytes. Chinese Microbiology and Immunology (Chinese) 1994; 14(6): 399-402.

[51]   Ben-Avi R, Farhi R, Ben-Nun A, *et al.* Establishment of adoptive cell therapy with tumor infiltrating lymphocytes for non-small cell lung cancer patients. Cancer Immunol Immunother 2018; 67(8): 1221-30.
[http://dx.doi.org/10.1007/s00262-018-2174-4] [PMID: 29845338]

[52]   Topalian SL, Muul LM, Solomon D, Rosenberg SA. Expansion of human tumor infiltrating lymphocytes for use in immunotherapy trials. J Immunol Methods 1987; 102(1): 127-41.
[http://dx.doi.org/10.1016/S0022-1759(87)80018-2] [PMID: 3305708]

[53]   Li B, Liu G, Hu HL, Ding JQ, Zheng J, Tong A. Biomarkers Analysis for Heterogeneous Immune Responses of Quiescent CD8+cells -A Clue for Personalized Immunotherapy. Biom J 2015; 1(3): 1-10.

[54]   Li B, Hu HL, Ding JQ, Yan D, Yang LM. Functional cell proliferation and differentiation by system modeling for cell therapy. International Journal of Latest Research in Science and Technology 2015; 4(2): 180-7.

[55]   Li B. Breakthroughs of 2015-Personalized Immunotherapy Based on Individual GWAS and Biomarkers. Biom J 2015; 1(8): 1-2.

CHAPTER 9

Development of Adoptive T-cell Immunotherapy-Future of Personalized Immunotherapy

Biaoru Li[1,2,*], Shanqing Tong[2], Xihan Zhang[2], Youming Zhu[2], Baoyu Wu[2] and **Deyuan Lu[2]**

[1] *Georgia Cancer Center and Department of Pediatrics, Medical College at GA, Augusta, GA 30912, USA*

[2] *Department of Microbiology, Shanghai Second Medical University, Shanghai, 200025, PRC*

Abstract: Lymphocytes play vital roles in surveillance of the formation and development of tumors as well as control of tumor disease. Employing the immune cells to recognize and destroy tumor cells is a central task of anticancer immunotherapy. Since 1987 cultured tumor-infiltrating lymphocytes (TIL) from the site of tumor tissue have been discovered more than 100-fold to kill tumor cells to compare cultured T-cell from peripheral blood, we have been studying TIL anti-tumor mechanism and clinical feasibility of immune-cell immunotherapy, especially functionally inducing TILs for immunotherapy purpose for more than two decades. At present, to make it a clinically feasible treatment, there have been increased reports in optimizing those procedures. Several standard protocols of laboratory performance and clinical treatments have been quickly developed in cancer immunotherapy. With using this standard protocol, cytotoxic T-cells are infused into cancer patients with cytokine help in recognizing, targeting, and destroying tumor cells. In the chapter, we review some of the significant successes of adoptive T-cell immunotherapy (AIT or ACT) and the significant obstacles that have been overcome to optimize ACT. Here, we also more focus on the study of research and development of T-cell inducing, culture and proliferation for adoptive immunotherapy, and eventually introduce clinical knowledge of lymphocytes application including feasible and affordable to treat patients.

Keywords: Adoptive immunotherapy (AIT), Adoptive cell therapy (ACT), CIK (cytokine-induced killer cells), LAK (lymphokine-activated killer), NK cells, Personalized immunotherapy, TIL (tumor-infiltrating lymphocyte).

INTRODUCTION

Adoptive T-cell immunotherapy of tumor diseases had birthed about thirty years when Steven Rosenberg had applied for tumor - infiltrating lymphocyte (TIL) to

* **Corresponding author Biaoru Li**: Georgia Cancer Center and Department of Pediatrics, Medical College at GA, Augusta, GA 30912, USA; Tel: 440-317-1443; E-mail: bli@augusta.edu

treat melanoma of patients in 1988 [1], and then we have used TIL to treat several hundreds of patients with solid tumors since 1990 [2]. T-cell immunotherapy has been developed so quickly that a few new procedures have come out since then.

Now, TIL and cytokine-inducing lymphocytes from peripheral blood mononuclear cells (PBMN), including lymphokine-activated killer (LAK) [3], cytokine-induced killer cells (CIK) [4], dendritic cells and cytokine-induced killer cells (DC-CIK) [5] have participated into adoptive T-cell immunotherapy. TIL, one of the best adoptive T-cell immunotherapies (AIT or adoptive cell therapy, ACT), has great profits that make it amenable for cancer treatment. For example, (I) the T-cell responses are specific, and thus specifically kill tumor cells; (II) the T-cells responses are powerful, undergoing to 1,000 fold clonal expansion after activation; (III) the T-cells can travel into the site of a tumor, suggesting a mechanism for the eradication of distant metastases; (IV) the T-cell responses have memory, maintaining therapeutic effect for many years after initial treatment [6, 7].

However, there are two obstacles to effective adoptive T-cell immunotherapy of tumor disease. (I) Despite these theoretical benefits, T-cell immunotherapy, actuarily, could not proceed until it was established that immune responses could specifically distinguish tumor cells from normal cells [8]. Unlike microbial pathogens, immune recognition of specific tumor-antigen on the surface of tumor cells is not very unclear since the cancer immunosurveillance hypothesis was previously raised [9]. Fortunately, human tumor-associated antigens (TAAs) was identified for a new interest in tumor immunology driven by tumor transplant into the mouse and provided definitive proof that specific anti-tumor responses could be generated under optimal conditions [10]. (II) The second obstacle to be addressed was to assay cytotoxicity of tumor-specific lymphocytes for different tumor diseases. According to several laboratories' reports, TIL cells with anti-tumor cytotoxic activity can be identified in tumor samples of more than 80% of patients with melanoma [11], but other tumor diseases are less frequent. However, it is now clear that TIL infiltration is "hallmarks" of cancer, allowing those killing tumor cells. Although the immune surveillance theory remains controversial and TILs actively mediating rejection of human tumor cells is kept debate, adoptive T-cell immunotherapy has conclusively shown that ACT can kill tumor cells under optimal culture in laboratories and right therapeutic conditions in clinics [12].

In order to draw a clear outline of adoptive T-cell immunotherapy, in the chapter, we will first present the history and development of different adoptive T-cells for immunotherapies and then introduce feasibility and affordability of different immune cells after a clinical trial of immunotherapy. Finally, we briefly present the future of adoptive T-cell immunotherapy.

HISTORY AND DEVELOPMENT OF IMMUNE THERAPY

To let us clearly review history and development of immunotherapy during the thirty years, which we are experiencing, we will divide the development into four sections: (I) development of TIL culture procedures for clinical application; (II) development of TILs clinical application; (III) development of TILs location administration; (IV) other immune cells' culture and clinical application.

1. Development of TIL Culture Procedures for Clinical Application

After 1987 Dr. Rosenberg discovered that TILs could be cultured with the aid of the cytokine IL-2 and induced TIL exhibited cytotoxic activity against melanoma cells *in vitro*, TILs isolated from tumor samples are earliest trials of ACT conducted at the surgical branch of the National Cancer Institute (NCI) in 1988 [13]. That early time, objective responses were observed in 11 of 20 patients with metastatic melanoma. Only 5 of the 29 (17%) were complete responses (CR) with the median duration of response as four months in these early studies [14].

For the purpose of optimal procedure of TIL isolation and proliferation, we have carefully studied those NCI had reported, and thus we modified the protocol and further set up to a new TIL culture and proliferation procedure. As our early report, our procedures modified are different from the NCI conventional approaches: (1) cold digestion of collagenase IV for overnight or 24 hours after tumor tissue were digested by different enzymes in early 1995 [15] as Table **1**; (2) we added a procedure for cleaning inhibiting cells during isolating TILs, such as filter and adhesive process after discovered TILs silent status from tumor tissue [16], now those inhibiting cells called as tumor microenvironment (TME) [17]; (3) we simplified several processes such as washes and centrifugation as out early publications after we found that TIL would be damaged by isolation performance [18].

Table 1. TIL proliferation rate under enzyme digestion.

Condition	Regular	Collagenase II	Collagenase IV	Hyaluronidase	Trypsin
Expansion Mean (37C°, 1h)	689	1375	1517	810	239
Expansion range (37C°, 1h)	(12-4210)	(15-12500)	(25-15000)	(7-2700)	(8-1250)
Expansion Mean (4C°, 24h)	896	1571	2707	792	139
Expansion range (4C°, 24h)	(7-10500)	(30-12500)	(210-21000)	(10-2500)	(10-1200)

Compared with those from NCI reports, the proliferation, activity, and cytotoxicity of TILs were much improved after modified. The TILs growth curve is long, and cytotoxicity against tumor cells is more potent than those obtained from traditional methods. For example, after setting up the new approach of isolation and culture for TILs, 83 cases of solid tumors were studied as our early publications. The proliferation observation showed that 65% of TILs had a proliferation of more than 1,000 folds Table **2**. ^{3}H-*TdR incorporation* peaked at 45-75 days Table **3**. Cytotoxicity against tumor cells could maintain 56 days. The phenotypes of TILs after inducing by IL-2 were CD3 80+21%, CD4 37+21%, CD8 44+18% and HLA DR 69+24%. CD3 and CD8 were higher than those before induction [19] (Table **4**).

Table 2. TIL expansion rate under cold enzyme digestion.

Total-Fold Expansion	Number of Cases	Percent (%)
500	6	24
1000	2	8
2000	6	24
3000	4	16
> 3000	7	28

Table 3 . TIL toxicity rate under cold enzyme digestion.

			A Common Approach (%)	Modified Approach (%)		
Effector:target	20	40	56 (days)	20	40	56(days)
5:01	37	41	12	28	41	38
10:01	32	31	17	31	27	34
25:01:00	41	38	12	57	50	47
50:01:00	56	54	16	48	52	60
100:01:00	62	64	10	71	68	79

Table 4. TIL phenotype change under cold enzyme digestion.

TIL Phenotype	Before Induction	After Induction
CD3 cells	23+8%	80+20%
CD4 cells	12+6%	37+21%
CD8 cells	13+8%	44+18%
HLA DR cells	31+20%	69+4.2%
Giemsa staining lymphocytes	83+6%	89+4.2%

Since then, we have used the TILs to treat several hundreds of patients with solid tumors, including publishing more than fifty papers [20]. We found that TILs can be used to solid-tumor disease by cytotoxicity assays in a laboratory and by optimal administration in clinics, while Rosenberg's approach to isolate TILs was only used in the clinical treatment of melanoma [21]. Although TILs used for solid tumor have been kept debating more than 30 years [22], now, after thirty years' development, fortunately, a few of laboratories have as similar data as our reports, so that TILs have been reported to be used for different solid tumors, such as pancreatic cancer, head and neck cancer, lung cancer, brain cancer and liver cancer under the optimal culture procedures and right therapeutic conditions [23 - 28].

Furthermore, cytokines are essential to the *in vitro* stimulation and expansion of TIL immunotherapy. Successful T-cell immunotherapy depends on optimal cytokines induction so that now several new methods regarding cytokines are being developed during the thirty years. For example, now inducing factors include adding IL2 and IL12, IL2 and Anti-CD3 and IL2 and Anti-CD3/CD28 during culture [29, 30].

Furthermost, TIL properties are effective indicators for immunotherapy, including differentiation state with phenotypes, ability to persist *in vivo*, and capacity to exert effector functions against cancer cells in the host. After more than thirty years' development, now we understand that a good response of T-cell immunotherapy depends on CD+8 cell population, which we have reported in our early publications [31], and population of memory T-cells, for which some clinical scientists have largely confirmed CD8+cell memory subsets such as CD45RA, CD45RO, and CD62L for effective treatment [32].

2. Development of TILs Clinical Application

Because only 17% CR was achieved for TIL administration in early studies from NCI, a significant breakthrough occurred with the addition of lymphodepletion before ACT as Fig. (**1**) [33].

For instance, the benefits of lymphodepleting-chemotherapy or body irradiation were added lymphodepletion increased response rates in stage IV melanoma patients to 49%, 52%, and 72% with three sequential protocols of increasing intensity total body irradiation [34]. Also, a group achieved in 20 of 93 patients treated, and 19 of these 20 responses have persisted for at least five years in a human. Besides clinical trial in melanoma from NCI, medical doctors utilized a lymphodepleting chemotherapy regimen (without body irradiation), leading to a response rate of 48% (4 complete response, 11 partial). These results represented a breakthrough in melanoma treatment [35].

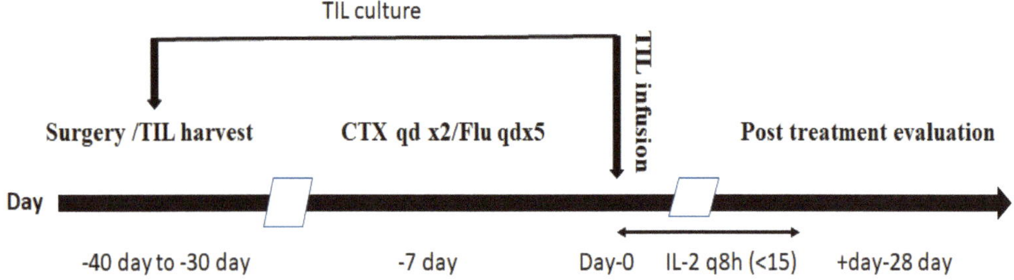

Fig. (1). TIL application with lymphodepletion.

In addition, after TIL isolation and expansion have been modified as our procedures published in 1995, we also set up combined procedures which integrated TIL with sensitive chemotherapy drugs, called as higher sensitive TIL and high sensitive drugs by CSA (chemotherapy sensitivity assay) of patient's tumor cell [2, 36] so that we had used both TIL immunotherapy and sensitive chemotherapy drugs tested by CSA to treat patients with solid tumors since the 1990s [2, 37] as Fig. (2).

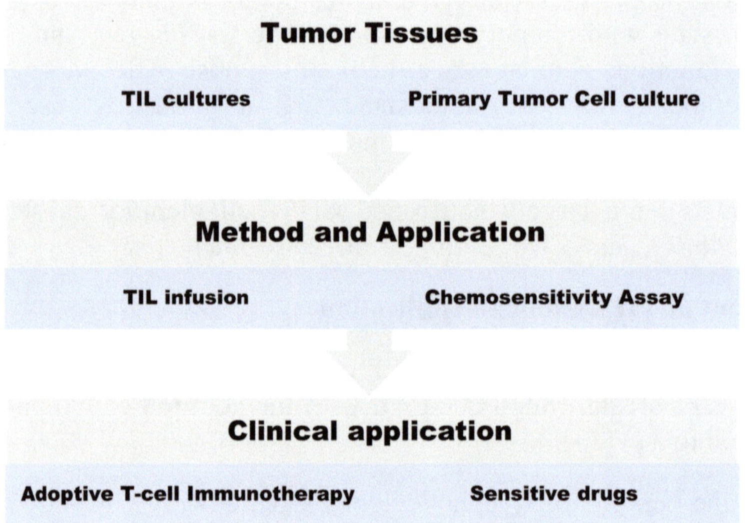

Fig. (2). TIL combined chemotherapy drugs. The culture of **(1)** TIL for T-cell immunotherapy and **(2)** the culture of primary tumor cells for CSA to determine chemotherapy for patients.

As Table **5**, we have reported total TIL proliferation ability from different solid tumors since 1995 [2, 38]. We also compared different ways to induce patients' remission with various solid tumors as our 22 publications from clinical reports in which some results are demonstrated from a group of clinical medical doctors as

Table **6** [2, 39]. Our results have confirmed that an excellent adoptive T-cell immunotherapy requires both preconditions: (1) optimal TIL culture, which can kill primary tumors cells in laboratories, and (2) right therapeutic conditions in clinics. According to our data, after we combined TIL and CSA drugs to solid tumors, the results demonstrated that those are much better than only TIL, IL2 and chemotherapy (efficiency rate included complete responses, partial responses, and stable disease, 5/5 under IL2, TIL and sensitive chemotherapy from a clinical trial) [2, 40]. However, our results cannot conclude that TIL combined with sensitive chemotherapy drugs as TILs support immune response to tumor cells and CSA drugs to kill tumor cells.

Table 5. TIL culture and proliferation.

Tumors	Cases	Useless Cases	TIL Expansion Fold				
			<500	<1000	<2000	<3000	>3000
Lung cancer	28	1	3	10	2	7	5
Liver cancer	13	1	2	1	7	1	1
Intestinal Ca	7	1	0	0	0	4	2
Bile duct Ca	2	0	0	0	1	0	1
Stomach Ca	6	1	1	0	0	2	2
Ovarian Ca	7	1	0	0	2	2	2
Melanoma	4	0	2	0	1	1	0
Brain Ca	7	1	3	2	1	0	0
Breast Ca	6	0	1	0	3	1	1
Sarcoma	1	0	1	0	0	0	0
Other	2	2	0	0	0	0	0
	83	8	13	13	17	18	14

Now, since discovering immune targeting therapy such as CTLA-4 Ab or PD-1 Ab to employ for clinical patients with advanced tumor diseases, TIL has also been discovered to be combined with the blockers of CTLA4 or PD1 to achieve promising results for some advanced tumor diseases [41]. For instance, some scientists reported that combining ACT with CTLA-4 blockade would allow more patients' response to TIL infusion. In a clinical grouping 13 advanced melanomas, patients received four doses of ipilimumab (3 mg/kg) beginning two weeks before tumor resection for TIL generation, then one week after resection, and 2 and 5 weeks after preconditioning chemotherapy and TIL infusion followed by IL-2.

Table 6. TIL application and combined therapy.

Approach	No. of Cases	No. of Data	No. of Efficiency
IL-2	20	20	4
IL-2+TIL	51	51	30
IL-2+TIL+Chemo	50	5	5

Their results, including progression-free survival (PFS) and overall survival (OS), demonstrated that there were five patients' objective responses (38.5%), four of whom continued in objective response at one year and one of which became a complete response at 52 months. Median progression-free survival was 7.3 months (95% CI 6.1–29.9 months). They concluded that Ipilimumab plus ACT was feasible and well-tolerated for metastatic melanoma [42]. Now several combination approaches have been registered to treat different tumor diseases in NCI so that the combined TIL with Ab blockers of immune suppression has demonstrated the efficacy of ACT in different solid tumor diseases [43].

3. TILs Clinical Location Administration

Although adoptive cell therapy using *ex vivo* activated autologous lymphocytes and in vein infusion has been considered as one of the promising approaches, immunotherapy alone and/or immunotherapy in vein infusion is not considered only efficient for clinical use at present. In order to enhance the therapeutic response of adoptive T-cell immunotherapy, various administrations of immunotherapies have been developed. In 1996, one of our colleagues, who used our cultured TILs, systemically studied TIL effects by different injection of TILs for 68 patients with ovarian cancers and other women malignant tumor diseases. After randomly divided three treatment groups, one with local injection, the second one in vein injection, and the third one within the vein and local injection, respectively. Their results demonstrated that the anticancer efficacy of the local group (85. 7%) was higher than that of vein group (48. 6%), but one-year' survival rate of the local group (66%) was lower than that of the vein group (80%). Comparative studies on circulating lymphocytes of cancer patients demonstrated that the increase of CD3+, CD8+, CD4+ T lymphocytes of vein group were higher than those of local group, but not different from that of vein infusion and local injection. These results suggest the possibility that in vein injection of TILs could induce immune with activation of cellular immunity to enhance the one-year's survival rate while anticancer efficacy of the local group was higher than that of vein group [40, 44].

Moreover, another group designed a study of local injection of autologous tumor-infiltrating lymphocytes with ten cases of recurrent malignant gliomas (7 cases of glioblastoma multiforme, two cases of anaplastic astrocytoma, and one case of anaplastic oligoastrocytoma). After they studied the advantages and disadvantages of local cell transfer therapy using *ex vivo* expanded autologous tumor-specific T lymphocytes for recurrent cases of malignant gliomas, their results demonstrated that five cases responded to this therapy (namely, one case showed complete remission, and four cases had a partial response). There were three cases of no change and two cases of progressive disease. The overall tumor response rate was 50%. Interestingly, no complications were noticed, except for two cases of minor local hemorrhage and eight cases of temporary fever. Their results support that local administration of T-cells is an effective treatment in recurrent malignant gliomas. Furthermore, these results demonstrated a high benefit and minor side effects after the clinical researches [45].

4. Immune Cell Therapy Beyond TILs

Since 1980s TILs, have been applied for personalized immunotherapy of tumor diseases, now, natural killer cells (NK cell), lymphokine-activated killer (LAK), cytokine-induced killer cells (CIK), dendritic cells and cytokine-induced killer cells (DC-CIK), called as non-specific immunotherapy, have been participated into adoptive immunotherapy in different phases of clinical trials. In order to develop the immune cells into personalized immunotherapy, after we introduce the basic knowledge of NK, LAK/CIK/DCCIK, we will present specific immunotherapy from the non-specific allogeneic immune cells and autologous immune cells.

Development and Application of NK cells

NK cells provide cell-mediated immune responses to tumor cells, which can recognize tumor cells in the absence of antibodies and MHC, allowing for much faster immune reaction. Their signaling proteins on cell membranes consist of inhibitory receptors and activating receptors killing the tumor cells absent self MHC and Ab. NK cells, normally, contain activating receptors (NKG2D, NCR, CD16) and inhibitory receptors (KIR, LIR, CD94/NKG2). Once tumor cells lose matching MHC molecules, which can bind inhibitory receptor on the surface of NK cells, NK cells can quickly kill tumor cells by the granule-mediated immune response (perforin and granzymes), Ab-mediated immune response (CD16) and cytokine-mediated immune response (IFNγ and TNFα) from the reaction of activating receptors [46]. Several studies have successfully exploited adoptive NK cells therapy against various tumors, especially hematological malignancies; however, NK cells were delayed being applied for anti-tumor adoptive immunotherapy because anti-tumor response of NK cells also faces some of the limitations. Three major limitations result in delaying clinical application of NK cell: (I) the poor ability of NK cells to reach tumor tissues limits their application as therapies for solid tumors; (II) NKG2D decreasing on the surface of NK cell leading to a decreased therapeutic response; (III) dendritic cells (DCs) and regulatory T (Treg) cells in the tumor microenvironment (TME) causing a major barrier to the effectiveness of adoptive NK cells therapy [47]. In order to overcome above problems, many strategies have been studied by adding immune stimulants to produce synergistic effects, or by genetically modifying NK cells themselves to be stronger, by vesicle structures secreted by NK cells known as an extracellular vesicle (EV) into the tumor sites for their applications in cancer therapies.

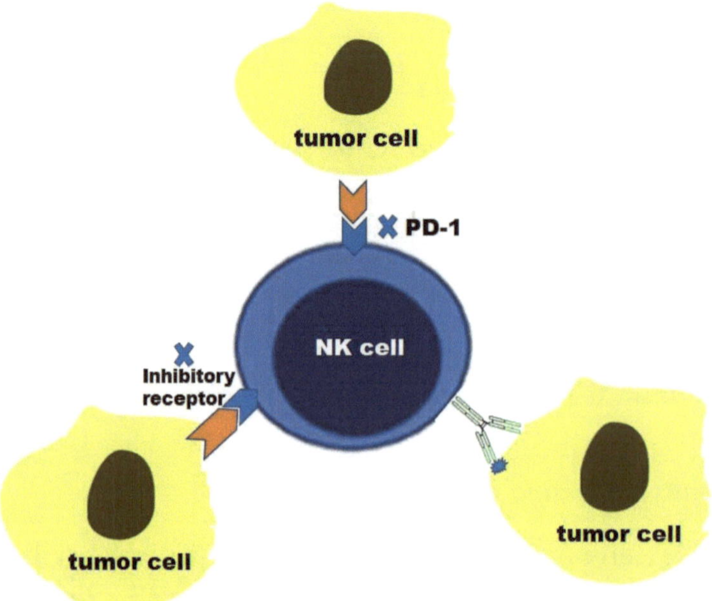

Fig. (3). NK modified with culture for increasing cytotoxicity or specific personalized immunotherapy. **A.** Blocking immune checkpoints to release the inhibition on NK Cells; **B.** using tumor-specific antibodies to mediate ADCC of NK Cells; **C.** multiple specific Killer-Engagers to stimulate NK Cell Activity.

5. Development of NK Cells Culture

IL-2, IL-15, IL-12, IL-21, and IL-18 have been confirmed to improve the anti-tumor function of NK cells and boost their proliferation *in vitro* and *in vivo*. IL2 is one of the most popular cytokines used to culture with tumor cytotoxicity for NK cell growth. Recently, IL-2 can be discovered to activate Treg cells which inhibit NK cell proliferation and cytotoxicity; three modified IL-2 was developed to replace the natural IL-2 [48]: (1) alternative forms of IL-2, called as "super-2", constructed affinity for the IL-2/15Rβ subunit present on NK cells with lower affinity for IL-2Rα subunit; (2) variants of IL-2, such as F42K, show decreased affinity *in vitro* for IL-2Rα; (3) reconstructed NKG2D binding protein with a mutated form of IL-2 stimulating IL-2 on cells bearing NKG2D only. Moreover, some scientists used IL15 and other interleukins to stimulates immature and mature NK cells [49].

Besides development of using growth factors to culture NK cells, other three ways as Fig. (**3**) are going to be developed for NK cell proliferation and specific application: (1) using blocking immune checkpoints to release the inhibition on NK cells; (2) using tumor-specific antibodies to mediate ADCC of NK cell; (3) using multiple specific Killer-Engagers to stimulate NK cell activity.

Using blocking inhibitory checkpoints is extremely popular to promote the activity of NK cells. The purpose of antibodies is to unblock a blocked immune response to increase anti-tumor activity. For example, PD-1 is an inhibitory receptor expressed on the surface of B-cells, T-cells, and NK cells. The designs of PD-1 antibodies, including nivolumab, pidilizumab, and pembrolizumab are going to be developed to inhibit PD-1 function so that it is worth developing an increase of NK cell cytotoxicity by PD-1 antibodies *in vivo* and *in the intro* by eliminating NK cell immunosuppression [50].

Monoclonal Ab (mAb) of tumor-specific antibodies is to promote NK cell ADCC through the binding of the IgG Fc part and its activating receptor CD16A expressed on NK cell. Some studies have focused on modifying mAb to enhance ADCC by increasing affinity for Fc receptors through mutagenesis or glycosylation. For example, scientists produced mAb 7C6 against MICA/B (Major Histocompatibility Complex Class-I chain-related gene A/B), which could prevent the extracellular domains of MICA and MICB from proteolytic shedding and mediated anti-tumor immunity by activation of NKG2D and CD16 on NK cells [51].

Using multiple specific killer-engagers to stimulate NK cell activity is an excellent way to stimulate NK cells. The multiple specific killer-engagers (such as bi-specific or tri-specific killer cell engagers) are designed moieties containing single-chain variable fragments (scFv) against both TAAs and activating receptors on NK cells to create an immunologic synapse between NK cells and tumor cells. CD16 is an active receptor of NK cell-dependent tumor cell killing molecules. It has been demonstrated that CD16-directed bi-specific (CD16×19) and tri-specific (CD16×19×22) scFv directly binding NK cells *via* CD16 for NK cells to kill lymphoid tumors [52].

6. Development of a Clinical Application for NK Immunotherapy

Adoptive transfer of NK cells with high yields and high quality is to improve the function of the immune system through infusing as Fig. (**4A**): (1) NK cells activated *ex vivo* or (2) chimeric antigen receptor (CAR) modified NK cells (3) VEs of NK cells alternatives to cell-based therapeutics. The three NK cells related to products have been demonstrated to be promising adoptive immunotherapy against tumor cells.

Autologous NK cells expanded *ex vivo* have been tested for treating patients with lymphoma, colon cancer, breast cancer and lung cancer in clinical trials, however, only very few of anti-tumor effect was observed for the autologous NK cells. The major reason was that the inhibitory receptors on autologous NK cells matched self MHC class I presented on tumor cells, inhibiting the activation of NK cells. In addition, autologous NK cells observed from cancer patients were in silent status, making NK cells restrict anti-tumor ability. NK cells had a clinical benefit by donor- *vs* .-recipient NK cell alloreactivity, which was mainly resulted from KIR ligand incompatibility.

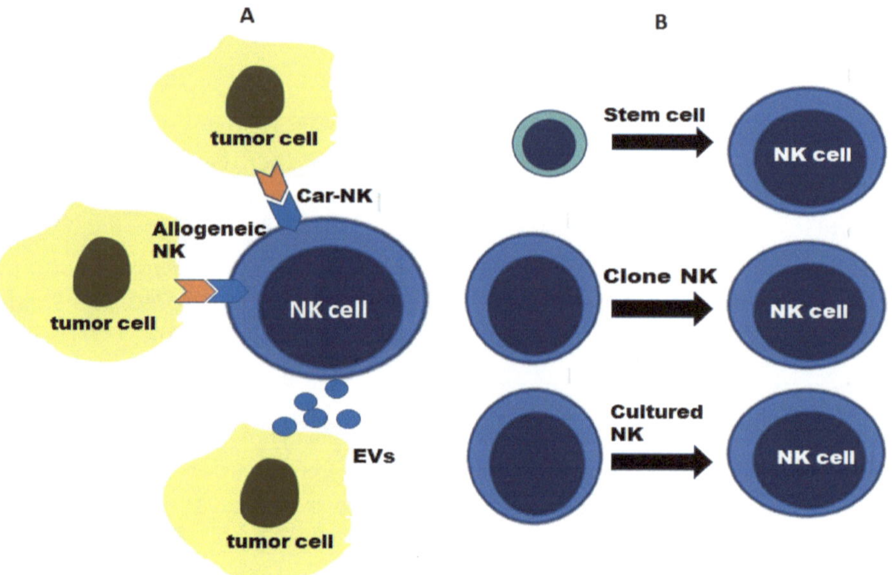

Fig. (4). NK clinical application. **A:** (I) NK cells activated *ex vivo* ; (II) chimeric antigen receptor (CAR) modified NK cells; (III) VEs of NK cells alternatives to cell-based therapeutics; **B** Allogeneic NK sources.

Now as Fig. (**4B**) [53], (I) adoptive NK immunotherapy of *ex vivo* activated allogeneic KIR/KIR ligand mismatched NK cells demonstrated responses to AML, melanoma, breast cancer, ovarian cancer, neuroblastoma, renal cell carcinoma, colorectal cancer, and hepatocellular cancer; (II) some clonal NK cell lines, such as NK-92, KHYG-1, HANK-1, NKG, NK-YS, YTS, YT, produce large numbers of cytotoxic NK cells for immunotherapy. Among them, NK-92 is the only cell line approved by the US FDA for use in the clinical trials; (III) NK cells for tumor lysis can be cultured from human pluripotent stem cells (hPSCs), including hematopoietic stem/progenitor cells (HSPC) from umbilical cord blood (UCB), induced pluripotent stem cells (iPSCs), and human embryonic stem cells (hESCs). The protocols for producing NK cells from hPSCs are based on NK cell cytokines (IL-3, IL-7, IL-15, SCF, FLT3L).

Genetic modification of NK cells with CAR constructs are going to be developed from sources of NK cells as described above, such as allogeneic primary NK cells, NK cell lines, and HPSCs. CAR-NK has adopted the basic structural framework of CAR-T, that is, chimeric antigen receptors mainly composed of an extracellular, hinge, transmembrane, and intracellular domains with transfection methods. The extracellular domain can bind tightly to tumor-associated antigens expressed on the surface of tumor cells, which determines the specificity of CAR structures. Single-chain variable fragments (ScFvs) are the most commonly used ectodomains for CARs. At present, CAR-NK cells have been evaluated for the treatment of hematological cancers and solid tumors in preclinical studies resulting in some good results. Although CAR-NK therapy is still under clinical evaluation, NK cells possess several advantages over T-cells in being engineered to express CARs and used for cancer treatment [54]: (I) NK cells are easy to be isolated and have a relatively short lifespan and thus the risk of overexpansion of transferred CAR-NK cells in patients is relatively low; (II) the cytokines secreted by NK cells mainly include IFN-γ and GM-CSF, safer than TNF-α and IL-6 which are released by activated CAR-T cells so that life-threatening cytokine release syndrome (CRS) is low; (III) CAR-NK cells could trigger the lysis of target cells in both CAR-dependent and CAR-independent manners killing tumor cells; (IV) CAR-NK therapy derived from PBMCs, NK cell lines, and hPSCs while CAR-T therapy is required to be autologous sources. If several obstacles are overcome, such as (I) GVHD, (II) non-specific binding of CARs to antigens expressed on normal tissues, (III) retroviral transduction weakens NK efficiency, (IV) CAR-NK binding epitope distance, those CAR-NK cells will play an important role in personalized immunotherapy.

Because NK cells can hardly relocate tumor tissues to kill tumor cells, resulting in poor therapeutic effects, and because GMP NK culture, NK cell preserving and transporting clinical-grade living immune cells is a high cost for clinical application, EVs, a nano-sized vesicle naturally secreted by many different types of cells including NK cells, have gradually been proposed and studied, providing a new cell-free immunotherapy method. EVs of NK cells usually consist of NK biomarkers (CD56) and lytic proteins such as FasL and perforin. Therefore, VEs of NK cells are considered as potential alternatives to cell-based therapeutics based on advantages [55] such as (1) passively diffuse into tumor tissues and (2) easy fusion between EVs and tumor cells based on an acidic environment of solid tumors caused by hypoxia and (3) EV ability to traverse biological barriers such as the blood-brain barrier (BBB) and the blood-tumor barrier (BTB); (4) EVs are stable at −80 °C, lasting up to 12 months.

7. Research and Development of Autologous Lymphocytes

Autologous lymphocytes isolated from peripheral blood mononuclear cells (PBMN) and induced by cytokines can be used for non-specific cell therapy. This is immunotherapy for "no"-specific anti-tumor immune response to reject and destroy tumor cells. Based on different types of inducing methods, the T-cells immunotherapy involved in PBMN lymphocytes is grouped as LAK cell, CIK cell, and DCCIK cell-mediated anti-tumor therapies. Although these non-specific cell therapies are not involved in personalized immunotherapy, we will further present techniques or mechanisms to modify peripheral lymphocytes for some potentials of personalized immunotherapy.

1. History and Development of LAK, CIK and DCCIK

Grimm and his colleagues first reported non-specific killer cells generated by culture of peripheral blood mononuclear cells (PBMC) with a high dose of interleukin-2 (IL-2), which was named as LAK (lymphokine-activated killer) in 1982 [56]. LAK cells contain a mixture of T cells and NK cells, both of which are not restricted by the major histocompatibility complex (MHC) against a broad range of tumor cells *in vitro*. Rosenberg's results showed very lower effects by using autologous LAK cells and IL-2 for patients in their early research [57]. In 1988, a large sample size of study with a total of 221 tumor patients demonstrated only 16 CR and 26 PR after combination treatment of LAK cells and IL-2 [58]. However, in another randomized clinical trial, the result suggested a trend toward improving survival when IL-2 was given together with LAK cells to melanoma patients but not occur in patients with renal cell carcinoma. Moreover, a randomized phase III trial of IL-2 with or without LAK cells in the treatment of patients with advanced renal cell carcinoma demonstrated that there was no difference in treatment response (P=0.61) and survival (P=0.67) between these two groups of treatments. Although LAK cell therapy seemed to kill some tumor cells effectively, high toxicity caused by a high dose of IL-2, resulting in severe hypotension, limited its clinical usage.

CIK (Cytokine Induced Killer) cells are obtained by PBMCs and then stimulated with a cocktail of IL-2, IFN-γ, an anti-CD3 monoclonal antibody in an *ex vivo* culturing process for approximately two weeks. CIK cells are a mixture of cells with non-MHC-restricted cytolytic activity, including CD3+CD56−T-cells and CD3+CD56+NK-T cells, and a relatively minor population of CD3−CD56+NK cells. Compared to standard IL-2 stimulated LAK cells, CIK cells have enhanced anti-tumor cytotoxic activity by over 70-fold. The lytic activity can be further enhanced by the addition of IL-1, IFN-γ, IL-7, IL-15, and other cytokines. At present, the total response rate (RR) under CIK treatment was 23.7% (91/384), while 161 patients (41.9%) had an SD, and 129 patients (33.6%) had progressive disease (PD). Only three patients had tumor volume decreased [59].

Dendritic cells (DCs) are professional antigen-presenting cells (APCs) to initiate an antigen-specific cytotoxic T lymphocyte response killing tumor cells. Cytokine-induced killer (CIK) cells contain a population of cytotoxic T lymphocytes (CTL) that are generated by incubation of peripheral blood lymphocytes with an anti-CD3 monoclonal antibody, IL-2, IFN-γ, and IL-1. DC/CIK cells show strong anti-tumor cytotoxicity under both *in vitro* and *in vivo* conditions. Although DCCIK has some promising results, the adoptive T-cell immunotherapy should be much studied in the laboratory and clinics [60].

2. The Strategy of Cytokine Inducing PBMN Lymphocyte for Personalized Immunotherapy

As described above, these ACT from LAK, CIK, and DCCIK is not involved in specific cell therapy or personalized immunotherapy. Here we introduce some strategies for personalized immunotherapy by using some techniques to rebuild the PBMN lymphocytes. These techniques, at least, include: (1) using tumor cells or tumor-associated Ag (TAA) to changing dendritic cells to stimulate PBMN lymphocytes; (2) using genomic data to define tumor-specific Ag mutant (or tumor-associated Ag) to produce specific-personalized immunotherapy; (3) using genetically modify normal lymphocytes by TCR and CAR-T to produce specific personalized immunotherapy;

In the early period, some scientists had studied *in vitro* generation of effector lymphocytes by a mixed lymphocyte-tumor culture (MLTC) system, followed by stimulation with the interleukin (IL)-2 and anti-CD3 antibody (IL-2/CD3) system to perform specific immunotherapy [61]. How to optimally present tumor Ag to CD+8 cells has been studied or will be studied to a large extent. For example, DCs, professional antigen-presenting cells (APCs) are differentiated with granulocyte-macrophage colony-stimulating factor (GM-CSF) and IL-4 cultured from PBMN and then antigenic peptides pulsed into cultured DCs (peptide-pulsed DC-activated killer, PDAK) with autologous lymphocyte to generate tumor-reactive effector lymphocytes [62]. Currently, using PDAK cells for HLA-A2 and

HLA-A24 patients with antigen-positive (CEA, Her-2, MAGE, MART, SART, WT-1) are going to research for different metastatic tumors. More recently, it was reported that tumor-derived RNA allowed DCs to stimulate anti-tumor CTL [63].

Using genomic data defining tumor-specific Ag mutant or tumor-associated Ag can be producing specific-personalized immunotherapy. For instance, genomic studies of melanoma TIL showed that T cells that mediated complete tumor regression recognized unique somatic mutations expressed by cancer and that reactivity against these unique mutations elicited more effective anti-tumor responses such as MART-1 [64]. These strong correlations led to the possibility that immunologic reactivity against unique somatic mutations in common epithelial cancers might also be useful targets for cancer immunotherapy. Moreover, the genomic sequence discovered that autologous T-cells that recognize epitopes encoded by a somatic mutation on many common epithelial cancers. These findings led to the first successful treatment of a patient with a bile duct cancer treated with her autologous T-cells that recognized a unique ERBB2IP mutation expressed by her tumor [65]. Following the administration of these specific anti-tumor cells, the patient exhibited a near-complete cancer regression of lung and liver metastases.

Genetically modify normal lymphocytes with receptors against tumor antigens have been successfully used in T cell receptors against the MART-1 for melanoma [66]. Moreover, some studies demonstrated that the treatment of patients with metastatic synovial cell sarcomas treated with T cells genetically engineered to express TCRs against the NYESO-1 (cancer testes antigen) could mediate cancer regression [67]. T-cells genetically engineered to express chimeric antigen receptors (CARs) against the CD-19 B cell antigen were shown to mediate complete regressions in patients with acute and chronic lymphocytic leukemia, follicular lymphomas, and aggressive diffuse large B cell lymphomas [68]. These achievements confirm genetically modifying normal lymphocytes led to autologous lymphocyte successful treatment of a patient with different hematologic malignancies and solid tumor diseases.

CURRENT CONSIDERATION AFTER COMPLETION OF CLINICAL TRIALS

Good immunotherapy should be high efficacy, low side-effect, and low economic cost for each patient with tumor disease. According to the consideration, these developments of immunotherapy in the future require the development of affordable treatment, bearable side-effect, and responsible effects for each patient in optimal cell culture and the right clinical treatment.

At present, there are two models to pay treatment for cell therapy in clinics, sipuleucel-T (antigen present-cell), and stem cell transplantation. sipuleucel-T approved by FDA has been successfully used for patients with prostate cancers [69]. Sipuleucel-T is composed of recombinant antigen protein (PAP), which must be incubated with the patient's isolated APCs *ex vivo*. The procedure starts at the physician's office or the blood-collection center or the laboratory, where blood containing the APCs is collected by leukapheresis. APCs isolated from the blood are reconstructed with a recombinant fusion protein antigen, which contains both PAP and GM–CSF. The activated antigen-loaded APCs are transported back to the infusion center and are infused into the patient. The cells shipped, cultured *in vitro* with tumor antigens, and shipped back to treatment centers of infusion back into the patient cost $93,000 per course [70]. Although sipuleucel-T is very effective, the high price may influence its long-term benefit to patients with prostate cancer. On the other hand, stem cell transplantation as same as adoptive T-cell therapy for hematologic malignancies and solid tumors has been performed mainly at academic medical centers with funding reimbursement. The reimbursed model of stem cell transplantation for the medical center relies on a diagnosis-related group (DRG), a bundled payment for costs during medication. The DRG-based reimbursement depends on the approval of treatment-specific reimbursement codes with about 36000-8800 dollars for autologous cells and 96000-204000 dollars for allogeneic cells [71]. Because of different protocols or codes, and thus, the true costs are difficult to determine. Of course, the costs of adoptive T cell therapy are also difficult to determine as stem cell transplantation. Adoptive T-cell therapy should be considered an affordable treatment for patients with their medical insurance, with responsible effects for each patient to compare to other therapies, and with bearable side-effect for each subject.

FUTURE OF ADOPTIVE T-CELL IMMUNOTHERAPY

It is certain that, under optimal culture in laboratories and right therapeutic conditions in clinics, ACT can induce regression of tumors, including hematologic malignancies and solid tumors. Once different results are confirmed to be very inspiring after clinical trials, new protocols of immunotherapy and personalized immunotherapy should be more optimized by decreasing side-effects and increasing efficacy in the next step. Current efforts of adoptive T-cell immunotherapy concentrate on setting up optimal T-cell culture in laboratories, selecting the right administration in clinics, considering affordability, and enhancing availability for patients.

CONSENT FOR PUBLICATION

Not applicable.

CONFLICT OF INTEREST

The authors declare no financial interests.

ACKNOWLEDGEMENTS

We have set up a TIL culture for clinical application for 30 years. DYL and SQD supervised BRL in early periods. XHZ, BYW, YMZ cooperated with BRL in the periods.

The mention of trade names or commercial products in this article is solely to provide specific information and does not imply recommendation.

REFERENCES

[1]   Rosenberg SA, Packard BS, Aebersold PM, *et al.* Use of tumor-infiltrating lymphocytes and interleukin-2 in the immunotherapy of patients with metastatic melanoma. A preliminary report. N Engl J Med 1988; 319(25): 1676-80.
[http://dx.doi.org/10.1056/NEJM198812223192527] [PMID: 3264384]

[2]   Li BR, Tong SQ, Zhang XH, Lu J, Gu QL, Lu DY. A new experimental and clinical approach of combining usage of highly active tumor-infiltrating lymphocytes and highly sensitive antitumor drugs for the advanced malignant tumor. Chin Med J (Engl) 1994; 107(11): 803-7.
[PMID: 7867384]

[3]   Finkelstein DM, Miller RG. Cell surface recognition determinants involved in triggering the lymphokine activated killer cell phenomenon: enhanced killing of modified "anti-self" targets by varying LAK culture conditions. J Otolaryngol 1990; 19(5): 294-8.
[PMID: 2262945]

[4]   Mohsenzadegan M, Peng RW, Roudi R. Dendritic cell/cytokine-induced killer cell-based immunotherapy in lung cancer: What we know and future landscape. J Cell Physiol 2019.
[http://dx.doi.org/10.1002/jcp.28977] [PMID: 31222740]

[5]   Ren PT, Zhang Y. Comparative investigation of the effects of specific antigen-sensitized DC-CIK and DC-CTL cells against B16 melanoma tumor cells. Mol Med Rep 2017; 15(4): 1533-8.
[http://dx.doi.org/10.3892/mmr.2017.6175] [PMID: 28260039]

[6]   Hamilton TC, Ozols RF, Longo DL. Biologic therapy for the treatment of malignant common epithelial tumors of the ovary. Cancer 1987; 60(8) (Suppl.): 2054-63.
[http://dx.doi.org/10.1002/1097-0142(19901015)60:8+<2054::AID-CNCR2820601518>3.0.CO;2-0]
[PMID: 2443236]

[7]   Khavari P. Cytotoxic cellular mediators of the immune response to neoplasia: a review. Yale J Biol Med 1987; 60(5): 409-19.
[PMID: 3321723]

[8]   Xiang B, Snook AE, Magee MS, Waldman SA. Colorectal cancer immunotherapy. Discov Med 2013; 15(84): 301-8.
[PMID: 23725603]

[9]   Choi BK, Kim SH, Kim YH, Kwon BS. Cancer immunotherapy using tumor antigen-reactive T cells. Immunotherapy 2018; 10(3): 235-45.
[http://dx.doi.org/10.2217/imt-2017-0130] [PMID: 29370726]

[10]   Ngiow SF, Loi S, Thomas D, Smyth MJ. Mouse Models of Tumor Immunotherapy. Adv Immunol 2016; 130: 1-24.

[http://dx.doi.org/10.1016/bs.ai.2015.12.004] [PMID: 26922998]

[11]   Rosenberg SA, Spiess P, Lafreniere R. A new approach to the adoptive immunotherapy of cancer with tumor-infiltrating lymphocytes. Science 1986; 233(4770): 1318-21.
[http://dx.doi.org/10.1126/science.3489291] [PMID: 3489291]

[12]   Muul LM, Spiess PJ, Director EP, Rosenberg SA. Identification of specific cytolytic immune responses against autologous tumor in humans bearing malignant melanoma. J Immunol 1987; 138(3): 989-95.
[PMID: 3100623]

[13]   Hinrichs CS, Rosenberg SA. Exploiting the curative potential of adoptive T-cell therapy for cancer. Immunol Rev 2014; 257(1): 56-71.
[http://dx.doi.org/10.1111/imr.12132] [PMID: 24329789]

[14]   Kawakami Y, Nishimura MI, Restifo NP, *et al.* T-cell recognition of human melanoma antigens. J Immunother Emphasis Tumor Immunol 1993; 14(2): 88-93.
[http://dx.doi.org/10.1097/00002371-199308000-00002] [PMID: 8280705]

[15]   Li BR, Tong SQ, Hu BY, *et al.* [Study on the influence of enzymatic digestion upon tumor-infiltrating lymphocytes]. Shi Yan Sheng Wu Xue Bao 1994; 27(1): 103-7.
[PMID: 8042406]

[16]   Li B, Tong SQ, Zhang XH, Zhu YM, *et al.* Research on TIL proliferation, phenotype and lethality of human malignant solid tumors; Modern Immunology. Chinese 1994; p. 05.

[17]   Li B, Shen DH. Preliminary Study on the Resting Status of Tumor-infiltrating Lymphocytes. Chinese Microbiology and Immunology (Chinese) 1994; 14(6): 399-402.

[18]   Li B, Tong SQ, Zhu YM. HU BW et al Establishment of a method for separation of tumor-infiltrating lymphocytes with high vitality; Journal of Immunology. Chinese 1994; p. 01.

[19]   Zhu YM, Zhang XH, Li B, Hu BY, *et al.* Removal of tumor-doped tumor cells in tumor-infiltrating lymphocyte culture Journal of Shanghai Jiaotong University (Medical Science Edition, Chinese) 1995; 02.

[20]   Li B, Ding JQ, *et al.* Tumor Tissue Recycling-A new combination therapy for solid tumor: experimental and Preliminarily clinical research. Anticancer 1999; 13(5): 1-6. *IN VIVO.*

[21]   Rosenberg SA, Dudley ME. Adoptive cell therapy for the treatment of patients with metastatic melanoma. Curr Opin Immunol 2009; 21(2): 233-40.
[http://dx.doi.org/10.1016/j.coi.2009.03.002] [PMID: 19304471]

[22]   Yamaue H, Tanimura H, Tsunoda T, *et al.* [Clinical application of adoptive immunotherapy by cytotoxic T lymphocytes induced from tumor-infiltrating lymphocytes]. Nippon Gan Chiryo Gakkai Shi 1990; 25(5): 978-89.
[PMID: 2391445]

[23]   Guo W. An experimental study of the anti-tumor activity of tumor-infiltrating lymphocytes (TIL) in human tongue carcinoma *in vitro* . Zhonghua Kou Qiang Yi Xue Za Zhi 1992; 27(5): 61-259. 318

[24]   Semino C, Martini L, Queirolo P, *et al.* Adoptive immunotherapy of advanced solid tumors: an eight year clinical experience. Anticancer Res 1999; 19(6C): 5645-9.
[PMID: 10697634]

[25]   Xiang B, Snook AE, Magee MS, Waldman SA. Colorectal cancer immunotherapy. Discov Med 2013; 15(84): 301-8.
[PMID: 23725603]

[26]   Ben-Avi R, Farhi R, Ben-Nun A, *et al.* Establishment of adoptive cell therapy with tumor infiltrating lymphocytes for non-small cell lung cancer patients. Cancer Immunol Immunother 2018; 67(8): 1221-30.
[http://dx.doi.org/10.1007/s00262-018-2174-4] [PMID: 29845338]

[27]   Lin Y, Okada H. Cellular immunotherapy for malignant gliomas. Expert Opin Biol Ther 2016; 16(10): 1265-75.
[http://dx.doi.org/10.1080/14712598.2016.1214266] [PMID: 27434205]

[28]   Zhang YX, Wang XY, Liu JB, Zhang SQ, Chen YR. [Effects of auto-tumor infiltrating lymphocytes induced by interleukin (IL)-12 with IL-2 on patients of primary hepatic carcinoma]. Zhonghua Yi Xue Za Zhi 2008; 88(14): 973-6.
[PMID: 18756970]

[29]   Mulder WM, Stukart MJ, Roos M, *et al.* Culture of tumour-infiltrating lymphocytes from melanoma and colon carcinoma: removal of tumour cells does not affect tumour-specificity. Cancer Immunol Immunother 1995; 41(5): 293-301.
[http://dx.doi.org/10.1007/BF01517217] [PMID: 8536275]

[30]   Tian YJ, Cui BX, Ma DX, Zhang Y, Hou F, Zhang WJ. [Effect of interleukin 21 and/or interleukin 12 on the antitumor activity of peripheral blood mononuclear cells in patients with endometrial cancer]. Zhongguo Yi Xue Ke Xue Yuan Xue Bao 2011; 33(3): 292-8.
[PMID: 21718613]

[31]   Wang JH, Tong SQ, Li B, *et al.* Immunological Character of TIL in Ovarian Carcinoma. Chin J Cancer Res 2000; 12(2): 99-104.
[http://dx.doi.org/10.1007/BF02983432]

[32]   Teo YWB, Linn YC, Goh YT, Li S, Ho LP. Tumor infiltrating lymphocytes from acute myeloid leukemia marrow can be reverted to CD45RA+ central memory state by reactivation in SIP (Simulated Infective Protocol). Immunobiology 2019; 224(4): 526-31.
[http://dx.doi.org/10.1016/j.imbio.2019.05.001] [PMID: 31072628]

[33]   Rohaan MW, van den Berg JH, Kvistborg P, Haanen JBAG. Adoptive transfer of tumor-infiltrating lymphocytes in melanoma: a viable treatment option. J Immunother Cancer 2018; 6(1): 102.
[http://dx.doi.org/10.1186/s40425-018-0391-1] [PMID: 30285902]

[34]   Goff SL, Dudley ME, Citrin DE, *et al.* Randomized, Prospective Evaluation Comparing Intensity of Lymphodepletion Before Adoptive Transfer of Tumor-Infiltrating Lymphocytes for Patients With Metastatic Melanoma. J Clin Oncol 2016; 34(20): 2389-97.
[http://dx.doi.org/10.1200/JCO.2016.66.7220] [PMID: 27217459]

[35]   Chandran SS, Somerville RPT, Yang JC, *et al.* Treatment of metastatic uveal melanoma with adoptive transfer of tumour-infiltrating lymphocytes: a single-centre, two-stage, single-arm, phase 2 study. Lancet Oncol 2017; 18(6): 792-802.
[http://dx.doi.org/10.1016/S1470-2045(17)30251-6] [PMID: 28395880]

[36]   Gu QL, *et al.* Phenotype and cytotoxic activity of infiltrating lymphocytes in gastrointestinal tumors. Journal of Shanghai Second Medical University (Chinese) 1996; 03.

[37]   Deng YD, Gu QL, Li B, *et al.* MTT colorimetric assay for LAK and TIL cell activity in cord blood Journal of Shanghai Jiaotong University (Medical Science Edition, Chinese) 1995; 02.

[38]   Hu BC, Li GW, Cheng W, Shen JK, *et al.* Clinical application of infiltrating lymphocytes in malignant brain tumors. Journal of Immunology (Chinese) 1997; 02.

[39]   Hua ZD, Lu J, Li HF, Li B, *et al.* Clinical study of tumor-infiltrating lymphocytes in ovarian cancer Chinese Journal of Obstetrics and Gynecology. Chinese 1996; p. 09.

[40]   Lu J, Hu LW, Hua ZD, Li B, *et al.* Analysis of the therapeutic effects of different therapeutic approaches for TIL. Journal of Chinese Tumor Biological Treatment (Chinese) 1996; 02.

[41]   Jie HB, Srivastava RM, Argiris A, Bauman JE, Kane LP, Ferris RL. Increased PD-1[+] and TIM-3[+] TILs during Cetuximab Therapy Inversely Correlate with Response in Head and Neck Cancer Patients. Cancer Immunol Res 2017; 5(5): 408-16.
[http://dx.doi.org/10.1158/2326-6066.CIR-16-0333] [PMID: 28408386]

[42]   Mullinax JE, Hall M, Prabhakaran S, *et al.* Combination of Ipilimumab and Adoptive Cell Therapy with Tumor-Infiltrating Lymphocytes for Patients with Metastatic Melanoma. Front Oncol 2018; 8: 44.
[http://dx.doi.org/10.3389/fonc.2018.00044] [PMID: 29552542]

[43]   Harada K, Abdelhakeem AAF, Ajani JA. A balancing act: dual immune-checkpoint inhibition for oesophagogastric cancer. Nat Rev Clin Oncol 2019; 16(1): 9-10.
[http://dx.doi.org/10.1038/s41571-018-0108-x] [PMID: 30291292]

[44]   Lu J, Hua ZD, Li HF, Li B, *et al. In vitro* study of ovarian cancer TIL[J]. Shanghai Medical Journal (Chinese) 1995; 06.

[45]   Tsuboi K, Saijo K, Ishikawa E, *et al.* Effects of local injection of *ex vivo* expanded autologous tumor-specific T lymphocytes in cases with recurrent malignant gliomas. Clin Cancer Res 2003; 9(9): 3294-302.
[PMID: 12960115]

[46]   Lakhtin VM, Lakhtin MV, Mironov AY, Aleshkin VA, Afanasiev SS. [Lectin populations of NK cells against tumors coupled to viral infections (review of literature)]. Klin Lab Diagn 2019; 64(5): 314-20.
[http://dx.doi.org/10.18821/0869-2084-2019-64-5-314-320] [PMID: 31185156]

[47]   Vitale M, Cantoni C, Pietra G, Mingari MC, Moretta L. Effect of tumor cells and tumor microenvironment on NK-cell function. Eur J Immunol 2014; 44(6): 1582-92.
[http://dx.doi.org/10.1002/eji.201344272] [PMID: 24777896]

[48]   Sim GC, Liu C, Wang E, *et al.* IL2 Variant circumvents ICOS+ Regulatory T-cell expansion and promotes NK cell activation. Cancer Immunol Res 2016; 4(11): 983-94.
[http://dx.doi.org/10.1158/2326-6066.CIR-15-0195] [PMID: 27697858]

[49]   Floros T, Tarhini AA. Anticancer cytokines: biology and clinical effects of interferon-alpha2, interleukin (IL)-2, IL-15, IL-21, and IL-12. Semin Oncol 2015; 42(4): 539-48.
[http://dx.doi.org/10.1053/j.seminoncol.2015.05.015] [PMID: 26320059]

[50]   Ohaegbulam KC, Assal A, Lazar-Molnar E, Yao Y, Zang X. Human cancer immunotherapy with antibodies to the PD-1 and PD-L1 pathway. Trends Mol Med 2015; 21(1): 24-33.
[http://dx.doi.org/10.1016/j.molmed.2014.10.009] [PMID: 25440090]

[51]   Johnston MP, Khakoo SI. Immunotherapy for hepatocellular carcinoma: Current and future. World J Gastroenterol 2019; 25(24): 2977-89.
[http://dx.doi.org/10.3748/wjg.v25.i24.2977] [PMID: 31293335]

[52]   Rothe A, Sasse S, Topp MS, *et al.* A phase 1 study of the bispecific anti-CD30/CD16A antibody construct AFM13 in patients with relapsed or refractory Hodgkin lymphoma. Blood 2015; 125(26): 4024-31.
[http://dx.doi.org/10.1182/blood-2014-12-614636] [PMID: 25887777]

[53]   Benson DM Jr, Bakan CE, Zhang S, *et al.* IPH2101, a novel anti-inhibitory KIR antibody, and lenalidomide combine to enhance the natural killer cell *versus* multiple myeloma effect. Blood 2011; 118(24): 6387-91.
[http://dx.doi.org/10.1182/blood-2011-06-360255] [PMID: 22031859]

[54]   Oberschmidt O, Kloess S, Koehl U. Redirected primary human chimeric antigen receptor natural killer cells as an "Off-the-Shelf Immunotherapy" for improvement in cancer treatment. Front Immunol 2017; 8: 654.
[http://dx.doi.org/10.3389/fimmu.2017.00654] [PMID: 28649246]

[55]   Raimondo F, Morosi L, Chinello C, Magni F, Pitto M. Advances in membranous vesicle and exosome proteomics improving biological understanding and biomarker discovery. Proteomics 2011; 11(4): 709-20.
[http://dx.doi.org/10.1002/pmic.201000422] [PMID: 21241021]

[56]   Rosenberg SA, Lotze MT, Muul LM, *et al.* Observations on the systemic administration of autologous

lymphokine-activated killer cells and recombinant interleukin-2 to patients with metastatic cancer. N Engl J Med 1985; 313(23): 1485-92.
[http://dx.doi.org/10.1056/NEJM198512053132327] [PMID: 3903508]

[57]   Rosenberg SA, Restifo NP, Yang JC, Morgan RA, Dudley ME. Adoptive cell transfer: a clinical path to effective cancer immunotherapy. Nat Rev Cancer 2008; 8(4): 299-308.
[http://dx.doi.org/10.1038/nrc2355] [PMID: 18354418]

[58]   Rosenberg SA, Yang JC, Sherry RM, *et al.* Durable complete responses in heavily pretreated patients with metastatic melanoma using T-cell transfer immunotherapy. Clin Cancer Res 2011; 17(13): 4550-7.
[http://dx.doi.org/10.1158/1078-0432.CCR-11-0116] [PMID: 21498393]

[59]   Chawla PC, Chawla A. The Promise of Oncoimmunology: Integrating Immunotherapy with Conventional Cancer Treatments. J Interv Oncol 2014; 3: 2.
[http://dx.doi.org/10.4172/2329-6771.1000124]

[60]   Zhao Y, Qiao G, Wang X, *et al.* Combination of DC/CIK adoptive T cell immunotherapy with chemotherapy in advanced non-small-cell lung cancer (NSCLC) patients: a prospective patients' preference-based study (PPPS). Clin Transl Oncol 2019; 21(6): 721-8.
[http://dx.doi.org/10.1007/s12094-018-1968-3] [PMID: 30374838]

[61]   Yamaguchi Y, Ohshita A, Kawabuchi Y, *et al.* Adoptive immunotherapy of cancer using activated autologous lymphocytes--current status and new strategies. Hum Cell 2003; 16(4): 183-9.
[http://dx.doi.org/10.1111/j.1749-0774.2003.tb00152.x] [PMID: 15147038]

[62]   Yamaguchi Y, Ohta K, Kawabuchi Y, *et al.* Feasibility study of adoptive immunotherapy for metastatic lung tumors using peptide-pulsed dendritic cell-activated killer (PDAK) cells. Anticancer Res 2005; 25(3c): 2407-15.
[PMID: 16080467]

[63]   Brabants E, Heyns K, De Smet S, *et al.* An accelerated, clinical-grade protocol to generate high yields of type 1-polarizing messenger RNA-loaded dendritic cells for cancer vaccination. Cytotherapy 2018; 20(9): 1164-81.
[http://dx.doi.org/10.1016/j.jcyt.2018.06.006] [PMID: 30122654]

[64]   Powell MR, Sheehan DJ, Kleven DT. Altered Morphology and Immunohistochemical Characteristics in Metastatic Malignant Melanoma After Therapy With Vemurafenib. Am J Dermatopathol 2016; 38(9): e137-9.
[http://dx.doi.org/10.1097/DAD.0000000000000619] [PMID: 27541173]

[65]   Tran E, Turcotte S, Gros A, *et al.* Cancer immunotherapy based on mutation-specific CD4+ T cells in a patient with epithelial cancer. Science 2014; 344(6184): 641-5.
[http://dx.doi.org/10.1126/science.1251102] [PMID: 24812403]

[66]   Morgan RA, Dudley ME, Wunderlich JR, *et al.* Cancer regression in patients after transfer of genetically engineered lymphocytes. Science 2006; 314(5796): 126-9.
[http://dx.doi.org/10.1126/science.1129003] [PMID: 16946036]

[67]   Robbins PF, Morgan RA, Feldman SA, *et al.* Tumor regression in patients with metastatic synovial cell sarcoma and melanoma using genetically engineered lymphocytes reactive with NY-ESO-1. J Clin Oncol 2011; 29(7): 917-24.
[http://dx.doi.org/10.1200/JCO.2010.32.2537] [PMID: 21282551]

[68]   Kochenderfer JN, Wilson WH, Janik JE, *et al.* Eradication of B-lineage cells and regression of lymphoma in a patient treated with autologous T cells genetically engineered to recognize CD19. Blood 2010; 116(20): 4099-102.
[http://dx.doi.org/10.1182/blood-2010-04-281931] [PMID: 20668228]

[69]   Christopher M. Pieczonka, Dimitrios Telonis, Vladimir Mouraviev, David Albala. Rev Urol 2015; 17(4): 203-10.
[PMID: 26839517]

[70] Perica K, Varela JC, Oelke M, Schneck J. Adoptive T cell immunotherapy for cancer. Rambam Maimonides Med J 2015; 6(1)e0004
[http://dx.doi.org/10.5041/RMMJ.10179] [PMID: 25717386]

[71] Khera N, Zeliadt SB, Lee SJ. Economics of hematopoietic cell transplantation. Blood 2012; 120(8): 1545-51.
[http://dx.doi.org/10.1182/blood-2012-05-426783] [PMID: 22700725]

CHAPTER 10

Gene Therapy and Genomic Editing-Development of Adoptive T-cell Immunotherapy

JianQing Ding[1], GuanXiang Qian[2], Shishu Chen[2] and Biaoru Li[1,*]

[1] *Department of Microbiology, Shanghai Second Medical University, Shanghai, 200003, PRC*

[2] *Department of Biochemistry, Shanghai Second Medical School, Shanghai, 200003, PRC*

[3] *Georgia Cancer Center and Department of Pediatrics, Medical College at GA, Augusta, GA 30912, USA*

Abstract: For several decades, clinical scientists and physicians have been studying gene-modified T-cells to treat tumor patients, called T-cell based gene therapy. However, T-cell based gene therapy has efficacy questions and side-effects so that these techniques limited to the clinical application quickly. Therefore the possibility of creating cell-based gene therapy is just like a dream for tumor patients. With the recent development of CRISPR technology and genomic decoding, it is becoming increasingly possible to engineer cells by gene-modification for patients with tumor diseases. Gene-editing systems based on CRISPR, as well as transcription activator-like effector nucleases (TALENs) and zinc-finger nucleases (ZFNs), are becoming valuable tools for the new generation tool of gene therapy. However, each of these systems to effectively apply for patients, including safe delivery and gene modification technologies, is still unknown. This chapter briefly introduces the history of gene therapy, the principle of gene editing with their non-viral and viral delivery methods. The chapter aims to discuss the latest developments in gene-editing technology and discuss their application to adoptive T cell immunotherapy.

Keywords: CRISPR/CAS9 (Clustered regularly interspaced short palindromic repeats), Gene editing, Genetic modification, Gene therapy, Personalized immunotherapy, T-cell Adoptive immunotherapy, TIL (tumor-infiltrating lymphocyte), Transcription activator-like effector nucleases (TALENs), Zinc-finger nucleases (ZFNs).

INTRODUCTION

Gene modification is a basic technique to study gene function and apply for translational medicine. Several decades before, molecular biologists have launched the gene modifications so that the function of the gene is revealed, and

* **Corresponding author Biaoru Li**: Georgia Cancer Center and Department of Pediatrics, Medical College at GA, Augusta, GA 30912, USA; Tel: 440-317-1443; E-mail: bli@augusta.edu

then gene therapy is employed for translational medicine regarding genes with their function additions and deletions of treatment [1]. For instance, after 1989 Rosenberg used vector Mo-MuLV to transduce TNF-α into TIL with a first clinical trial for T-cell immunotherapy in human, we had begun to study cell-based gene therapy using Mo-MuLV for TIL since 1994. Our researches focused on three goals [2]: (I) the optimal transducing efficiency, (II) the clinical application of gene therapy, (III) studying how to avoid clinical side-effect. Our early results demonstrated that TILs cultured during 9 day-25 days have optimally proliferated phase after transduction, comparing groups of culture in <9 days and > 25 days, including TIL survival most extended as Table **1**.

Table 1. Effect of transducing time on proliferation rate and life-span of transduced TIL.

Groups	Date of Transducing (days)	Average Expansion	Average Life-Span
1	<9	282	12.5
2	9-25	1624	31.2
3	>25	136	12

Table 2. FACS phenotype change of transduced TIL.

Cell Phenotype	Before Transducing (%)	After Transducing (%)
CD3	95.69	95.58
CD4	15.29	8.34
CD8	76.49	76.43
CD16CD56	2.33	3.28
CD28	17.41	17.5

We collected 1×10^6 TIL and analyzed the phenotypes by FACs. The results showed no significant difference as Table **2**, with a considerable increase of TNF-α tittering in the culture medium.

After we set up a transduced TIL technique by TNF-α, we performed a first clinical trial in China. A female patient with 50 years old was diagnosed as primary and advanced stomach cancer with metastatic and multiple liver tumors by the gastrointestinal scope and CT examination. Under informed consent, surgeons cut out the stomach carrying the primary tumor. The metastatic hepatic tumor was used to study treatment efficiency with a settled catheter into the liver artery. 20 days late after surgery, 2.4×10^9 TILs were injected into the liver catheter; one month late, 2.8×10^9 transduced TIL was second injected into the liver catheter by the hepatic artery. Every two months, morphological imaging such as ultrasonic and CT were examined to study the efficacy of metastatic liver cancer. The results of the first month after transduced TIL treatment showed as Table **3** with partial response in tumor mass in CT as our early publication [3].

Table 3. CEA and AKP change of transduced TIL.

Item of Examination	Before Therapy	After Therapy
CEA	178.9 ng/ml	49.44 ng/ml
AKP	276 U/ml	149 U/ml

Although we achieved a good result, a safety question still influenced the technology development and clinical application; therefore, the possibility of clinical application for genetic modifications was just a dream for some genetic and tumor diseases. Recently, the new generation of gene modifications performed by the investigator has revolutionized the study for its various diseases. Especially This leads to the possibility of genetic modification to treat genetic diseases. For example, transcription activator-like effector nucleases (TALENs) and zinc-finger nucleases (ZFNs) were emerging in gene editing system, the recent development of CRISPR technology (Clustered regularly interspaced short palindromic repeats) are becoming valuable tools for biomedical research, drug discovery and development, and even gene therapy as Fig. (**1**) [4]. Moreover, for safety reasons, protein levels, without DNA and RNA modification, of the three delivery systems are also quickly researched for functional modification as our publication [47] and Table **4**.

Table 4. DNA, RNA and protein level genetic modification.

Level	DNA/RNA			Protein		
Modified Methods	ZFNs	TALENs	CRISPR/Cas-9	ZFNs	TALENs	CRISPR/Cas-9
Function	gene-edition	gene-edition	gene-edition	gene-affinity	gene-affinity	gene-affinity
Techniques	Viral vectors			chemical (ZnCl2, L-arg)	chemical (cys-D-arg)9	HDR (mutation)
	Non-Viral vectors			physical (cold shock, repeat)	physical (1M NaOH, SFM)	

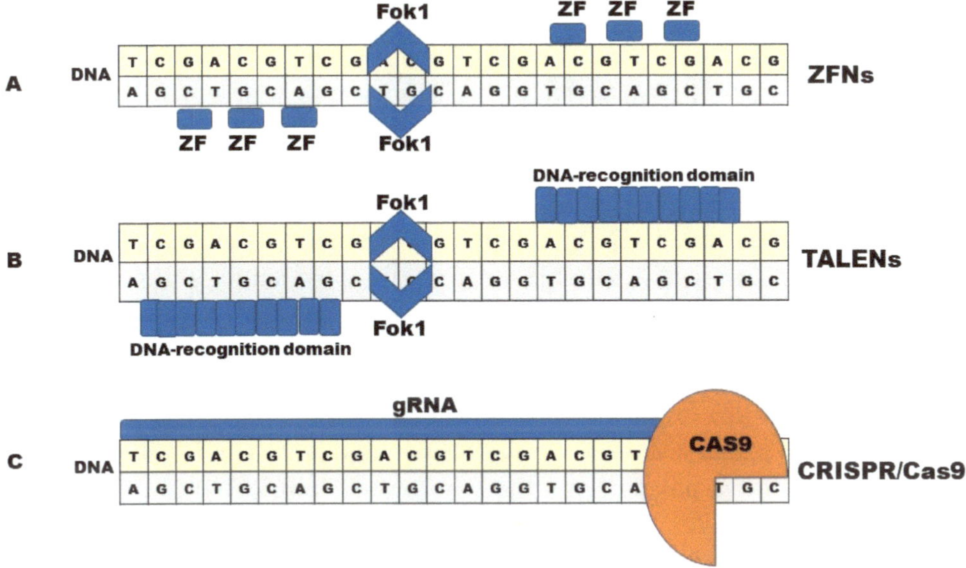

Fig. (1). Genetic modification and gene editing for personalized immunotherapy.
A is zinc-finger nucleases, **B** is transcription activator-like effector nucleases (TALENs). **C** is CRISPR/CAS9
(Clustered regularly interspaced short palindromic repeats)

In addition, enzymes of specific digestion at the genomic level are increasingly
studied as Table **5** [5, 6]. In order to address gene-editing techniques for adoptive
T-cell immunotherapy, this chapter will introduce the clinical development of
different gene therapy and gene editing, the background of T-cell immunotherapy
by using gene-editing techniques and then discuss the current application of
adoptive T-cell immunotherapy by using gene-editing techniques.

DEVELOPMENT OF VECTORS OF CLINICAL GENE THERAPY

After maturing in molecular cloning, gene transfer techniques have given
scientists the possibility for clinical therapies with many genetic and tumor
diseases since the late 1980s [7]. Because first clinical trials were initiated for
children with severe combined immune deficiency (SCID) due to mutations in the
adenosine deaminase (ADA) gene [8], the child has the concurrent treatment of
ADA injections impairing the success of gene therapy, and thus, limit the
technique development. After two decades' development, the "return of gene
therapy" has considered a major scientific breakthrough since 2009 [9]. Typically,
the concept of gene therapy includes *ex vivo* gene therapy, which is transferring
the gene into cells that had been removed from the patient and *in vivo* gene
therapy, which is directly infusing gene into the patient [10]. Clinically, *ex vivo*

gene therapy with their techniques consist of viral vectors or non-viral process into hematopoietic stem cells (HSCs) and primary lymphocytes [11]. For transferring techniques of clinical application, viral delivery utilizes a viral vector such as AAVs, lentiviruses, and adenoviruses to encapsulate a gene, in RNA or DNA form, to facilitate efficient delivery [12]. Non-viral delivery includes physical methods (electroporation, micro-fluidic-based technologies), nanomaterial-based methods (cationic lipids, and cell-penetrating peptides), and self-assembled nanoparticle [13]. Although *ex vivo* transfection enables the use of physical methods that are not suitable very well for systemic application, viral vectors are commonly used to transfer genes into cells and tissue which have been achieved during the past decade. Now viral vector systems can provide useful tools to deliver genetic and genome-editing systems for both translational and clinical applications *in vitro, ex vivo,* and *in vivo.* Moreover, retroviral vectors, adenoviral vectors, and AAV vectors have been extensively studied in preclinical models, and thus, they have been tested in several clinical trials. Clinically, retroviral and lentiviral vectors will be first considered *ex vivo* delivery systems into HSCs or primary lymphocytes to express therapeutic genes with relatively high transfection efficiency stably.

Table 5. Genome-editing nucleases.

Nuclease Domain	Property	Type of DSB	Associated Reagents
FokI	Type IIS, dimeric, non-specific nuclease	3-nt 5′ overhang	ZFNs, TALENs, Cas9-FokI
I-TevI	GIY-YIG, monomeric, site-specific	2-nt 3′ overhang	ZFEs, TALENs, MegaTev, TevCas9
PvuII	Type IIP, homodimeric, site-specific	Blunt end	I-SceI-PvuII, ZF-PvuII, PvuII-LHE
Recombinase	Serine recombinase (Sin recombinase); invertase Gin	Not applicable	ZF-recombinase, TALE-recombinase
Cas9	Type II CRISPR/Cas family	Blunt end	CRISPR/Cas9, CRISPRi, Cas9-FokI
Cpf1	Monomeric	5-nt 5′ overhang	CRISPR/Cpf1
Meganuclease	LAGLIDADG family, monomeric or dimeric; very specific	4-nt 3′ overhang	MegaTAL, TALE-I-SceI, MegaTev

BACKGROUND OF GENE EDITING FOR ADOPTIVE T-CELL IMMUNOTHERAPY

Most adoptive T-cell immunotherapy is to use autologous T-cells collected from peripheral blood mononuclear cells (PBMN) or from tumor tissue of patients, which called tumor-infiltrating lymphocyte (TIL). According to some reports of clinical laboratories, cell manufacturing of TIL is challenging to approach enough numbers of lymphocyte, enough quality resulting in poor effective treatment. Besides, even if patients achieve successful collection, they still need to wait several weeks to months for cell manufacturing and quality control. For these reasons, some scientists study ready-made T-cells obtained from allogeneic donor T-cells, to solve the problem of T-cell collections and long-term manufacture process. Allogeneic donor T-cells have two questions that need to be addressed: Graft *versus* Host Disease (GVHD) [14] and T-cell immunosuppression [15], called as T-cell silence, in the tumor microenvironment (TME). Based on the two issues as introduced above, using gene-editing technologies can address the two questions regarding T-cell GVHD and immune silence in TME so that gene-editing technologies can be developed for adoptive T-cell therapies. The application of gene editing to immunotherapy can potentially allow for finer tuning of the immune response, performing a more specific activity, increasing immune cell function, and playing more potential for ready-made use. Several gene-editing technologies have recently been applied to T-cell immunotherapy, and the most powerful is the clustered regularly interspaced short palindromic repeats (CRISPR)-CRISPR-associated 9 (Cas9) platform. The following parts present the gene-editing strategy and discuss how we can apply for adoptive T-cell immunotherapy.

APPLICATION OF GENE EDITING FOR T-CELL IMMUNOTHERAPY

1. Gene Editing of T-cells as a Universal Donor

As described above, the use of allogeneic T cells immunotherapy is limited by GVHD, which is mainly initiated by T cell receptor (TCR) activation. In order to resolve the question, universal donors of ready-made (now named as off-th--shelf) T-cells have been broadly researched by TCR construction for T-cell immunotherapy so that gene-editing technologies could be used to generate a universal T cell that could be infused to any unmatched recipient as Fig. (**2**). For instance, scientists working in MD Anderson Cancer Center generated a ZFN able to specifically knock out the endogenous TCR, blocking their ability to recognize recipient peptides resulting in GVHD [16]. Disruption of the T-cell receptor alpha chain (TRAC) gene has also been achieved using TALEN technology in CD19 CAR T cells (UCART19) [17]. Two children patients with relapsed B-ALL were treated with UCART19 because both patients experienced CAR-mediated disease control and developed GVHD [18]. Several new preclinical studies have been reported using CRISPR technology to both increases the application of CAR T-cells and enhance CAR T cell activity [19]. In a recent report from a group, multiplex genome editing was achieved using the CRISPR/Cas9 system to disrupt

TCR alpha simultaneously, and beta chains (TRAC and TRBC) in NY-ESO1 TCR engineered T cells. Optimization of sgRNA delivery resulted in >95% disruption of TCR expression, and this disruption significantly impaired allogeneic activity *in vitro* [20]. CRISPR technology was employed to target the TRAC locus so that a CD19 CAR construct was engineered with flanking homology domains that resulted in the integration of the CAR gene within the TRAC locus. The primary advantage of this technology is site-specific integration of the CAR gene, which eliminates the possibility of an integration event that leads to the disruption of an essential gene, as well as endogenous promoter-driven expression. Moreover, integration of the CAR19 gene into the TRAC locus allowed for a more physiological regulation (TCR-like) of CAR function, leading to better antitumor activity than standard CAR engineering [21].

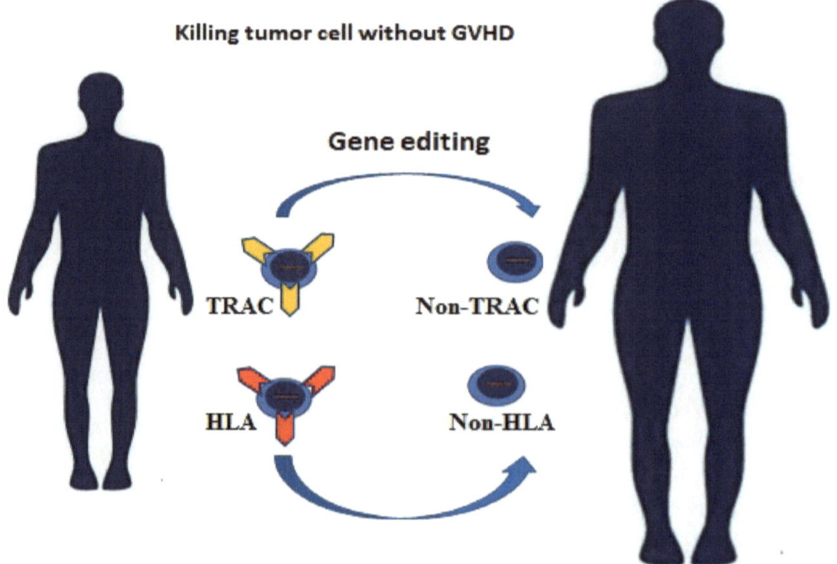

Fig. (2). TRAC and HLA depletion of allogeneic T-cell to T-cell ready-made immunotherapy.

A requirement for the development of universal T cells is to prevent donor T cell rejection. TCR-negative universal T cells could be rejected by recipient T cells through recognition of non-self HLA. Elimination of HLA molecules from T cells using gene-editing technologies like ZFN or CRISPR-Cas9 has been studied as a mechanism of this rejection [22, 23]. Moreover, new generation enzyme (such as meganucleases) has been used to knock out beta-2-microglobulin (together with the TCR) to obtain HLA class I negative T cells so that T-cell immunotherapy can make avoid T cell-mediated rejection [24].

2. Biomarker Depletion of Allogeneic Stem Cell to Support CAR-T Biomarker of Non-Specific Targets

Antigen-directed immunotherapies such as CAR-T or antibody-drug conjugates (ADCs) to some diseases (such as acute myeloid leukemia, AML) are associated with severe toxicities due to the lack of specific targetable antigens that can distinguish leukemic cells from normal myeloid cells or myeloid progenitors [25]. For example, CD33 expressed on both normal and malignant myeloid cells, and its expression is found in>90% adult and childhood AML blasts and on leukemia stem cells [26]. Both in preclinical and clinical studies, anti-CD33 therapy using CART33 or mAbs, such as Lintuzumab (SGN33) and Gemtuzumab Ozogamicin (GO), have shown a good response in a subset of AML [27 - 30]. Despite such good responses in preclinical and clinical AML studies, anti-CD33 therapies were not in routine use in AML patients until recently for several reasons. In preclinical models, hematopoietic toxicities, including cytopenia and reduction in myeloid progenitors, were observed [31 - 33]. Myelosuppression was associated with severe impairment of immune and clotting functions due to severe neutropenia and thrombocytopenia,

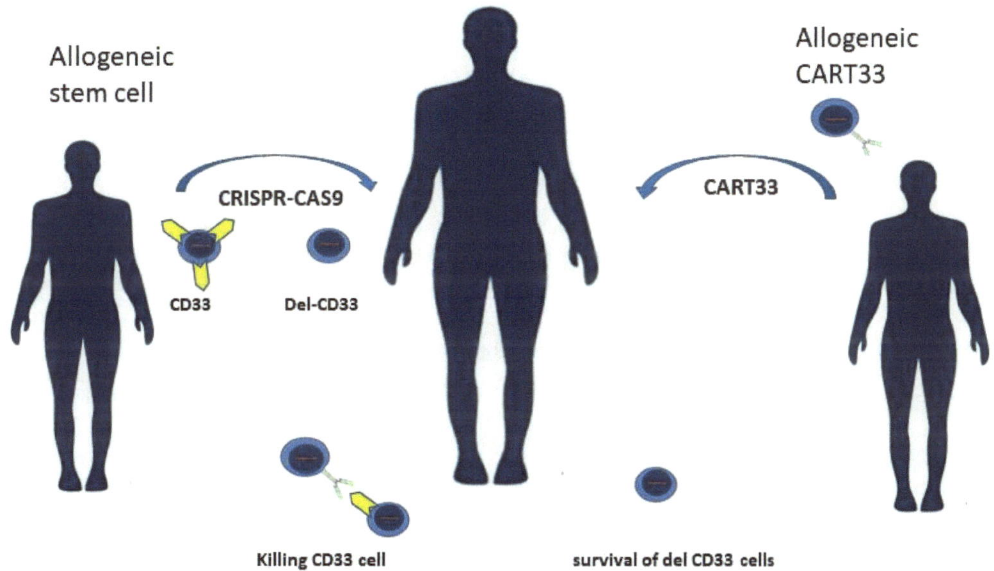

Fig. (3). CD33 depletion of allogeneic stem cell to support CAR-T 33 non-specific targets.

respectively. According to the strategy, a group reported an approach to treat AML by targeting the lineage-specific myeloid antigen CD33 [33 - 36]. They combined CD33-targeted CAR-T cells or the ADC Gemtuzumab Ozogamicin with the transplantation of hematopoietic stem cells that have been engineered to ablate CD33 expression using genomic engineering methods. Their results demonstrated that highly efficient genetic ablation of CD33 antigen using CRISPR/Cas9 technology in human stem/progenitor cells (HSPC) so that the evidence that the deletion of CD33 in HSPC doesn't impair their ability to engraft and to repopulate a functional multilineage hematopoietic system *in vivo*. Whole-genome sequencing and RNA sequencing analysis revealed no detectable off-target mutagenesis and no loss of functional p53 pathways [37 - 39]. They further modeled a post-remission marrow with minimal residual disease and showed that the transplantation of CD33-ablated HSPCs with CD33-targeted immunotherapy leads to leukemia clearance. As Fig. (**3**), engraftment has not any myelosuppression because multilineage descendants of CD33-ablated HSPCs can be recovered.

The strategy can contribute to the advancement of targeted immunotherapy so that they can develop into other malignancies. For example, a group from Baylor has designed a method to engineer CAR T cells to target T-cell antigens. A major curb in the design of T-cell immunotherapies targeting T-cells is fratricidal, resulting in their cytotoxicity activated by antigens they themselves express. In a recent report, the authors used CRISPR/Cas9 editing to knockout CD7, an antigen unique to T cells, and then engineered CD7-deplete cells to express a CAR targeting CD7 [40]. These CD7 CAR T-cells demonstrated efficacy *in vitro*, confirming the feasibility of this platform. The immunodeficiency resulting from pan-T cell depletion, however, would remain a significant barrier to the clinical translation of this strategy.

3. Depletion of Immunosuppression for T-cell Function

In normal T-cell physiology, naturally-occurring "off signals" exist to ensure appropriate control of the robust and cascading T-cell response. These inhibitory signals terminate T-cell activation and inhibit further effector functions, avoiding possible side effects as autoimmunity or uncontrolled inflammation. Several studies have demonstrated that increased expression of these inhibitory molecules such as PD-1, CTLA-4, TIM-3, and LAG-3) in T cells permits immune evasion by tumor cells [41], and thus, therapies have been developed that specifically block this inhibitory signal to prevent T-cell immunosuppression. The design has demonstrated impressive success in both solid tumors [42, 43] and hematologic malignancies [42]. However, although the design can re-activate antitumor T cells, checkpoint inhibitors can also lead to autoimmunity by dis-inhibiting self-reactive T cells [43]. Now CAR and TCR T-cells used in the ACT are subject to studying immunosuppression within tumors and TME. Therefore gene-editing technologies have been applied to adoptive T-cell immunotherapy to interfere networks controlling T-cell exhaustion. As discussed above, gene editing techniques with TCR and HLA class I knock out in CAR T-cells [44] combined disrupted PD-1 in CD19 CAR T-cells. These results demonstrated enhanced anti-leukemia activity in a xenograft model of BALL, suggesting that genetic disruption of checkpoint molecules may enhance CAR T-cell activity. Further development of this technology allows the integration of several sgRNAs into the CAR lentiviral gene vector to achieve high-efficiency multiplex gene editing using single electroporation. This system demonstrated high fidelity in the disruption of up to four genes (TCR, HLA, PD-1, and CTLA-4) to generate universal CAR T-cells resistant to two inhibitory pathways [45]. Several clinical trials have studied the safety of using CRISPR/Cas9 technology to knockout exhaustion immunosuppression biomarkers. Some groups are studying the gene-editing system to block PD-1, CTLA-4, TIM-3, and LAG-3.

In addition, using CRISPR gene editing T-cells is also both to delete expression of PD-1 and to change native TCR, which is T-cell engineered using lentiviral vectors to express a transgenic T-cell receptor-targeted to tumor antigens. This strategy removes two barriers to the success of engineered cell therapies with keeping potent and highly effective antigen targeting [46].

CONCLUSION

CART19 is now an FDA-approved drug, and several CARTs are being studied so that a new generation of T-cell therapies emerge in the near future. The development of technologies that allow surgical gene-editing has opened new ways for the engineering of T-cells. CRISPR-Cas9, TALEN, and ZENs allow efficient and relatively simple gene knockout and are being applied to the new generation of universal T-cells, exhaustion-resistant T cells, and decrease on-target toxicity of redirected T-cells. The translational medicine results and data from early clinical trials are promising. Although clinical experience with these technologies, such as CRISPR-Cas9 is good, they still are required to confirm safety and efficacy. Several trials are ongoing so that early results will be available in the next few years. Furthermost, for safety reasons, the protein level of the three delivery systems without DNA and RNA modification is also quickly studied for functional modification as our publication [47]. The rapid development of T-cell therapies and gene-editing technology generates an opportunity to successfully treat more patients with tumor diseases using engineered T-cell products.

CONSENT FOR PUBLICATION

Not applicable.

CONFLICT OF INTEREST

The authors declare no financial interests.

ACKNOWLEDGEMENTS

During the early period, JQD, BL, and GXQ under the guidance of SSC, set up first cell-based gene therapy, as described in the chapter. BL further study more than 25 years for TIL immunotherapy, including setting up single-cell methods to analyze genomic profiles including CD3+, CD3+CD8+ from liver cancer during 1999-2007 in Case Western Reserve University and then BL set up bioinformatics analysis from a single cell. The research was previously supported by National Cancer Institute IRG-91-022-09, USA (to BL).

The mention of trade names or commercial products in this article is solely to provide specific information and does not imply recommendation.

REFERENCES

[1]   Shudo K. From cancer prevention to cancer treatment. Yakugaku Zasshi 2000; 120(10): 987-95.
        [http://dx.doi.org/10.1248/yakushi1947.120.10_987] [PMID: 11082709]

[2]   Li B, Wei X, Qian GX, Zhang XH, Dong SQ, Chen SS. Methodology of TNF gene transduction of tumor-infiltrating lymphocytes. J Shanghai Sec Med Uni 1995; 15: 3.

[3]   Ding JQ, Qian GX, Li B, Wei X, Zhu YM, Liang H, *et al.* A preliminary study of tumor necrosis factor gene transduction of tumor-infiltrating lymphocytes Application. Chinese J Cancer Biotherapy 1995. 01

[4]   Chen KY, Knoepfler PS. To CRISPR and beyond: the evolution of genome editing in stem cells. Regen Med 2016; 11(8): 801-16.
        [http://dx.doi.org/10.2217/rme-2016-0107] [PMID: 27905217]

[5]   Guha TK, Edgell DR. Applications of Alternative Nucleases in the Age of CRISPR/Cas9. Int J Mol Sci 2017; 18(12): 1-13.
        [PMID: 29186020]

[6]   Liu J, Gaj T, Yang Y, *et al.* Efficient delivery of nuclease proteins for genome editing in human stem cells and primary cells. Nat Protoc 2015; 10(11): 1842-59.
        [http://dx.doi.org/10.1038/nprot.2015.117] [PMID: 26492140]

[7]   Kamarck ME, Barbosa JA, Kühn L, Peters PG, Shulman L, Ruddle FH. Somatic cell genetics and flow cytometry. Cytometry 1983; 4(2): 99-108.
        [http://dx.doi.org/10.1002/cyto.990040202] [PMID: 6354642]

[8]   Sheridan C. Gene therapy finds its niche. Nat Biotechnol 2011; 29(2): 121-8.
        [http://dx.doi.org/10.1038/nbt.1769] [PMID: 21301435]

[9]   Castanotto D, Rossi JJ. The promises and pitfalls of RNA-interference-based therapeutics. Nature 2009; 457(7228): 426-33.
        [http://dx.doi.org/10.1038/nature07758] [PMID: 19158789]

[10]   Lipinski C, Hopkins A. Navigating chemical space for biology and medicine. Nature 2004; 432(7019): 61-855.
        [http://dx.doi.org/10.1038/nature03193]

[11]   Li B, Ding J, Larson A, Song S. Tumor tissue recycling--a new combination treatment for solid tumors: Experimental and preliminary clinical research. *In Vivo* 1999; 13(5): 433-8.
[PMID: 10654199]

[12]   Joung J, Konermann S, Gootenberg JS, *et al.* Genome-scale CRISPR-Cas9 knockout and transcriptional activation screening. Nat Protoc 2017; 12(4): 828-63.
[http://dx.doi.org/10.1038/nprot.2017.016] [PMID: 28333914]

[13]   Yin H, Kanasty RL, Eltoukhy AA, Vegas AJ, Dorkin JR, Anderson DG. Non-viral vectors for gene-based therapy. Nat Rev Genet 2014; 15(8): 541-55.
[http://dx.doi.org/10.1038/nrg3763] [PMID: 25022906]

[14]   Bryant AR, Perales MA. Advances in *ex vivo* T Cell Depletion - Where Do We Stand? Adv Cell Gene Ther 2019; 2(1)e29
[http://dx.doi.org/10.1002/acg2.29] [PMID: 31106295]

[15]   Li B, Shen DH. Preliminary study on the resting status of tumor-infiltrating lymphocytes. Chinese Microbiology and Immunology (Chinese) 1994; 14(6): 399-402.

[16]   Torikai H, Reik A, Liu PQ, *et al.* A foundation for universal T-cell based immunotherapy: T cells engineered to express a CD19-specific chimeric-antigen-receptor and eliminate expression of endogenous TCR. Blood 2012; 119(24): 5697-705. [one of the first reports of Zinc-finger nucleases to generate TCR knockout in T cells.].
[http://dx.doi.org/10.1182/blood-2012-01-405365] [PMID: 22535661]

[17]   Poirot L, Philip B, Schiffer-Mannioui C, Le Clerre D, Chion-Sotinel I, Derniame S, *et al.* Multiplex Genome-Edited T-cell Manufacturing Platform for "Off-the-Shelf" Adoptive T-cell Immunotherapies. Cancer research 2015; 75(18): 3853-64.

[18]   Qasim W, Zhan H, Samarasinghe S, Adams S, Amrolia P, Stafford S, *et al.* Molecular remission of infant B-ALL after infusion of universal TALEN gene-edited CAR T cells. Sci Transl Med 2017; 9(374) the first report on the use of TALEN-edited CART19 for BALL
[http://dx.doi.org/10.1126/scitranslmed.aaj2013]

[19]   Singh N, Shi J, June CH, Ruella M. Genome-editing technologies in adoptive T cell immunotherapy for cancer. Curr Hematol Malig Rep 2017; 12(6): 522-9.
[http://dx.doi.org/10.1007/s11899-017-0417-7] [PMID: 29039115]

[20]   Ren J, Liu X, Fang C, Jiang S, June CH, Zhao Y. Multiplex Genome Editing to Generate Universal CAR T Cells Resistant to PD1 Inhibition. Clin Cancer Res. 2017; 23(9): 66-2255. The important paper describing the generation and the activity of PD-1 knocked-out T cells.
[http://dx.doi.org/10.1158/1078-0432.CCR-16-1300]

[21]   Eyquem J, Mansilla-Soto J, Giavridis T, van der Stegen SJ, Hamieh M, Cunanan KM, *et al.* Targeting a CAR to the TRAC locus with CRISPR/Cas9 enhances tumor rejection. Nature 2017; 543(7643): 7-113. Seminal report on the specific insertion of the CAR19 gene in the TCR locus.

[22]   Torikai H, Reik A, Soldner F, *et al.* Toward eliminating HLA class I expression to generate universal cells from allogeneic donors. Blood 2013; 122(8): 1341-9. [Interesting work aimed at reducing rejection of universal T cells by the knockout of HLA.].
[http://dx.doi.org/10.1182/blood-2013-03-478255] [PMID: 23741009]

[23]   Ren J, Zhang X, Liu X, Fang C, Jiang S, June CH, *et al.* A versatile system for rapid multiplex genome-edited CAR T cell generation. Oncotarget. 2017 Important paper describing the generation of multiplex knock out in T cells.
[http://dx.doi.org/10.18632/oncotarget.15218]

[24]   ASGCT 19th Annual Meeting: Abstracts. Molecular therapy: The journal of the American Society of Gene Therapy 2016; 24(Suppl 1): S1- S304.

[25]   Alcantara M, Tesio M, June CH, Houot R. CAR T-cells for T-cell malignancies: challenges in distinguishing between therapeutic, normal, and neoplastic T-cells. Leukemia 2018; 32(11): 2307-15.

[http://dx.doi.org/10.1038/s41375-018-0285-8] [PMID: 30315238]

[26]   Morgan RA, Yang JC, Kitano M, Dudley ME, Laurencot CM, Rosenberg SA. Case report of a serious adverse event following the administration of T cells transduced with a chimeric antigen receptor recognizing ERBB2. Mol Ther 2010; 18(4): 843-51.
[http://dx.doi.org/10.1038/mt.2010.24] [PMID: 20179677]

[27]   Lamers CH, Sleijfer S, van Steenbergen S, *et al.* Treatment of metastatic renal cell carcinoma with CAIX CAR-engineered T cells: clinical evaluation and management of on-target toxicity. Mol Ther 2013; 21(4): 904-12.
[http://dx.doi.org/10.1038/mt.2013.17] [PMID: 23423337]

[28]   Dotti G, Gottschalk S, Savoldo B, Brenner MK. Design and development of therapies using chimeric antigen receptor-expressing T cells. Immunol Rev 2014; 257(1): 107-26.
[http://dx.doi.org/10.1111/imr.12131] [PMID: 24329793]

[29]   Davila ML, Riviere I, Wang X, *et al.* Efficacy and toxicity management of 19-28z CAR T cell therapy in B cell acute lymphoblastic leukemia. Sci Transl Med 2014; 6(224)224ra25
[http://dx.doi.org/10.1126/scitranslmed.3008226] [PMID: 24553386]

[30]   Kalos M, Levine BL, Porter DL, *et al.* T cells with chimeric antigen receptors have potent antitumor effects and can establish memory in patients with advanced leukemia. Sci Transl Med 2011; 3(95)95ra73
[http://dx.doi.org/10.1126/scitranslmed.3002842] [PMID: 21832238]

[31]   Porter DL, Levine BL, Kalos M, Bagg A, June CH. Chimeric antigen receptor-modified T cells in chronic lymphoid leukemia. N Engl J Med 2011; 365(8): 725-33.
[http://dx.doi.org/10.1056/NEJMoa1103849] [PMID: 21830940]

[32]   Laing AA, Harrison CJ, Gibson BES, Keeshan K. Unlocking the potential of anti-CD33 therapy in adult and childhood acute myeloid leukemia. Exp Hematol 2017; 54: 40-50.
[http://dx.doi.org/10.1016/j.exphem.2017.06.007] [PMID: 28668350]

[33]   Kung Sutherland MS, Walter RB, Jeffrey SC, *et al.* SGN-CD33A: a novel CD33-targeting antibody-drug conjugate using a pyrrolobenzodiazepine dimer is active in models of drug-resistant AML. Blood 2013; 122(8): 1455-63.
[http://dx.doi.org/10.1182/blood-2013-03-491506] [PMID: 23770776]

[34]   Jurcic JG. What happened to anti-CD33 therapy for acute myeloid leukemia? Curr Hematol Malig Rep 2012; 7(1): 65-73.
[http://dx.doi.org/10.1007/s11899-011-0103-0] [PMID: 22109628]

[35]   Kenderian SS, Ruella M, Shestova O, *et al.* CD33-specific chimeric antigen receptor T cells exhibit potent preclinical activity against human acute myeloid leukemia. Leukemia 2015; 29(8): 1637-47.
[http://dx.doi.org/10.1038/leu.2015.52] [PMID: 25721896]

[36]   Gill S, Tasian SK, Ruella M, *et al.* Preclinical targeting of human acute myeloid leukemia and myeloablation using chimeric antigen receptor-modified T cells. Blood 2014; 123(15): 2343-54.
[http://dx.doi.org/10.1182/blood-2013-09-529537] [PMID: 24596416]

[37]   Gomes-Silva D, Srinivasan M, Sharma S, *et al.* CD7-edited T cells expressing a CD7-specific CAR for the therapy of T-cell malignancies. Blood 2017; 130(3): 285-96.
[http://dx.doi.org/10.1182/blood-2017-01-761320] [PMID: 28539325]

[38]   Carbone DP, Reck M, Paz-Ares L, *et al.* CheckMate 026 Investigators. First-Line Nivolumab in Stage IV or Recurrent Non-Small-Cell Lung Cancer. N Engl J Med 2017; 376(25): 2415-26.
[http://dx.doi.org/10.1056/NEJMoa1613493] [PMID: 28636851]

[39]   Reck M, Rodríguez-Abreu D, Robinson AG, *et al.* KEYNOTE-024 Investigators. Pembrolizumab *versus* Chemotherapy for PD-L1-Positive Non-Small-Cell Lung Cancer. N Engl J Med 2016; 375(19): 1823-33.
[http://dx.doi.org/10.1056/NEJMoa1606774] [PMID: 27718847]

[40] Eggermont AM, Chiarion-Sileni V, Grob JJ, *et al.* Prolonged Survival in Stage III Melanoma with Ipilimumab Adjuvant Therapy. N Engl J Med 2016; 375(19): 1845-55.
[http://dx.doi.org/10.1056/NEJMoa1611299] [PMID: 27717298]

[41] Wolchok JD, Kluger H, Callahan MK, *et al.* Nivolumab plus ipilimumab in advanced melanoma. N Engl J Med 2013; 369(2): 122-33.
[http://dx.doi.org/10.1056/NEJMoa1302369] [PMID: 23724867]

[42] Brahmer JR, Tykodi SS, Chow LQ, *et al.* Safety and activity of anti-PD-L1 antibody in patients with advanced cancer. N Engl J Med 2012; 366(26): 2455-65.
[http://dx.doi.org/10.1056/NEJMoa1200694] [PMID: 22658128]

[43] Topalian SL, Hodi FS, Brahmer JR, *et al.* Safety, activity, and immune correlates of anti-PD-1 antibody in cancer. N Engl J Med 2012; 366(26): 2443-54.
[http://dx.doi.org/10.1056/NEJMoa1200690] [PMID: 22658127]

[44] Ansell SM, Lesokhin AM, Borrello I, *et al.* PD-1 blockade with nivolumab in relapsed or refractory Hodgkin's lymphoma. N Engl J Med 2015; 372(4): 311-9.
[http://dx.doi.org/10.1056/NEJMoa1411087] [PMID: 25482239]

[45] Yousefi H, Yuan J, Keshavarz-Fathi M, Murphy JF, Rezaei N. Immunotherapy of cancers comes of age. Expert Rev Clin Immunol 2017; 13(10): 1001-15.
[http://dx.doi.org/10.1080/1744666X.2017.1366315] [PMID: 28795649]

[46] Ren J, Zhang X, Liu X, *et al.* A versatile system for rapid multiplex genome-edited CAR T cell generation. Oncotarget 2017; 8(10): 17002-11.
[http://dx.doi.org/10.18632/oncotarget.15218] [PMID: 28199983]

[47] Li B, Zhu X, Hossain MA, *et al.* Fetal hemoglobin induction in sickle erythroid progenitors using a synthetic zinc finger DNA-binding domain. Haematologica 2018; 103(9): e384-7.
[http://dx.doi.org/10.3324/haematol.2017.185967] [PMID: 29622657]

CHAPTER 11

Genetically Modified T-cells Affinity to Tumor Cells-Development of Adoptive T-cell Immunotherapy

Shen Li[1], Supriya Perabekam[2], Emmanuelle Devemy[2] and Biaoru Li[2,3,*]

[1] *Division of Surgical Oncology, Massachusetts General Hospital Cancer Center and Harvard Medical School, Boston, MA, 02114, USA*

[2] *Rush Medical Center, Chicago, IL, USA*

[3] *Georgia Cancer Center and Department of Pediatrics, Medical College at GA, Augusta, GA 30912, USA*

Abstract: T-cells play an essential role in the cell-mediated immune response to tumor cells, while tumor cells in tumor sites take many strategies to evade the host immune response, including creating many immune-suppressive factors from tumor microenvironment (TME) or decreasing expression of immunogenicity of target antigens. To resolve the evasion of tumor cells from T-cells attacking, some strategies such as genetically modified T-cells altering the specificity of the T-cell receptor (TCR) or introducing antibody-like recognition of chimeric antigen receptors (CARs) have made significant advances. The modified TCR T-cells or CAR T-cells have been administered to cure B-cell lymphoma or B-lymphocyte leukemia in clinical trials successfully. We have been going to study the specificity and safety of T-cell adoptive immunotherapy for more than 30 years so that our experiences to apply for genetically modified T-cell more focus on the specificity and safety of these therapies. Moreover, the strategies using genetically modified T-cell immunotherapy need face challenges for immunogenicity from different types of tumors. The chapter will introduce T-cell specific affinity between T-cell and tumor cells such as TCR and CAR T-cells, discuss challenges from the selection of antigen targets, and address safety issues to clinical development. All in all, T-cell adoptive immunology regarding TCR and CAR T-cell improves the clinical application.

Keywords: Chimeric antigen receptors (CARs) T-cells, Personalized immunotherapy, T-cell Adoptive immunotherapy, TIL (tumor-infiltrating lymphocyte), Tumor microenvironment (TME), T-cell receptor (TCR) T-cells.

---

* **Corresponding author Biaoru Li**: Georgia Cancer Center and Department of Pediatrics, Medical College at GA, Augusta, GA 30912, USA; Tel: 440-317-1443; E-mail: bli@augusta.edu

INTRODUCTION

Since Steven Rosenberg had applied for tumor-infiltrating lymphocyte (TIL) to treat patients with melanoma in 1987 [1], T-cell immunotherapies of tumor diseases have birthed about thirty years. We have also studied TIL, and thus, administered TIL to treat solid tumors for several hundreds of tumor patients since the early 1990s [2]. T-cell immunotherapy has been developed so quickly that a few new methods have come out since then. However, there are some obstacles to effective adoptive T-cell immunotherapy of tumor disease. For example, T-cell immunotherapy, actuarily, could not proceed until it was established that immune responses could specifically distinguish tumor cells from normal cells [3]. T-cells have a function of immune surveillance; any target cell that is identified as non-self is eliminated [4]. The target cells include not only virally infected cells but also tumor cells, which acquire antigenicity, and therefore, immunogenicity can produce through the neoantigens (tumor-specific Ag or tumor-associated Ag) that can be recognized as non-self [5]. However, tumor cells have developed a mechanism to escape and suppress the immunogenicity, which leads to T-cell a failure to initiate antitumor immunity, and consequently facilitates tumor cells' development [6]. The mechanism of tumor cells includes a decrease of the expression of antigens, which evade host immunity, and tumor cells suppressing host immune response through the synthesis of different inhibiting factors, which block T-cell function. Following Research and Development (R&D) of immune therapy, increasing numbers of new therapies are being developed to apply for the T-cells to tumor cell targeting response through genetic modification of immune cells [7]. The chapter will focus on the development of treatment strategies that use genetically modified T-cell immunotherapies. The strategies of immunotherapy administer patients with a specific-molecule of T-cell to tumor cells expressing specific antigens by genetically modified T-cell immunotherapies. For instance, the T-cell receptor (TCR) of one clone T-cells can distinguish from other T-cells by the presence of T cell receptors (TCRs) on the cell surface [8]. TCR is a multi-subunit transmembrane complex that mediates the antigen-specific activation of T-cells [9]. TCR is composed of two different polypeptide chains, the TCR α, and β chains, as Fig. (**1A**). Both chains have an N-terminal variable region and a constant region. The chains are linked by a disulfide bond, with each receptor providing a single antigen-binding site. The TCR confers antigenic specificity on the T-cell, by recognizing an antigen ligand consisting of a short contiguous amino acid sequence of a protein that is presented on the target cell by a major histocompatibility complex (MHC I) molecule as Fig. (**1B**) [10]. Accessory affinity molecules expressed by T-cells, such as CD4 for MHC class II and CD8 for MHC class I, are also involved. TCR interacts with this ligand affinity for both the MHC molecule and the antigen peptide. Signal transduction is through the

CD3 complex, which consists of four different CD3 proteins that form two heterodimers (CD3δε and CD3γε) and one homodimer (CD3ζζ) [11]. The following affinity to their cognate peptides presented by MHC class I molecules, and hence, naive CD8+T-cells proliferate quickly and acquire phenotypic and functional properties leading to those to act as effector T-cells to killing tumor cells. For instance, CD8+T-cells eliminate tumor cells expressing the antigen through apoptosis-inducing ligands or the release of lytic granules. In addition, long-term memory T-cells are generated that can self-renew, keeping fast expansion in the presence of the target antigen and providing a sustained response to the same antigen upon re-exposure [12]. In conclusion, the function of T-cells is employed by the specificity of the TCR as a conductor for the adaptive immune response.

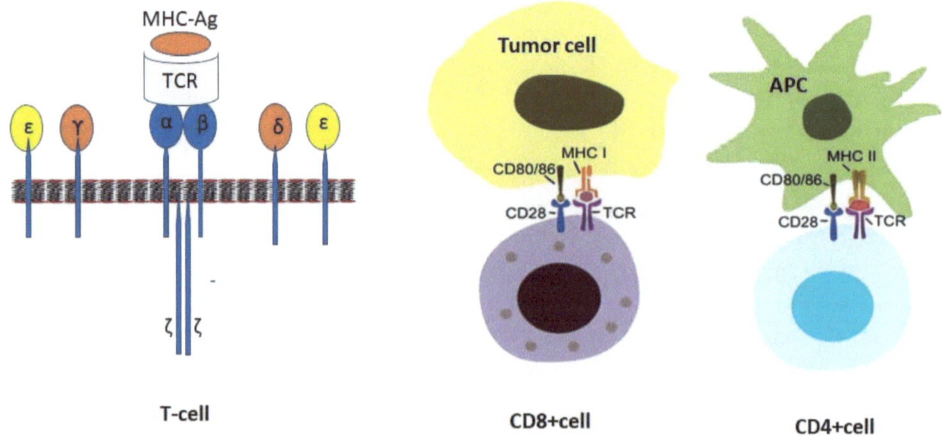

Fig. (1). T-cells and CD8+cell and CD4+cell Membrane Signaling Protein. Fig. (**1A**) demonstrates T-cells membrane signaling molecules, and Fig. (**1B**) shows the difference between CD8+ and CD4+ cells.

In order to make a clear understanding of adoptive T-cell immunotherapy with genetical modification for specific affinity, in the chapter, we will first introduce history and development of genetical modification for immunotherapy and then present availability of T-cells with different phases of a clinical trial of TCR T-cell and CAR T-cell immunotherapy as reported in publications. Finally, we will discuss the future of adoptive TCR T-cell and CAR T-cell immunotherapy.

HISTORY AND DEVELOPMENT OF TCR AND CAR IMMUNE THERAPY

A study on T-cell specific affinity to tumor cells regarding TCR T-cell and CAR T-cell of T-cell adoptive immunology is over 30 years. First chimeric TCR for T-cell specific affinity by anti-TNP mRNA cloning into TCR v-chain and c-chain to targeting cell was reported in 1989 [13]. According to the evidence reported in PNAS, in 1989, Dr. Shen (Fig. **2A**) had tried to design DHBsAb from Duck Hepatitis B Virus (DHBV) to clone into CD3 of TIL forming DHBsAb-CD3 CAR T-cells as same as current design of CAR T-cells. As we know, DHBV from Chinese duck is the same family as the hepatitis B virus (HBV) from humans as Fig. (**2B**). DHBV has a similar structure and function of HBV such as a small DNA virus in a diameter of 42 nm. The viral envelope is made up of the host cell lipid, with viral surface antigens (DHBsAg) [14]. The icosahedral nucleocapsid is composed of the virus core antigen (DHBcAg) and surrounds the DNA genome and viral polymerase. Because DHBsAg has almost as homologous sequences as those of HBsAg, it has similar function and structure of HBsAg to confer specific affinity of the virus to the duck hepatic cell containing DHBV infection as human hepatitis B virus-related to hepatic cancer [15], we began to study TIL with chimeric DHBsAb targeting HBsAg of hepatic cancer cells (HCC) infected by HBV as Fig. (**3**). Although we achieved a successful result for DHBV-LSP inducting animal model of hepatic necrosis as reported in 1989 [16] and successfully set up TIL culture and clone technique as reported in 1995 [17], we failed to achieve DHBsAb-CD3 chimeric TILs to specific affinity both DHBV and HBV infected HCC cells due to knowledge limitation of CD3 and TCR structure in that early period [18].

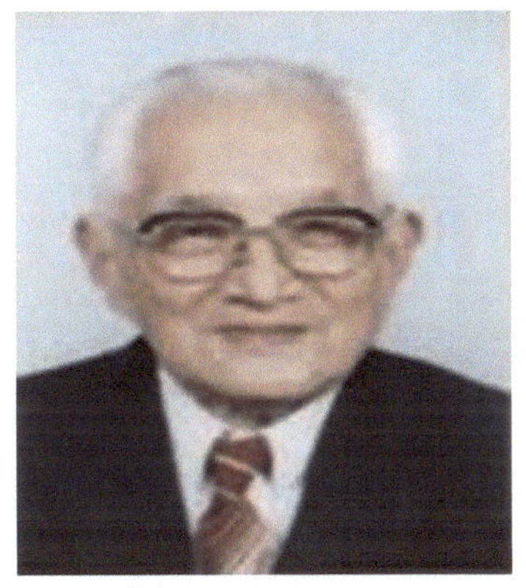

Shen, Dinghong
(1910-2011)

A

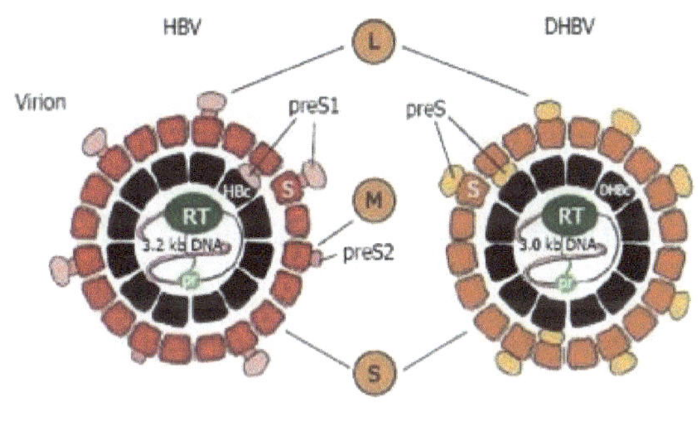

B

Fig. (2). T-cells affinity to hepatic cancer cells. Fig. (**2A**) Dr. Shen first designed the DHBV-LPS model to induce hepatic cell necrosis (1986) and chimeric DHBsAb-CD3 TIL affinity HBV HCC (1989); Fig. (**2B**) structure of DHBV and HBV.

After successfully reported synthetic immunoglobulin/TCR chimeric molecule with antibody-like specificity in 1987-1989, Irving and Weiss further discovered that CD8 and the CD3ζ chain could independently mediate T-cell activation of the endogenous TCR [19] so that CARs consist of an extracellular domain for tumor antigen recognition and one or more intracellular signaling domains that mediate T-cell activation. The antigen-binding single-chain variable fragment (scFv) consists of the variable heavy (VH) and variable light (VL) chains of an antibody, fused by a peptide spacer of ~15 residues in length [20]. An intracellular signaling molecule comprised of the TCR CD3ζ signaling chain or more intracellular signaling domains of another immune receptor. The immune receptor-tyrosin--based-activation-motif (ITAM) contains protein sequences, tandem costimulation domains such as the 4-1BB or CD28 signaling modules. First-generation CARs contain CD3ζ alone, while second-generation chimeric receptors incorporate a costimulatory endodomain (4-1BB/CD3ζ) and third-generation chimeric receptors with CD28/4-1BB/CD3 ζ as Fig. (**4**). Now all CAR T-cells generally consist of 3 parts: an ectodomain containing an scFv for recognition of specific antigen, a transmembrane domain, and an endodomain including a CD3 ζ chain with 3 immunoreceptor tyrosine-based activation motifs (ITAMs). The main advantage of using CAR-based approaches for cancer immunotherapy is that the scFv is derived from an antibody with specific affinities, including following several orders of magnitude from modified TCR [21 - 23].

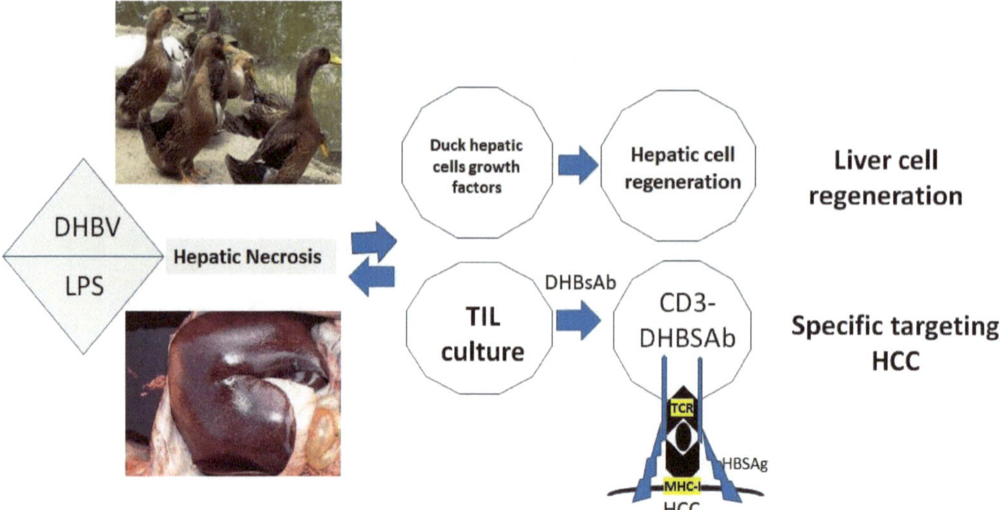

Fig. (3). T-cells chimeric affinity to hepatic cancer cells by DHBsAb-CD3.

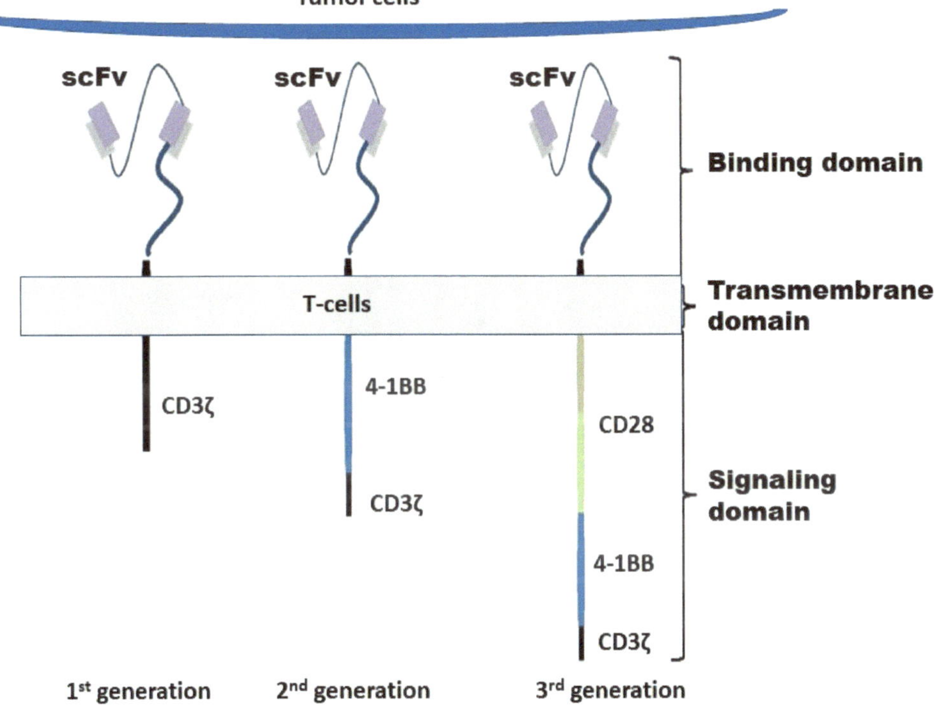

Fig. (4). Three generations of CAR-T-cell.

As described above, although CAR was first studied in the late 1980s, these synthetic chimeric antigen receptors were not confirmed to effective treatment before 2006 [24]. The initial results had shown 50% antitumor effects (4 of 8 children with metastatic neuroblastoma) using a single infusion of first-generation CAR T-cells containing CD3ζ alone, by which patients showed short survival after first-generation CAR T-cell treatment because CAR T-cells did not further proliferate *in vivo*. Moreover, CD28 and 4-1BB signaling domains into CARs can be discovered to recapitulate functional costimulation leading to the potency of engineered T-cells. CD137 (4-1BB) signaling domain was demonstrated as a critical determinant of survival and proliferation of CAR T-cells. 4-1BB with CD3 ζ is better than CD28 costimulation or CD3ζ signaling alone in CAR T-cells [25, 26]. The 4-1BB/CD3ζ delivered by lentiviral vector transduction was first found that these CAR T-cells are capable of on-target chronic lymphocytic leukemia (CLL) with clinical significance, so that these designs lead to producing autologous CD19 CAR-T cells to treat B-cell lymphoma [27, 28]. Recent trials of CAR T-cells have also developed in different hematological malignancies.

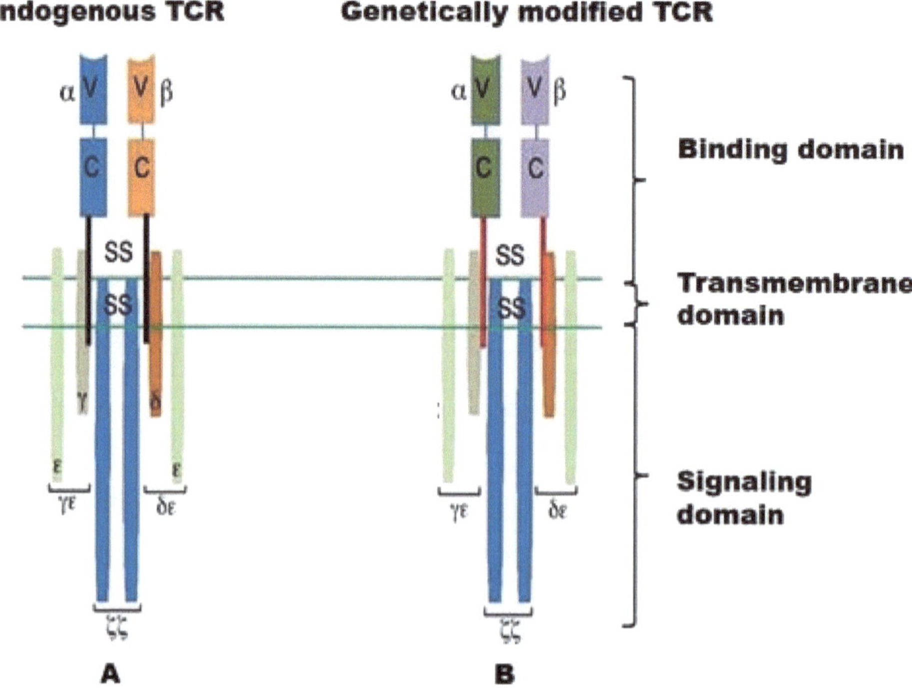

Fig. (5). TCR-genetically modified T-cell. Fig. (**5A**) is natural TCR, and Fig. (**5B**) is genetically modified TCR T-cell.

CAR T-cell therapy has shown excellent results against hematological malignancies; however, its effect against solid tumors is unsatisfactory by comparison of TCR T-cells. After several years' effort, TCR engineered T-cells have demonstrated better responses against solid tumors than those of CAR engineering T-cells. TCRs depend on their interaction with peptide-major histocompatibility complex (MHC), complexes formed by peptide bound to MHC [29]. Intracellular antigens are cut up into peptide chains and displayed by MHC molecules to form peptide-MHCs. CD8+T-cell produce peptide-MHCs by ribosomal translation products, which are cleaved into peptide chains by proteolysis at cytoplasm and functional peptides, are bound to MHC class I, which are expressed on all nucleated cell surface. On the other side, antigen-presenting cells (APCs) internalize foreign proteins by endocytosis and cleave them into peptide chains to bind to MHC class II. T-cell receptors from T-cells so that they can be matched to human leukocyte antigen (HLA) alleles of patients, allowing these peptide-MHC class I binding and killing cancer cells [30].

As Fig. (**5**) A to B, TCR-engineered T cell has TCR consisting of an α chain and a β chain, each containing a variable domain (v) and a constant domain (c), as well as an unlabeled transmembrane domain and 6 CD3 chains for T-cell activation. MHC Class I consists of an α chain with 3 domains a1, a2, a3, and a β2-microglobulin, presenting peptides derived from proteolysis of intracellular proteins [31]. Now several genetically modified TCR has been researched as Fig. (**6**).

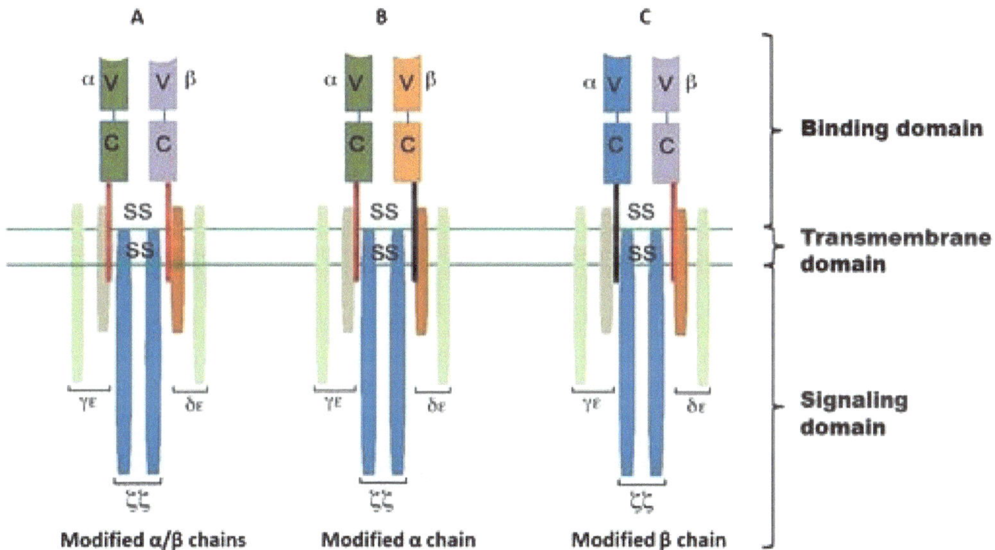

Fig. (6). Different TCR-genetically modified T-cells. Fig. (**6A**) has genetically modified α/βTCR T-cells, and Fig. (**6B**) has genetically modified a chain T-cell, and Fig. (**6C**) is genetically modified /βTCR T-cells.

The different structures of CAR T-cells and TCR T-cells are shown in Fig. (**7**). CAR T-cells employ antibody-antigen recognition machinery that consists of an scFv derived from an antibody to bind to antigens on the target cell's surface, which activates immune responses along with transmembrane domains and costimulatory domains within T-cells. However, most proteins are expressed inside cells, while only about 28% is expressed on the cell surface so that antigens are limited by CAR-T-cell targets [32]. According to a recent study, the full-length TCR T-cells have greater sensitivity than CAR T-cells, although CARs are expressed at higher densities. This higher sensitivity of TCR T-cells can enable the quick killing of tumor cells, although these increases the risk of "on-target, off-tumor" toxicity. TCR T-cells are shown the release of fewer amounts of cytokines after treatment, and thus, cytokine release syndromes (CRS) should be lower by TCR T-cell therapy than those of CAR T-cell therapy [33]. Furthermore, TCR T-cells have been discovered to administer in both solid tumors and hematological cancers successfully. Now results of genetically modified TCR T-cells have been confirmed that good therapy is involved in MHC complexes to specifically target the antigens expressed by tumor cells while higher densities expressed by CAR T-cells have found to better administer in hematological cancers such as B-cell lymphoma and B-lymphocyte leukemia [34] as Fig. (7).

GENERATION OF CLINICALLY EFFECTIVE TCR T-CELL AND CAR T-CELLS

The production of CAR T-cells and TCR T-cells involves four steps: (I) cell collection from a patient, (II) T-cell enrichment with the removal of other cells, (III) transgene delivery, and (IV) *ex vivo* expansion [35]. As Table **1**, one of the critical manufacturing is efficient isolation of T-cells from leukapheresis. Leukapheresis products from cancer patients consist of a heterogeneous population of cells including T-cells, myeloid cells, natural killer cells, erythroid cells, and malignant cells. The application of positive and negative selection methods can enrich T-cells to exclude autologous peripheral blood mononuclear cells and leukemia cells. Thus, efficient T-cell purification and tumor cell purging will improve the safety and potency of cellular products for adoptive transfer therapies [36].

In order to achieve durable clinical responses to cell-based gene therapies, permanent transgene expression is often required. Murine gamma-retroviruses and lentiviruses are two available clinical gene therapy vector systems that afford long-term CAR and TCR transgene expression. Considerable clinical evidence shows that retroviral vectors are safe when expressed in human T-cells [37]. In contrast, lentiviral vectors, especially third-generation self-inactivating vectors, have a lower risk of insertional mutagenesis, which may be attributed to the absence of strong enhancer elements present in oncogenic murine gamma-retroviruses. Lentiviral vectors also have substantially higher efficiency for genetically engineering human T-cells [38, 39]. It may be possible to develop clinically feasible cellular manufacturing processes based on guided integration of antigen receptor transgenes into specific loci using viral and non-viral methods.

Clinical studies are currently being conducted to evaluate the safety and efficacy of CAR T-cells and TCR T-cells, including leukapheresis, T-cell enrichment with purity and quantity, transgene delivery with vector selection, and *ex vivo* expansion under GMP condition [40]. Differences in CAR T-cells and TCR T-cells are shown in Table **1**.

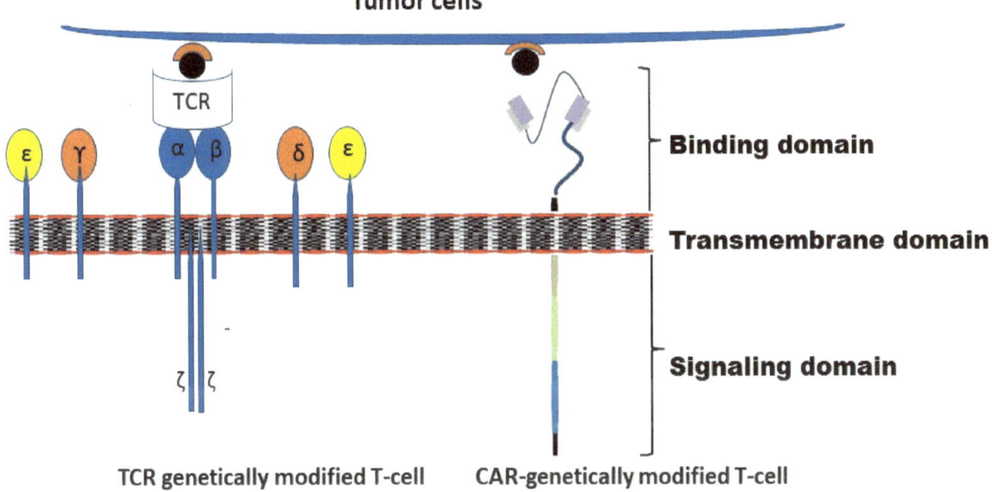

Fig. (7). Difference between TCR-genetically modified T-cells and CAR-genetically modified T-cells.

Table 1. TIL, CAR-T-cells and TCR T-cells.

	TIL	TCR	CAR
First efficacy	1987	2006	2013
Production method	Isolation of T cells from tumors and expansion *ex vivo*	Isolation of peripheral T cells *via* apheresis and *ex vivo* transduction with a TCR against the tumor antigen	Isolation of peripheral T cells *via* apheresis and *ex vivo* transduction with a CAR against the tumor antigen
Target	MHC-peptide complex	MHC-peptide complex	Non-MHC cell surface proteins
Lymphodepleting preparative regimen	Yes	Yes	Yes
Supportive IL-2	Yes	Varying	No
Specificity	Polyclonal	Monoclonal	Monoclonal
Main toxicity	Lymphodepleting regimen	Lymphodepleting regimen	Lymphodepleting regimen
	IL-2 mediated (chills, fever, edema)	"On-target, off-tumor"	"On-target, off-tumor"
	Seldom autoimmune	CRS	CRS
			Neurological

Restrictions	Heterogeneous infusion product	MHC-restricted	Currently only effective for the treatment of hematological malignancies.
	Low toxicity	Toxicity	Toxicity

CLINICAL TRIALS OF TCR T-CELL AND CAR T-CELL

Although a few clinical successes are reported by CAR T-cells administration, they are not all effective in some patients. A certain level of CAR T-cell expansion and persistence is necessary to induce tumor regressions, but the predictive indicators associated with remarkable proliferation and persistent clinical responses are mostly unknown. Major questions are how to enhance the potency and sustain the function of CAR T-cells *in vivo* and how to increase the resistance of CAR T-cells in TME [41]. Efficacy of CAR T-cells are like those of TIL treatment, the majority of subjects responding to CAR T-cell therapy displayed well *in vivo* expansion of CAR T-cells. The levels of CAR T-cell expansion and function *in vivo* are directly related to the proliferative capacity of those cells during *ex vivo* culture [42]. According to a recent report, the antitumor activity and toxicity of CD19 CAR T-cells in non-Hodgkin's lymphoma (NHL) patients were associated with the polyfunctional nature of the pre-infusion cellular product. Additional predictive indicators of response to anti-CD19 CAR T-cell therapy include a high frequency of CD3+CD8+CD27+CD45RO− lymphocytes at the time of collection and transcriptomic signatures of early memory T-cell differentiation [43]. Predictive biomarkers can be utilized by physicians to prescribe CAR T-cell therapy only to the responding population of the patient, and therefore, eliminating the unnecessary expense and risk of immune-related adverse events for non-responders [44]. In the future, genomic mechanisms of the antitumor activity of CAR T-cells at the cellular and molecular level may increase CAR T-cells utilization for patients. On the other hand, clinical TCR T-cell therapy relies on tumor antigens expressed in tumor cells. Human tumor antigens are classified into two main types: shared tumor-associated antigens (TAAs) and tumor-specific antigens (TSA). TAA includes (I) cancer-testis (CT) antigens overexpressed antigens, (II) differentiation antigens, and (III) oncofetal antigen while TSA includes neoantigens and onco-viral antigens such as HBV, EBV, CMV and human papillomavirus (HPV) E6/E7 protein. CT antigens are protein antigens with normal expression restricted to adult testicular germ cells aberrantly activated and expressed in different types of human cancer. At least a group of antigens has been found to elicit spontaneous humoral and cell-mediated immune responses in cancer patients, raising the possibility that these antigens could produce TCR T-cell targets as Table **2** [45]. According to several data from researches, CT antigens are expressed in different types of tumor diseases, which also exist a period during times of spermatogenesis and placenta. Normally they are silent in adult tissues, and therefore, they are activated once the mechanism of transcription is stimulated in different tumor types. Although many types of tumor diseases express CT antigens at a high level and corresponding normal tissues lower express at a low level, they are a sometimes high expression in normal tissues. In a MAGE-A3 trial, TCR targeted at MAGE-A3 unexpectedly cross-reacted with the related peptide, MAGE-A12, which is expressed in the brain, resulting in the death of two in nine patients with severe mental damage [46].

Table 2. Cancer-testis antigen-related with adult cancers.

Tumor Type	Antigen	Association
Melanoma	MAGEA1, MAGEA2, MAGEA3, MAGEA4	Tumor thickness and metastasis
NSCLC	MAGEA1, MAGEA3, MAGEA4, MAGEA10, MAGEC1	Advanced tumor type, nodal and pathologic stages as well as pleural invasion
Pancreatic cancer	MAGEA3	Poor survival
Hepatocellular carcinoma	MAGEC1	Reduced overall survival
Multiple myelomas	MAGEA1, MAGEA3, MAGEA4, MAGEC1	Stage and risk status of the disease
Serous ovarian carcinomas	MAGEA4	Inverse correlation between expression and patient survival
Melanoma	NY-ESO1	Thicker primary lesions and a higher frequency of metastatic disease

Differentiation antigens are encoded by genes that express in a tissue-specific manner. The proteins are normally produced in very low quantities but whose production is dramatically increased in tumor cells, activating an immune response. An example of such a protein is tyrosine, which is required for melanin production. Normally tyrosinase is produced in minute quantities, but its levels are very much elevated in melanoma cells. They have also shared antigens between tumor cells and corresponding normal cells, unlike overexpressed antigens. Most of these antigens, including gp100 (glycoprotein), MART-1 (melanoma antigen), and tyrosinase, are recognized by T-cells, which are mainly found in melanomas and normal melanocytes [47, 48].

The oncofetal antigen is the third important tumor antigens, such as alpha fetal protein (AFP) and carcinoembryonic antigen (CEA) [49, 50]. These proteins are normally produced in the early stages of embryonic development and disappear by the time the immune system is fully developed at adults, and thus, self-tolerance does not develop against these antigens. CEA is often highly expressed in colon cancer and other tumor diseases in clinical biomarker analyses, including

NSCLC (non-small cell lung cancer) in which CEA is identified as one biomarker of lung adenocarcinoma.

Table 3. Target Antigens related to common tumor diseases for clinical trials.

Target Ag	Common Tech	Common Tumor-1	Common Tumor-2	Common Tumor-3	Common Tumor-4
CD19	CARS	B-cell lymphoma	B-cell leukemia	NHL	DLBCL
CD20	CARS	MCL	FL	DLBCL	
CD22	CARS	B-cell lymphoma	ALL		
CD30	CARS	NHL	HL		
CD33	CARS	AML	CML		
NY-ESO	TCRS	NSCLC	Ovarian cancer	Melanoma	Multiple myeloma
MAGE-A10	TCRS	NSCLC	Urinary bladder cancer	Head and neck cancer	Melanoma
PRAME	TCRS	AML	MDS		
AFP	TCRS	HCC			
CEA	TCRS	GI tumor			
HER2	TCRS	Breast tumor			
MART-1	TCRS	Melanoma			
WT1	TCRS	Lung cancer	AML	ALL	Other solid tumors
MAGE-A4	TCRS	Melanoma			
MAGE-A3	TCRS	Melanoma			
MAGE-A10	TCRS	Melanoma			
gp100	TCRS	Melanoma			
P53	TCRS	epithelial tumor			
KRASG12V	TCRS	Lung cancer			
HBV	TCRS	HCC			
HPVE6	TCRS	Cervical cancer	Head and neck cancer		
HPVE7	TCRS	Cervical cancer	Head and neck cancer		
CMV	TCRS	GBM			
EBV	TCRS	HL			
Thyroglobulin	TCRS	DTC			

(Table 3) cont.....

HA1	TCRS	Hematologic malignancy			
Tyrosinase	TCRS	TAA-positive cancer cells			
IMA-201	TCRS	TAA-positive cancer cells			

Targeting such differentiation Ag, CT Ag, and oncofetal Ag could be likely to induce "on-target, off-tumor toxicity" on normal cells in important human organs. The first trials of TCR-T-cell therapy against MART-1 protein used 2 different proteins that were class I MHC-restricted but that were targeting similar epitopes [51]. Other toxicity consists of erythematous skin rash, anterior uveitis, and hearing loss observed in patients using TCR T-cells [52]. Lethal cardiac toxicity was also observed in undergoing trials against MART-1 [53]. Now TCR T-cells should be studied to reach immune response enough to kill tumor cells while the threshold has been controlled below "on-target, off-tumor" toxicity. Because of the "on-target, off-tumor" toxicity by targeting antigens, clinical researchers should more focus on specific affinity tumor cells without corresponding normal cells so that TCR products can be safely used for patients.

As Table **3**, because CAR-T cells have been proved efficiency in treating B-cell hematological malignancies published on ClinicalTrials.gov, several groups are going to attempt to use CAR-T cells administration against non-CD19 CAR T-cells; therefore, it is possible that CAR-T cells might be widely available for most of the hematological malignancies, maybe also including solid tumor treatment in the future. As shown in Table **3**, more than 300 clinical trials for TCR T-cells published on ClinicalTrials.gov, more than half of the antigens targeted are CT antigens and some for target NY-ESO-1 because the NY-ESO-1-specific TCR-T cells have been most thoroughly examined and tested in terms of therapeutic potentials in synovial cell sarcoma, melanoma and myeloma [54, 55]. More important, clinical scientists should resolve specific affinity to tumor cells, avoiding nonspecific affinity corresponding to normal cells for clinical safety.

COMPANY PRODUCTS OF CAR T-CELL AND TCR T-CELL

CAR T-cells and TCR T-cells represent one of the most promising advancements in adoptive T-cell immunotherapy. With the support of NIH and the National Cancer Institute, a few companies with their different phases for CAR T-cells and TCR T-cells are advancing their research and engineering potential cures for different tumor diseases.

At least ten CAR T-cell companies reported by the news are going to develop their products so that a few clinical projects have been approved by the FDA. This commercial success will secure more capital for these companies to fuel their pipelines and allow their companies to develop further new technologies that can impact even more patients [56].

TCR T-cell companies are also quickly advanced so that at least six commercial companies are developed to produce TCR T-cells with their platforms such as Adaptimmune, Bellicum Pharmaceutical, Kite Pharma, Medigene, Immatics, TCR2 Therapeutics [57].

1. **Adaptimmune** develops high-affinity products, including CT antigens by MAGE-A4, MAGE-A10, and NY-ESO-1 and AFP TCRs. They also support the preclinical screening program consisting of molecular analysis, systematical identifying peptides, and target cancer cell peptide to exclude cross-reactivity with normal cells.

2. **Bellicum Pharmaceutical** develops a switch technology for TCR T-cell therapy called CaspaCIDe. This technology involves transforming T-cells coding caspase-9 and chemically induced dimerization (CID) protein with specially designed domain allowing for the binding of rimiducid. When a patient is experiencing severe side effects due to "on-target, off-tumor" toxicity, rimiducid is introduced and dimerizes CID proteins. The dimerization of CID proteins initiates a signaling cascade that activates caspase-9, finally leading to apoptosis of T cells to decrease side effects.

3. **Kite Pharma** is to produce MAGE-A3/MAGE-A6 targeting and some neoantigens. They also set up the TCR-GENErator platform to screen and identify TCRs.

4. **Medigene** is to extend viral vector-mediated transfer to infuse genes that code for specific TCRs into T-cells. Its TCR-T platform delivers TCR T-cells recognizing various tumor antigens, including common antigens shared by tumors and neoantigens specific to each individual patient.

5. **Immatics Company** has developed ACTengine approach to genetically engineering T-cell to express exogenous TCR upon lentiviral transduction. Their specific exogenous TCRs with optimal affinity can be used for high throughput screening (HTS). They have developed three products: IMA-201, IMA-202, and IMA-203. They have developed bispecific TCR molecules that could be easily synthesized in mammalian host cells, and that contain two domains: T-cell recruiting antibody domain that targets immunomodulating T-

cell surface proteins, such as CD3, and a specific TCR domain that targets and binds to tumor antigens presented by class I MHC complexes. Their products can prevent "on-target, off-tumor" toxicity.

6. **TCR2 Therapeutics** has a unique TRuC platform to screen TCRs without HLA matching, including tumor scFv, single-domain antibody, and an antigen-binding fragment of TCR. Their products do not require HLA matching because their products consist of a complete TCR system with both TCR and CD3 complex. They also have some innovations such as T-cells to more effectively kill tumor cells and products with avoiding "on-target, off-tumor" toxicity.

FUTURE OF CAR T-CELL AND TCR T-CELL

CAR T-cells for T-cell adoptive immunotherapy are going into a new era after approved by FDA to CD19 CAR T-cells for the treatment of ALL and DLBCL [58 - 60]. CAR T-cell therapy will be entering dominant trend in T-cell adoptive immunotherapy for other hematological malignancies. The capacity of CAR T-cells to overcome Ag evasion, proliferate *in vivo* and move to tumor sites, synergize with the endogenous immune response, and persist in long-term *in vivo* may allow this CAR T-cells to effective antitumor treatment in hematological malignancies. Large studies are currently being involved in the safety and reliability of CAR T-cells for hematological malignancies besides CD19-positive B-cell malignancies. In the future, following the emergence of a new generation of GMP techniques, novel cell engineering approaches combine with genome profiles, and gene editing technologies for some strategies such as individualized tumor biomarkers and new tumor antigens, we believe that CAR T-cells will soon become safe and cost-effective for hematological malignancies.

On the other hand, TCR T-cells are going to be undertaken future clinical application in six sections: (1) TCR T-cell specific affinity; (2) TCR T-cell without "on target, off-tumor" toxicity; (3) TCR T-cell combination treatment; (4) TCR T-cell with gene-editing technique to block inhibiting factors; (5) TCR T-cell with CAR T-cells targeted against vascularized cells and factors; (6) some engineered T cells with some enzymes to increase functions of T-cell killing tumor cells.

1. TCR T-cell specific affinity is now subject to being studied some challenges for TCRs to specific affinity to some tumor antigens. For example, several methods are involved in those applied by (I) a new generation of primary tumor cell culture to identify personalized tumor Antigen affinity from an individual patient, (II) humanized mouse model for identification of affinity for a tumor antigen and (III) genomic profiles to define individualized tumor biomarkers

and neoantigens by neoantigen-specific TCRs such as TraCeR and single-cell at both bulk and single-cell levels including computational methods with TCR-seq for reconstructing TCRs and identifying immunogenic neoantigens for analyses of the diversity, dynamics, and clonality of T cells though its cost is still a relatively expensive method. In the near future, the TCR-neoantigen system should be developed for a new generation of TCR T-cell treatment [61].

2. Furthermore, the affinity of TCRs should be made avoid to their "on target, off-tumor" toxicity toward normal body cells so that several strategies have been used to patients, such as (I) local injection of TCR T-cells and (II) combined CAR T-cells to the TCR-T cell, in which a separate CAR containing an scFv targeting an antigen on normal tissue but not on tumor tissue is fused to an inhibitory cytoplasmic domain. This approach also enables TCR-T cells to distinguish between tumor cells and normal cells with the same antigen [62].

3. TME can inhibit specific affinity molecules, such as intercellular adhesion molecule, costimulatory ligands, or T-cell specific chemo-attractants. Cancer-associated fibroblasts and extracellular matrix components [vascular endothelial growth factor (VEGF), interleukin 10 (IL-10), and prostaglandin E2] can induce expression of FAS-ligand, and therefore, can mediate the apoptosis of FAS-positive CD8 effector T-cells. In TME, under situations of hypoxia, tumor cells can increase expression of the glucose transporter GLUT1, maintaining a high metabolic rate and proliferation to decrease T-cell antitumor activity. In addition, tumor cells often increase the expression of coinhibitory ligands (checkpoint inhibitors), including PD-1 ligand 1 (PD-L1), PD-1 ligand 2 (PD-L2), and B7 proteins that produce costimulatory signals when binding to CD28 on T-cells. Cytotoxic T-lymphocyte antigen-4 (CTLA-4), a homolog of CD28 but has greater binding affinities than CD28 and is expressed mainly by activated T-cells, can inhibit activation of T-cells when binding to ligand B7 on APCs. The PD-1 induces apoptosis of antigen-specific T-cells and reduces apoptosis of regulatory T cells when binding to PD-L1. CTLA-4 blockade and PD-1 blockade were proved to be effective in enhancing T-cell activation. CTLA-4 blocker (ipilimumab), PD-1 blocker (nivolumab and pembrolizumab), and PD-L1 inhibitors (atezolizumab) as Fig. (**8**) are going to be studied to combine with TCR T-cell treatment to increase TCR T-cell efficacy [63].

4. Gene editing technologies such as TALEN (transcription activator-like effector nuclease) and CRISPR/Cas9 system to remove genes in T-cells coding for coinhibitory-ligand-binding are also going to combine with TCR T-cell therapy such as (TALEN)-mediated PD-1 gene to change T-cells' resistance to PD--mediated cell death in tumor tissues. TCR T-cell therapy is likely to be more effective in advanced tumors, although the cost is likely to be another issue for

patients to treat TCR T-cells with immunotherapy by gene editing to PD-1 gene [64].

5. CAR-T cells are going to engineer T-cells with CARs targeted against vascularized cells and factors such as VEGFR-2 protein, which is overexpressed in tumor endothelial cells. TCR T-cells have been discovered to T-cell easy to traffic to tumor endothelial cells after CARs targeted against vascularized cells [65].

6. In addition, some approaches are to use to transduce engineered T cells with some enzyme genes such as CYP4B1 or Casp9, which increase functions of TCR T-cell killing tumor cells [66].

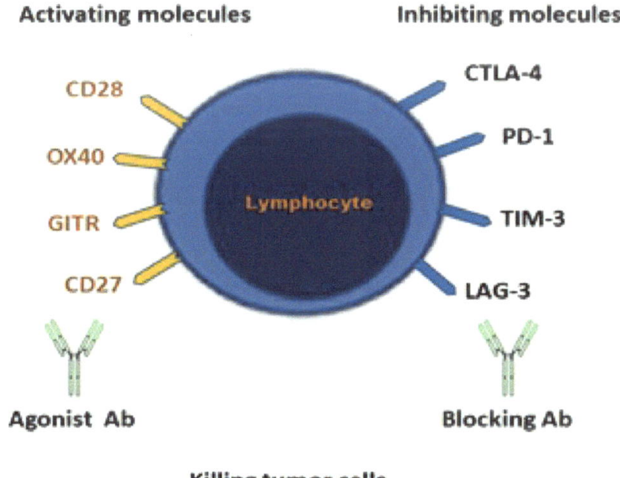

Fig. (8). T-cells Targeting Signaling. Inhibitory molecules such as CTLA-4, PD-1, TIM-3, and LAG-3 can be blocked to decrease T-cell exhaustion to kill tumor cells, and activating molecules such as CD28 can be used to stimulate T-cell function for kill tumor cells.

Overall, CAR T-cell and TCR T-cell have been rapidly developing, and consequently, they should become a promising strategy against various types of cancers in the future.

CONSENT FOR PUBLICATION

The authors declare no financial interests.

CONFLICT OF INTEREST

The authors declare no financial interests.

ACKNOWLEDGEMENTS

We had set up TIL isolation methods with a clinical application (1989-2004) when we worked in Dept. of Microbiology, Shanghai Second Medical University, and the single-cell level of genomic profiles for biomarker targeting, including CD3+, CD3+CD8+ during 1995-2007. Shen DH was the advisor of Li B before thirty years, who designed the first CAR T-cell model using the single chain of mAb mRNA response to duck hepatitis B virus surface Ag (DHBV HBsAg) cloning into CD3 of TIL to treat human hepatic cancer. ED and SP supported phage display under the leaders of Drs. Preisler and Smith in Rush Cancer Institute (1996-2000). SL designed the chapter for clinical purposes.

The mention of trade names or commercial products in this article is solely to provide specific information and does not imply recommendation.

REFERENCES

[1]   Topalian SL, Muul LM, Solomon D, Rosenberg SA. Expansion of human tumor infiltrating lymphocytes for use in immunotherapy trials. J Immunol Methods 1987; 102(1): 127-41.
[http://dx.doi.org/10.1016/S0022-1759(87)80018-2] [PMID: 3305708]

[2]   Li B, Tong SQ, Zhang XH, Zhu YM, *et al.* Research on TIL proliferation, phenotype, and lethality of human malignant solid tumors. Modern Immunology 1994; p. 05.

[3]   Xiang B, Snook AE, Magee MS, Waldman SA. Colorectal cancer immunotherapy. Discov Med 2013; 15(84): 301-8.
[PMID: 23725603]

[4]   Blankenstein T, Coulie PG, Gilboa E, Jaffee EM. The determinants of tumour immunogenicity. Nat Rev Cancer 2012; 12(4): 307-13.
[http://dx.doi.org/10.1038/nrc3246] [PMID: 22378190]

[5]   Pinzon-Charry A, Maxwell T, López JA. Dendritic cell dysfunction in cancer: a mechanism for immunosuppression. Immunol Cell Biol 2005; 83(5): 451-61.
[http://dx.doi.org/10.1111/j.1440-1711.2005.01371.x] [PMID: 16174093]

[6]   Cohen CJ, Zhao Y, Zheng Z, Rosenberg SA, Morgan RA. Enhanced antitumor activity of murine-human hybrid T-cell receptor (TCR) in human lymphocytes is associated with improved pairing and TCR/CD3 stability. Cancer Res 2006; 66(17): 8878-86.
[http://dx.doi.org/10.1158/0008-5472.CAN-06-1450] [PMID: 16951205]

[7]   Tendeiro Rego R, Morris EC, Lowdell MW. T-cell receptor gene-modified cells: past promises, present methodologies and future challenges. Cytotherapy 2019; 21(3): 341-57.
[http://dx.doi.org/10.1016/j.jcyt.2018.12.002] [PMID: 30655164]

[8]   Cohen CJ, Li YF, El-Gamil M, Robbins PF, Rosenberg SA, Morgan RA. Enhanced antitumor activity of T cells engineered to express T-cell receptors with a second disulfide bond. Cancer Res 2007; 67(8): 3898-903.
[http://dx.doi.org/10.1158/0008-5472.CAN-06-3986] [PMID: 17440104]

[9]   de Witte MA, Coccoris M, Wolkers MC, *et al.* Targeting self-antigens through allogeneic TCR gene

transfer. Blood 2006; 108(3): 870-7.
[http://dx.doi.org/10.1182/blood-2005-08-009357] [PMID: 16861342]

[10]   Bridgeman JS, Hawkins RE, Bagley S, Blaylock M, Holland M, Gilham DE. The optimal antigen response of chimeric antigen receptors harboring the CD3ζ transmembrane domain is dependent upon incorporation of the receptor into the endogenous TCR/CD3 complex. J Immunol 2010; 184(12): 6938-49.
[http://dx.doi.org/10.4049/jimmunol.0901766] [PMID: 20483753]

[11]   Eshhar Z, Waks T, Gross G, Schindler DG. Specific activation and targeting of cytotoxic lymphocytes through chimeric single chains consisting of antibody-binding domains and the γ or ζ subunits of the immunoglobulin and T-cell receptors. Proc Natl Acad Sci USA 1993; 90(2): 720-4.
[http://dx.doi.org/10.1073/pnas.90.2.720] [PMID: 8421711]

[12]   Dudley ME, Yang JC, Sherry R, *et al.* Adoptive cell therapy for patients with metastatic melanoma: evaluation of intensive myeloablative chemoradiation preparative regimens. J Clin Oncol 2008; 26(32): 5233-9.
[http://dx.doi.org/10.1200/JCO.2008.16.5449] [PMID: 18809613]

[13]   Gross G, Waks T, Eshhar Z. Expression of immunoglobulin-T-cell receptor chimeric molecules as functional receptors with antibody-type specificity. Proc Natl Acad Sci USA 1989; 86(24): 10024-8.
[http://dx.doi.org/10.1073/pnas.86.24.10024] [PMID: 2513569]

[14]   Liu Q, Jia RY. [Research on the gene structure of duck hepatitis B virus and its encoding proteins]. Bing Du Xue Bao 2012; 28(6): 681-8.
[PMID: 23367570]

[15]   Locarnini S, Littlejohn M, Aziz MN, Yuen L. Possible origins and evolution of the hepatitis B virus (HBV). Semin Cancer Biol 2013; 23 (6 Pt B): 561-75.
[http://dx.doi.org/10.1016/j.semcancer.2013.08.006] [PMID: 24013024]

[16]   Li B, Tong SQ, Lu DY, *et al.* DHBV induced acute hepatic cell necrosis in a duck-An experimental model for fulminant hepatitis. Acta Shanghai Second Medical University 1990; 10(3): 189-93.

[17]   Li BR, Tong SQ, Zhang XH, Lu J, Gu QL, Lu DY. A new experimental and clinical approach of combining usage of highly active tumor-infiltrating lymphocytes and highly sensitive antitumor drugs for the advanced malignant tumor. Chin Med J (Engl) 1994; 107(11): 803-7.
[PMID: 7867384]

[18]   Cai X, Zheng W, Pan S, *et al.* A virus-like particle of the hepatitis B virus preS antigen elicits robust neutralizing antibodies and T cell responses in mice. Antiviral Res 2018; 149: 48-57.
[http://dx.doi.org/10.1016/j.antiviral.2017.11.007] [PMID: 29129705]

[19]   Irving BA, Weiss A. The cytoplasmic domain of the T cell receptor zeta chain is sufficient to couple to receptor-associated signal transduction pathways. Cell 1991; 64(5): 891-901.
[http://dx.doi.org/10.1016/0092-8674(91)90314-O] [PMID: 1705867]

[20]   Embleton MJ, Gorochov G, Jones PT, Winter G. In-cell PCR from mRNA: amplifying and linking the rearranged immunoglobulin heavy and light chain V-genes within single cells. Nucleic Acids Res 1992; 20(15): 3831-7.
[http://dx.doi.org/10.1093/nar/20.15.3831] [PMID: 1508667]

[21]   Wong GK, Heather JM, Barmettler S, Cobbold M. Immune dysregulation in immunodeficiency disorders: The role of T-cell receptor sequencing. J Autoimmun 2017; 80: 1-9.
[http://dx.doi.org/10.1016/j.jaut.2017.04.002] [PMID: 28400082]

[22]   Siemionow M, Klimczak A. Immunodepletive anti-alpha/beta-TCR antibody in transplantation of composite tissue allografts: Cleveland Clinic research experience. Immunotherapy 2009; 1(4): 585-98.
[PMID: 20635989]

[23]   Dos Santos NR, Ghysdael J, Tran Quang C. The TCR/CD3 complex in leukemogenesis and as a therapeutic target in T-cell acute lymphoblastic leukemia. Adv Biol Regul 2019; 74100638

[http://dx.doi.org/10.1016/j.jbior.2019.100638] [PMID: 31378701]

[24]   Kershaw MH, Westwood JA, Parker LL, *et al.* A phase I study on adoptive immunotherapy using gene-modified T cells for ovarian cancer. Clin Cancer Res 2006; 12(20 Pt 1): 6106-15.
[http://dx.doi.org/10.1158/1078-0432.CCR-06-1183] [PMID: 17062687]

[25]   Park JR, Digiusto DL, Slovak M, *et al.* Adoptive transfer of chimeric antigen receptor re-directed cytolytic T lymphocyte clones in patients with neuroblastoma. Mol Ther 2007; 15(4): 825-33.
[http://dx.doi.org/10.1038/sj.mt.6300104] [PMID: 17299405]

[26]   Lamers CH, Sleijfer S, Vulto AG, *et al.* Treatment of metastatic renal cell carcinoma with autologous T-lymphocytes genetically retargeted against carbonic anhydrase IX: first clinical experience. J Clin Oncol 2006; 24(13): e20-2.
[http://dx.doi.org/10.1200/JCO.2006.05.9964] [PMID: 16648493]

[27]   Till BG, Jensen MC, Wang J, *et al.* Adoptive immunotherapy for indolent non-Hodgkin lymphoma and mantle cell lymphoma using genetically modified autologous CD20-specific T cells. Blood 2008; 112(6): 2261-71.
[http://dx.doi.org/10.1182/blood-2007-12-128843] [PMID: 18509084]

[28]   Finney HM, Lawson AD, Bebbington CR, Weir AN. Chimeric receptors providing both primary and costimulatory signaling in T cells from a single gene product. J Immunol 1998; 161(6): 2791-7.
[PMID: 9743337]

[29]   Friedmann-Morvinski D, Bendavid A, Waks T, Schindler D, Eshhar Z. Redirected primary T cells harboring a chimeric receptor require costimulation for their antigen-specific activation. Blood 2005; 105(8): 3087-93.
[http://dx.doi.org/10.1182/blood-2004-09-3737] [PMID: 15626734]

[30]   Golubovskaya V, Berahovich R, Xu S, Harto H, Wu L. Major Highlights of the CAR-TCR Summit, Boston, 2016. Anticancer Agents Med Chem 2017; 17(10): 1344-50.
[http://dx.doi.org/10.2174/1871520617666170110151900] [PMID: 28071584]

[31]   Sun ZJ, Kim KS, Wagner G, Reinherz EL. Mechanisms contributing to T cell receptor signaling and assembly revealed by the solution structure of an ectodomain fragment of the CD3 epsilon gamma heterodimer. Cell 2001; 105(7): 913-23.
[http://dx.doi.org/10.1016/S0092-8674(01)00395-6] [PMID: 11439187]

[32]   Uhlén M, Fagerberg L, Hallström BM, *et al.* Proteomics. Tissue-based map of the human proteome. Science 2015; 347(6220): 1260419-11260419.
[http://dx.doi.org/10.1126/science.1260419] [PMID: 25613900]

[33]   Xu Y, Yang Z, Horan LH, *et al.* A novel antibody-TCR (AbTCR) platform combines Fab-based antigen recognition with gamma/delta-TCR signaling to facilitate T-cell cytotoxicity with low cytokine release. Cell Discov 2018; 4(1): 62.
[http://dx.doi.org/10.1038/s41421-018-0066-6] [PMID: 30479831]

[34]   Rabinovich GA, Gabrilovich D, Sotomayor EM. Immunosuppressive strategies that are mediated by tumor cells. Annu Rev Immunol 2007; 25(1): 267-96.
[http://dx.doi.org/10.1146/annurev.immunol.25.022106.141609] [PMID: 17134371]

[35]   Ruella M, Xu J, Barrett DM, *et al.* Induction of resistance to chimeric antigen receptor T cell therapy by transduction of a single leukemic B cell. Nat Med 2018; 24(10): 1499-503.
[http://dx.doi.org/10.1038/s41591-018-0201-9] [PMID: 30275568]

[36]   Scholler J, Brady TL, Binder-Scholl G, *et al.* Decade-long safety and function of retroviral-modified chimeric antigen receptor T cells. Sci Transl Med 2012; 4(132)132ra53
[http://dx.doi.org/10.1126/scitranslmed.3003761] [PMID: 22553251]

[37]   Hacein-Bey-Abina S, Garrigue A, Wang GP, *et al.* Insertional oncogenesis in 4 patients after retrovirus-mediated gene therapy of SCID-X1. J Clin Invest 2008; 118(9): 3132-42.
[http://dx.doi.org/10.1172/JCI35700] [PMID: 18688285]

[38]   Montini E, Cesana D, Schmidt M, *et al.* The genotoxic potential of retroviral vectors is strongly modulated by vector design and integration site selection in a mouse model of HSC gene therapy. J Clin Invest 2009; 119(4): 964-75.
[http://dx.doi.org/10.1172/JCI37630] [PMID: 19307726]

[39]   Naldini L, Blömer U, Gallay P, *et al. In vivo* gene delivery and stable transduction of nondividing cells by a lentiviral vector. Science 1996; 272(5259): 263-7.
[http://dx.doi.org/10.1126/science.272.5259.263] [PMID: 8602510]

[40]   Stroncek DF, Ren J, Lee DW, *et al.* Myeloid cells in peripheral blood mononuclear cell concentrates inhibit the expansion of chimeric antigen receptor T cells. Cytotherapy 2016; 18(7): 893-901.
[http://dx.doi.org/10.1016/j.jcyt.2016.04.003] [PMID: 27210719]

[41]   Anderson KG, Stromnes IM, Greenberg PD. Obstacles posed by the tumor microenvironment to T cell activity: a case for synergistic therapies. Cancer Cell 2017; 31(3): 311-25.
[http://dx.doi.org/10.1016/j.ccell.2017.02.008] [PMID: 28292435]

[42]   Porter DL, Levine BL, Kalos M, Bagg A, June CH. Chimeric antigen receptor-modified T cells in chronic lymphoid leukemia. N Engl J Med 2011; 365(8): 725-33.
[http://dx.doi.org/10.1056/NEJMoa1103849] [PMID: 21830940]

[43]   Kalos M, Levine BL, Porter DL, *et al.* T cells with chimeric antigen receptors have potent antitumor effects and can establish memory in patients with advanced leukemia. Sci Transl Med 2011; 3(95)95ra73
[http://dx.doi.org/10.1126/scitranslmed.3002842] [PMID: 21832238]

[44]   Maude SL, Frey N, Shaw PA, *et al.* Chimeric antigen receptor T cells for sustained remissions in leukemia. N Engl J Med 2014; 371(16): 1507-17.
[http://dx.doi.org/10.1056/NEJMoa1407222] [PMID: 25317870]

[45]   De Smet C, Lurquin C, van der Bruggen P, De Plaen E, Brasseur F, Boon T. Sequence and expression pattern of the human MAGE2 gene. Immunogenetics 1994; 39(2): 121-9.
[http://dx.doi.org/10.1007/BF00188615] [PMID: 8276455]

[46]   Terra LF, Teixeira PC, Wailemann RA, *et al.* Proteins differentially expressed in human beta-cell--enriched pancreatic islet cultures and human insulinomas. Mol Cell Endocrinol 2013; 381(1-2): 16-25.
[http://dx.doi.org/10.1016/j.mce.2013.07.004] [PMID: 23891624]

[47]   Bakker AB, Schreurs MWJ, de Boer AJ, *et al.* Melanocyte lineage-specific antigen gp100 is recognized by melanoma-derived tumor-infiltrating lymphocytes. J Exp Med 1994; 179(3): 1005-9.
[http://dx.doi.org/10.1084/jem.179.3.1005] [PMID: 8113668]

[48]   Kawakami Y, Eliyahu S, Sakaguchi K, *et al.* Identification of the immunodominant peptides of the MART-1 human melanoma antigen recognized by the majority of HLA-A2-restricted tumor infiltrating lymphocytes. J Exp Med 1994; 180(1): 347-52.
[http://dx.doi.org/10.1084/jem.180.1.347] [PMID: 7516411]

[49]   Tsang KY, Zaremba S, Nieroda CA, Zhu MZ, Hamilton JM, Schlom J. Generation of human cytotoxic T cells specific for human carcinoembryonic antigen epitopes from patients immunized with recombinant vaccinia-CEA vaccine. J Natl Cancer Inst 1995; 87(13): 982-90.
[http://dx.doi.org/10.1093/jnci/87.13.982] [PMID: 7629885]

[50]   Wang X, Wang Q. Alpha-fetoprotein and hepatocellular carcinoma immunity. Can J Gastroenterol Hepatol 2018; 20189049252
[http://dx.doi.org/10.1155/2018/9049252] [PMID: 29805966]

[51]   Ping Y, Liu C, Zhang Y. T-cell receptor-engineered T cells for cancer treatment: current status and future directions. Protein Cell 2018; 9(3): 254-66.
[http://dx.doi.org/10.1007/s13238-016-0367-1] [PMID: 28108950]

[52]   van den Berg JH, Gomez-Eerland R, van de Wiel B, *et al.* Case report of a fatal serious adverse event

upon administration of T cells transduced with a MART-1-specific T-cell receptor. Mol Ther 2015; 23(9): 1541-50.
[http://dx.doi.org/10.1038/mt.2015.60] [PMID: 25896248]

[53]   Kunert A, Straetemans T, Govers C, *et al.* TCR-engineered T cells meet new challenges to treat solid tumors: choice of antigen, T cell fitness, and sensitization of tumor milieu. Front Immunol 2013; 4: 363.
[http://dx.doi.org/10.3389/fimmu.2013.00363] [PMID: 24265631]

[54]   McCormack E, Adams KJ, Hassan NJ, *et al.* Bi-specific TCR-anti CD3 redirected T-cell targeting of NY-ESO-1- and LAGE-1-positive tumors. Cancer Immunol Immunother 2013; 62(4): 773-85.
[http://dx.doi.org/10.1007/s00262-012-1384-4] [PMID: 23263452]

[55]   Tan MP, Gerry AB, Brewer JE, *et al.* T cell receptor binding affinity governs the functional profile of cancer-specific CD8+ T cells. Clin Exp Immunol 2015; 180(2): 255-70.
[http://dx.doi.org/10.1111/cei.12570] [PMID: 25496365]

[56]   Feins S, Kong W, Williams EF, Milone MC, Fraietta JA. An introduction to chimeric antigen receptor (CAR) T-cell immunotherapy for human cancer. Am J Hematol 2019; 94(S1): S3-9.
[http://dx.doi.org/10.1002/ajh.25418] [PMID: 30680780]

[57]   Zhang J, Wang L. The Emerging World of TCR-T Cell Trials Against Cancer: A Systematic Review. Technol Cancer Res Treat 20191: 18.
[http://dx.doi.org/10.1177/1533033819831068] [PMID: 30798772]

[58]   Turtle CJ, Hanafi LA, Berger C, *et al.* CD19 CAR-T cells of defined CD4+:CD8+ composition in adult B cell ALL patients. J Clin Invest 2016; 126(6): 2123-38.
[http://dx.doi.org/10.1172/JCI85309] [PMID: 27111235]

[59]   Neelapu SS, Locke FL, Bartlett NL, *et al.* Axicabtagene ciloleucel CAR T-cell therapy in refractory large B-cell lymphoma. N Engl J Med 2017; 377(26): 2531-44.
[http://dx.doi.org/10.1056/NEJMoa1707447] [PMID: 29226797]

[60]   Schuster SJ, Svoboda J, Chong EA, *et al.* Chimeric antigen receptor T cells in refractory B-cell lymphomas. N Engl J Med 2017; 377(26): 2545-54.
[http://dx.doi.org/10.1056/NEJMoa1708566] [PMID: 29226764]

[61]   Obenaus M, Leitão C, Leisegang M, *et al.* Identification of human T-cell receptors with optimal affinity to cancer antigens using antigen-negative humanized mice. Nat Biotechnol 2015; 33(4): 402-7.
[http://dx.doi.org/10.1038/nbt.3147] [PMID: 25774714]

[62]   Marabelle A, Kohrt H, Caux C, Levy R. Intratumoral immunization: a new paradigm for cancer therapy. Clin Cancer Res 2014; 20(7): 1747-56.
[http://dx.doi.org/10.1158/1078-0432.CCR-13-2116] [PMID: 24691639]

[63]   Leach DR, Krummel MF, Allison JP, Sleppy CR, Castleman AW. Enhancement of antitumor immunity by CTLA-4 blockade. Science 1996; 271(5256): 1734-6.
[http://dx.doi.org/10.1126/science.271.5256.1734] [PMID: 8596936]

[64]   Menger L, Sledzinska A, Bergerhoff K, *et al.* TALEN-mediated inactivation of PD-1 in tumor-reactive lymphocytes promotes intratumoral T-cell persistence and rejection of established tumors. Cancer Res 2016; 76(8): 2087-93.
[http://dx.doi.org/10.1158/0008-5472.CAN-15-3352] [PMID: 27197251]

[65]   Huang J, Liang J, Tang Q, *et al.* An active murine-human chimeric Fab antibody derived from Escherichia coli, potential therapy against over-expressing VEGFR2 solid tumors. Appl Microbiol Biotechnol 2011; 91(5): 1341-51.
[http://dx.doi.org/10.1007/s00253-011-3335-y] [PMID: 21604194]

[66]   Di Stasi A, Tey SK, Dotti G, *et al.* Inducible apoptosis as a safety switch for adoptive cell therapy. N Engl J Med 2011; 365(18): 1673-83.
[http://dx.doi.org/10.1056/NEJMoa1106152] [PMID: 22047558]

CHAPTER 12

System Modeling of T-cell Function-Development of Adoptive T-cell Immunotherapy

Biaoru Li[1,2,*], George Liu[2,3] and Jie Zheng[4]

[1] *Georgia Cancer Center and Department of Pediatrics, Medical College at GA, Augusta, GA 30912, USA*

[2] *Department of Biochemistry, Case Western Reserve University School of Medicine, Cleveland, OH, USA*

[3] *USDA, ARS, ANRI, Bovine Functional Genomics Laboratory, Beltsville Agricultural Research Center (BARC) – East, Beltsville, MD, USA*

[4] *School of Computer Engineering, Nanyang Technological University, 639798, Singapore*

Abstract: When primary-cells, including non-genetically modified and genetically modified T-cells to produce a special substance, are infused into patients, these performances would be defined as cell therapy. An excellent cell performance with its optimal proliferation for cell therapy should maintain its functional feature and efficacy *in vivo* with ethical acceptance and safe application. Because the efficacy of cell therapy maybe will be decreased *in vivo* special microenvironment after infusion, moreover, because cell therapy with these genetically modified T-cells would be faced by a safe challenge in clinics, a functional induction/inhibition of some genes' expressions used in T-cell growth without genetic modification has been increasingly studied. Here, T-cell therapy based on system biology for an induction/inhibition of special function and maintaining a special function *in vivo* microenvironment is called as functional cell therapy. Nowadays, following research and development (R&D) of T-cell proliferatively engineering techniques and system modeling by this computational simulation performance, the novel techniques of T-cell culture based on genomic analysis and supported by system biology will be increasingly studied for adoptive T-cell therapy so that oncologists can safely and effectively utilize the new strategy for personalized immunotherapy.

Keywords: CD8+cells, Gene expression signature (GES), Heterogeneous responses, Network, Personalized immunotherapy, Quantitative pathway, Tumor-infiltrating lymphocytes (TILs), Tumor microenvironment (TME).

* **Corresponding author Biaoru Li**: Georgia Cancer Center and Department of Pediatrics, Medical College at GA, Augusta, GA 30912, USA; Tel: 440-317-1443; E-mail: bli@augusta.edu

INTRODUCTION

Cells that are cultured directly from clinical specimens are known as primary cells [1]. The primary cells isolated from living tissues can be cultured *ex vivo* or *in vivo* environments. Now, the primary-cell culture technique can be used for stem cells, lymphocytes, cancer stem cells, and so on [2]. Accompanying with the research and development (R&D) of leukocytes (including T-cell, macrophage and other leukocytes) for adoptive cell immunotherapy of tumor disease, stem cells for regenerative medicine, and erythroid cell for treatment of different anemia, primary cell culture technique regarding T-cells, macrophage, stem cells and other leukocytes harvested from clinical specimens is going to play an increasingly important role in modern cell therapy [3]. Although the *ex vivo* culture of stem cells and T-cells have a well-established model by genetic modification such as Induced Pluripotent Stem cells (IPS cells), these genetically modified cells have safety challenges for their clinical applications [4]. Moreover, even if non-genetically modified human cells would be expanded very well *ex vivo*, the efficacy of the non-modified human cells would be decreased *in vivo* tumor microenvironment (TME) after infusion back to patients. Fortunately, when the human genome was decoded after 2004, it will give scientists and physicians a new idea to develop some new models to increase or decrease gene expression during primary cell culture [5]. Furthermore, many genomic databases from primary cells have been registered within Gene Expression Omnibus (GEO), such as database from a stem cell into different terminal cells or the genomic database from T-cell, macrophages, and leukocytes. Furthermost, gene regulations related to network and bioinformatics platforms related to system modeling and drug bank have been increasingly researched. Based on the R&D of cell proliferation of primary cell culture, relied on gene expression related system biology, we have set up a new strategy contributing to personalized immunotherapy.

CONCEPT FOR PRIMARY CELL PROLIFERATION WITH ITS CELL THERAPY

Following R&D of techniques of primary cell culture and application of cell therapy, history of cell therapy experiences through three stages in more than one hundred years: (I) cellular therapy, (II) cell therapy, and (III) functional cell therapy.

Cellular therapy-called as live cell therapy early refers to various procedures in which cells or tissue from animal embryos, fetuses, or organs were injected into human beings. The first recorded attempt was at cellular therapy in 1912 when German physicians attempted to treat hypothyroid children with thyroid cells [6]. In 1970, Dr. Kühnau began to use cellular therapy to treat cancer patients in

Tijuana, Mexico [7]. It is also claimed to build the immune system and help patients with Down's syndrome, Alzheimer's, and AIDS [8]. In 1987, Australian researchers reported on a result studied for children with Down's syndrome who received cellular therapy with similar children who did not. The study demonstrated no evidence between the two groups [9]. The first malpractice case involving cellular therapy was filed for Dr. Cousens for a Clostridium perfringens infection (gas gangrene) [10]. After then, live cell therapy from animal sources into human beings has been almost completely discontinued.

Cell therapy-the modern cellular therapy, now called cell therapy, early applied for bone marrow transplantation [11]. The first breakthrough was performed by Dr. Dausset in 1952, who won Nobel Prize in Physiology/Medicine (1980) by discovering an HLA antigen, an immunological rejection, and thus set up allogeneic bone marrow transplantation by HLA match test [12]. Now, cell therapy broadly describes the process of introducing a group of human cells such as stem cells, T-cell, macrophages, or other leukocytes into patients [13]. In the chapter, we concentrate on T-cell immunotherapy, although we will briefly introduce some functions for macrophage and leukocyte regarding functional adoptive T-cell therapy. As we all know, cell therapy can be divided into Autologous Cell Therapy and Allogeneic Cell Therapy. Autologous cell therapy may be harvested from a patient and then introduced back into the same patient [14]. This autologous method is the priority due to the non-immunologic matching assay requirement. Allogeneic cell therapy approach involves the harvesting of cells from one or universal donors followed by large scale expansion after immunologic matching [15]. This allogeneic approach utilizes cell types that do not elicit immune responses on implantation; therefore, they have the potential to treat hundreds of patients from a single manufactured lot of cells. The allogeneic cell therapy adapts to the manufacturing because the product can be readily available in a cell bank [16].

Functional cell therapy-if a cell needs to produce a special substance, genetically modified human cells are routinely performed to produce the special substance called cell-based gene therapy as Fig. **(1A)** [17]. This kind of cell therapy has severe challenges in clinical safety. For example, twenty-three years ago, we had used a retroviral vector carrying the TNF-α gene to transduce into tumor-infiltrating lymphocytes (TIL) to treat a patient with an advanced liver tumor. We performed a very prudent protocol for the patient treatment due to safety challenges. Currently, some challenges still remain in genetically modified human cells for cell-based gene therapy: (A) long-term culture with the genetically modified primary cell is limited to reach enough cell number for therapeutic efficacy; (B) safety question still cannot be completely resolved to transduced immune-cells [18]. After 2004, decoded human gnomic profiles give scientists and physicians a new chance to develop some new strategies for cell therapy. Up to date, workflows from genomic profiles to system modeling with functionally cell engineering have been increasingly studied [19]. For instance, while data of genomic profiles are observed from a cell, some pathways will be mined to discover activity or inhibition of pathological or physiological change of the cell. Because of numerous distinct pathways co-exist within a cell, this collection of pathways is called a network regarding the change. Computational reconstruction of the pathological or physiological network (or simulation) allows in-depth insight into the molecular mechanisms called as system modeling. The system modeling can identify significant genes linking different compounds or drugs by a quantitative integrated network and topology model (significant genes previously called as therapeutic targeting identification, TI, and here called as gene expression signature, GES) [20, 21]. Hitherto, this knowledge has been applied to create functional cell engineering for cell therapy. Here, the cell using the new culture and proliferation to inhibit/induce several proteins is called as functionally modified cells. Cell therapy with a special function and keeping the function in the tumor microenvironment is called functional cell therapy (Fig. **1B**). Nowadays, the system modeling with analysis of targeting compounds has to be used in personalized immunotherapy [22].

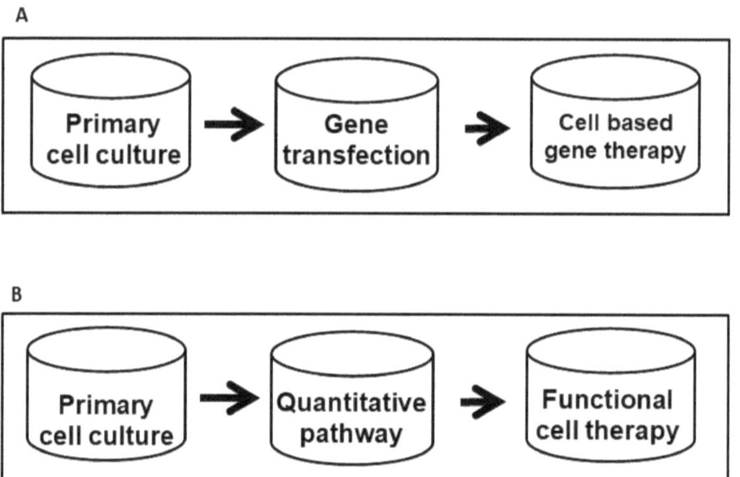

Fig. (1). Primary cell functional modification for personalized immunotherapy. Fig. (**1A**) cell-based gene therapy and Fig. (**1B**) is a functional modification for functional cell therapy.

Before we introduce experimental and clinical results with functional cell therapy, several ideas such as bioprocess of functional cell therapy and background of functional cell therapy regarding a system of immunosurveillance (T-cell, macrophage and other leukocytes) will be first presented.

CELL BIOPROCESSING RELATED WITH FUNCTIONAL CELL-PROLIFERATION

The primary cell culture of clinical purpose is named as cell bioprocessing. Cell bioprocessing is a process from primary cell isolation to expansion until the expanded cell harvest, all of which belong to the cell engineering process, including the quality and quantities of therapeutic cells [23]. Therapeutic cell manufacturing processes can be divided into upstream processes and downstream processes. The upstream process is defined as the entire process from early cell isolation and cultivation until the final harvest, including the availability of GMP grade fetal bovine serum [24]. The downstream bioprocessing focuses on the final harvest with their subsequent processes such as the concentration of the harvested cells, clarification of the harvested cells, formulation of the cells into an appropriate solution for bio-preservation and filling cells into the final container for fresh delivery or cryopreservation, storage, and delivery to clinics [25]. Once cell therapy is required for a patient, it must be shipped under appropriate conditions to the clinical site, prepared for delivery to the patient, and then administered by a trained medical doctor or trained medical center [26]. We experienced those for more than two decades, including using basic cell culture facilities and using cGMP facilities (current Good Manufacturing Practice). Most of the bioprocessing to produce functional T-cells is involved in upstream, including inducing and inhibiting genes during the culture stage once patients' genomic profiles are analyzed, system modeling is established, and inhibitor or activator is discovered for TIL from an individual patient.

BACKGROUND OF FUNCTIONAL CELL THERAPY

Optimal immune cells of cell therapy should have two therapeutic abilities: (1) cells such as macrophage and T-cell have the capacity to directly kill tumor cells; (2) cells releasing soluble factors to interact with other cells in TME with further keeping functions for a period *in vivo*. Up to now, lymphocyte, macrophages/monocyte, and granular leukocyte have been all reported to be feasible in cell therapy as Table **1**. Because functional T-cell immunotherapy supports immune mechanisms to kill tumor cells and interact with other cells, here we also introduce macrophage and other leukocytes for the background of functional cell immunotherapy [27].

Table 1. Comparison of leukocyte cell therapy for tumor disease.

Cell Types	Names	Animal Trial	Human Trial	Pros	Cons
T-cell and NK cell	LAK/DC/CIK	Yes	Yes	Culture easy	Non-specific
				Enough cell number	Middle effect
	NK	Yes	Yes	Culture easy	Non-specific
				Enough cell number	Middle effect
	TIL	Yes	Yes	Higher specific	Difficult culture
				Higher effect	Cell number limitation
Macrophage	TAM1	Yes	Yes	Higher effect	Difficult culture
					Cell number limitation
Leukocyte	TAN1	Yes	Yes	Culture easy	Not-many human data
				Enough cell number	
	CKA	Yes	Initiating	Non-culture	Screening efficacy of donor
				Enough cell number	Not many human data

1. T-cell

In the late 1980s, Rosenberg and his colleagues initially apply for T-cell cytotoxic responses to kill cancer cells (called adoptive T-cell therapy). One of the best immune cells is a tumor-infiltrating lymphocyte (TIL) from tumor sites, demonstrating capable of killing melanoma cells with encouraging clinical results [28]. After more than two decades of development, the cell culture and induction have been developed from IL-2 into anti-CD3 with other growth factors [29]. These cultured T-cells are then transferred back into the patient along with the exogenous administration of IL-2 to boost their anti-cancer activity further. Although TIL has been reported to successfully treat malignant melanoma with an advantage of higher population CD8+cell by TCR (T-cell receptor) recognizing tumor-Ag associated MHC-I peptide complex [30], TIL therapy has several challenges: (1) efficacy of TIL therapy is different from different tumors, for example, most of the laboratories reported only efficacy in malignant melanoma [31]; (2) cell bioprocessing standard is varied, such as to isolate TIL in a different location in tumor mass, varied expand methods and changeable harvest of cell number; (3) biopharmaceutical and clinical/commercial quantities of therapeutic cells is not easy to estimate different patients with diseases. We have been studying TILs with experiences of treatment of several hundred clinical patients for more than two decades. In 1994, we discovered that the efficacy of TIL therapy was related to obtaining from location and enzyme digestion in different tumor structures so that we set up a modified method with cold enzyme digestion and with isolating TIL from fixed tumor locations [32]. Our data demonstrated that TILs have a very good response to some solid tumors, especially in lung cancer (NSCLC) and liver cancer, although brain tumor and kidney cancer still have faced some challenges [33]. Recently, we utilized genomic analysis to study TIL features in a liver tumor, and thus, our results show TIL is inhibited in both tumor tissue and TME, such as hepatic sinus so that we concluded that TIL immune would be influenced by multiple factors in TME [34]. Genetically modified techniques have been largely developed in T-cells, such as genetic modification of tumor antigen by HLA-A2 MART-1, engineered T-cells with higher affinity by TCR and CAR-T techniques and engineered T-cell with some special substance by TNF-α, TGF-β, IL-2, IL12 and IFN-γ [35]. In 1995 we successfully utilized retroviral vector to transduce TNF-α into TIL for a patient with liver tumor [36]. Although retroviral vectors work very well for genetic modification, as described above, the safety of transduced T-cells is still unknown. Due to T-cell efficacy and safety issues for transduced T-cell of clinical application, we begin to study the new strategy by analysis of genomic profiles. After more than twenty years of efforts, we have successfully uncovered the genomic database of CD3+cell and CD8+cell from TILs by single-cell technique. We also established system modeling related T-cell engineering to study inducing or inhibiting genes [37] so that system modeling can be developed into personalized immunotherapy.

2. Macrophage

Macrophages are a major component infiltrating into TME. During the neoplastic progression, macrophage, dendritic cells, and TILs are attracted to the tumor site and initiate the immune response against tumor cells. Activated macrophage presents tumor Ag to T-cell, which is then activated to kill tumor cells [38]. In 1998, culture human macrophages were achieved in hydrophobic plastic, gas-permeable bags, so that this process enables the collection of non-adherent macrophages. Now DCCIK (Dendritic Cells Cytokine Induced Killer) has well performed to dendritic cell acting T-cells' cytotoxic effect to tumor cells with cell therapy.

In most clinical trials, macrophages activated by interferon-gamma (IFNγ) remain unknown. *In vitro*, macrophages are as efficient as monocyte-derived dendritic cells (MDDCs) in stimulating cytotoxic T lymphocyte (CTL) clones or circulating CTL precursors. However, tumor cells are often capable of escaping the immune function. Because of macrophage is "polarization," macrophage in tumor tissue (tumor-associated macrophage, TAM) also contributes to tumor progression by growth factors and neovascularization. After several years' study, macrophages can be divided into two groups, M1-macrophages exposed in IFN-γ have antitumor activity, and M2-macrophages activated by IL-4 or IL-13 have oriented to tissue repair, tissue remodeling, and immune regulation [39]. Most of the evidence has demonstrated M1 switch to M2 under local hypoxia, low glucose level, and low pH with regulating by CCL families, TGF-β, VEGF, PDGF, and M-CSF. This switch eventually appears tumor dissemination and invasion characteristics [40]. A recent study revealed that activation of macrophages by the infusion of antibodies against CD40 might induce macrophage-mediated tumor regression in both a mouse model for pancreatic cancer and patients with pancreatic cancer [41]. IL-6 stimulates tumor macrophage infiltration in ovarian cancer, and this action can be inhibited by the neutralizing anti-IL-6 antibody (siltuximab) in clinical studies [42]. Since TGF-β is responsible for tumor infiltration by macrophages, depletion of TGF-β has been shown to enhance tumor vaccine efficacy [43]. Because CCL2 plays a major role in the recruitment of TAMs, anti-CCL2 would be a blocking step in preventing this recruitment. As shown above, if we can use system modeling related with cell engineering T-cells to induce genes with M1 antitumor mechanism and to inhibit M2 genes helping-tumor function in TME, functional T-cell with *in vitro* inducing M1 genes or *in vitro* inhibiting M2 genes based on system modeling will be encouraged for future application *in vivo*.

3. Other Leukocytes

Traditionally, granulocyte mainly functions as a response to different infections. Now, tumor-associated neutrophil (TAN) and CKA (granulocyte with cancer-killing activity, CKA) were discovered in tumor disease [44], so that cell therapy extends cell-based immunotherapy from T-cell and macrophage into granulocyte. The two kinds of granulocytes have been involved in clinical researches. TAN can be further divided into two types, TAN1 with an antitumor function and TAN2 with a pro-tumorigenic function. Antitumor activities of N1 include expression of more immuno-activating cytokines and chemokines, lower levels of arginase, and lower levels of TGF-β with capability killing tumor cells *in vitro* [45]. As we know above, therapeutic targeting identification from a quantitative network with its genomic analysis is a very good tool to block TGF-β for functional cell therapy *in vitro* and *in vivo*, such as inducing N1 *in vitro* or inhibiting N2 *in vivo* from therapeutic targeting identification. CKA is second discovered for some scientists to study granulocyte's antitumor cells [46]. Some scientists used spontaneous regression/complete resistant (SR/CR) mice to uncover leukocytes infiltration (by innate immunity) into tumor tissue to regress tumor mass. If we can use system modeling for T-cell engineering to produce proteins interacting CKA, functional T-cell based on system modeling will be increased to kill tumor cells *in vivo*.

EXPERIMENTAL STUDY OF FUNCTIONAL T-CELL THERAPY

After describing concepts, cell bioprocess, and background of functional cell therapy as above, in order to study functional T-cell therapy, we should address two questions: "quiescent TIL CD3+ and CD8+cell" with their genomic profiles and "heterogeneous response" of TIL CD8+cells to react with tumor cells.

We have studied quiescent T-cells from tumor tissue since 1995, which is a small cell size with a lack of spontaneous proliferation and low metabolic rate in TME [47]. Because quiescent T-cells are very few before culture, we set up a single-cell technique to isolate TIL CD3+ and TILCD3+CD8+cells in which those have already contacted tumor cells from tumor tissue, and then, we performed single-cell genomics analysis to study their genomic profiles related with their networks [48]. After more than ten years efforts including published about ten papers, our studies have concluded [49]: (I) TIL CD8+cells are an actively maintained quiescent status in TME as compared to the default status in the absence of the stimulating signals; (II) CD8+cells maintain the quiescent status by activating several regulatory pathways; and (III) these activated signaling pathways finally inhibit cell cycling from maintaining the quiescent state of TIL. Now, some scientists have supported the genomic profiles of the T-cell quiescent status-related network. For example, lung-Krüpple-like factor (LKLF, a zinc finger-containing transcription factor) has been discovered to maintain T cell quiescence [50]; Tob (nuclear protein) was uncovered to have anti-proliferative activities by blocking T cell receptor (TCR) engagement in the presence of either CD28 co-stimulation or IL-2 [51].

We further studied the "heterogeneous response" of CD8+cells by which T-cells should produce different genomic profiles from different patients according to goals of "heterogeneous response" of TIL CD8+cells. As we know, GWAS of T-cells has confirmed that CD8 T-cells, personally, mediated complete tumor regression, such as recognizing MART-1 mutations for melanoma, NYESO-1 for metastatic synovial cell sarcomas, ERBB2IP mutation for bile duct cancer and CD-19 for chronic lymphocytic leukemia [68 - 72]. Genetically modified T-cells related to immunologic reactivity against somatic mutations or abnormal expression have supported "individually heterogeneous immune response" for cancer personalized immunotherapy [52, 53, 68 - 72]. In order to study the heterogeneous immune response at the gene expression level, we performed *in silico* analyses of gene expression signatures (GES) obtained from transcriptome data of quiescent CD8+cells harvested by single-cell technique; thus we set up CD8+cell related quiescent networks. According to the aims, we researched individual "heterogeneous" immune responses, including selecting specific therapeutic targeting molecules/stimulating agents (without genetically modified T-cell) to compare a pair of individual "heterogeneous" immune responses from liver cancer.

Our researches, after we uncovered TIL quiescent genes from a pair of CD8+cell from TILs of two patients with liver cancer as reports [53, 73], include (I) mRNA expression was confirmed by quantitative real-time PCR [54]; (II) the differentially expressed genes used for network construction [55 - 57], all datasets with the regulatory connectivity and calculated betweenness of each protein (node) within these networks; (III) topology study of genomic signatures used by Degree Centrality (DC) and Betweenness Centrality (BC) established as an important quantity to characterize the communications between each pair of nodes [58]; (IV) discovering "gene expression signatures, GES" identified as "topological significance" [59]; (V) experimental confirmation [60] by cell growth inhibition, quiescent gene expression, inhibition assay and TIL cytotoxic activity with workflow from I to IV as above [61, 62].

Our results demonstrated that eight candidate genes of TIL CD8+cell from a pair of two liver cancer patients have individual "heterogeneous" immune responses. After measuring mRNA level change by Q-rtPCR obtained from quiescent CD8+cells of the two liver tumor specimens, eight candidate genes were subtly different, as summarized in Table **2** and Figs. (**2A** and **2B**). Five genes (Myc, Tob, ERF, Ets-2 repressor factor, REST and TGF-β) had a high level of gene expression in specimen-1, and seven genes (KLF2, Ski, Sno-A, Myc, Tob, ERF and REST) were confirmed a high level of gene expression in Specimen-2.

Table 2. Change of gene expression level.

Gene list	Specimen 1	Specimen 2
c-Myc	3.075	5.263
Tob1	1.144*	2.548
REST	0.720*	5.679
ERF	4.926	0.945*
KLF2	0.461*	3.712
Ski	3.038	3.642
Sno-A	1.617	6.646
TGFB1	1.644	1.501

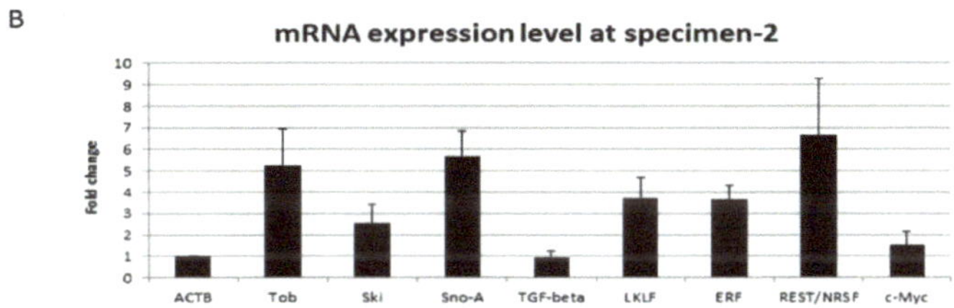

Fig. (2). mRNA expression level from two quiescent CD8 cells.

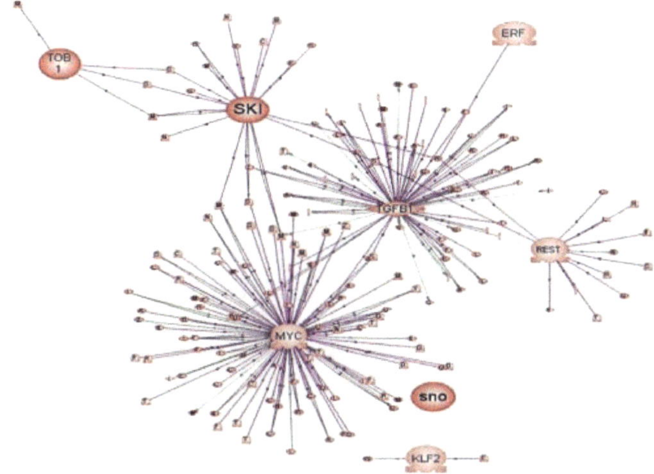

Fig. (3). Network of common pathways from quiescent CD8 cells.

Although mRNA level from quiescent TIL CD8+cells obtained from the two liver tumor specimens are subtle change, in order to study individual "heterogeneous" immune responses in the system biology, three networks were constructed, universal group (all of eight quiescent genes), specimen-1 (five quiescent genes) and specimen-2 (seven quiescent genes). In the universal group, all eight seed proteins discovered can produce a total of 196 nodes in the network of quiescent CD8 cells, including eight seed-proteins and 188 neighbors (Fig. **3**). As Fig. (**3**), one of eight seed proteins, Sno-A, has not any links resulting in non-involvement in the network analysis (*i.e.,* there was no *in silico* evidence of interactions).

TGFB1, one of seed protein, is a growth factor. Tob, one of the seed is membrane expression protein, and the other four of them (c-MYC, REST, ERF, and KLF2) are transcription factors located at the nucleus obtained from the networks.

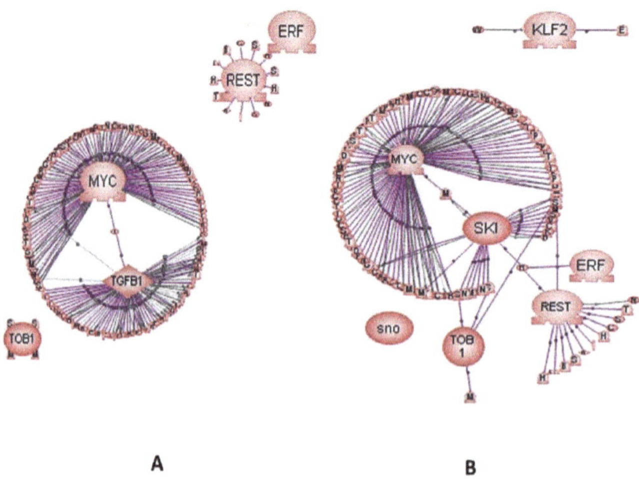

A   B

Fig. (4). Network and layout of the individual network.

In order to study heterogeneous responses in the networks for personalized therapeutic targeting, we further analyzed networks from specimen-1 and specimen-2, respectively. Five seed proteins from specimen-1 will produce a network containing five seed proteins and 155 neighbors derived from direct interaction Fig. (**4**). As Fig. (**4A**), TGFB1, one of seed protein, is the growth factor. Tob, one of the seed is membrane expression protein, and the other three of them (c-MYC, REST, ERF) are transcription factors located at the nucleus obtained from the networks. Similar to specimen-1, we studied networks from specimen-2, which contain seven seed proteins. Eventfully, 107 neighbors of a total of 114 proteins were constructed as Fig. (**4B**). Again, Sno-A, a seed protein, had no links in this network analysis, as shown in Fig. (**3**). Although only four proteins are different between these two samples, *i.e.,* TGFB1 in specimen-1 and Ski, Sno and KLF2 in specimen-2, resulting networks Fig. (**4A**) *vs.* Fig. (**4B**) have shown some differences. The results revealed that only very few genes change, maybe resulting in a large change of networks in a different individual.

Eight quiescent genes are further used by topology from both specimens with 196 nodes, including eight seed proteins and 188 non-seed proteins. The results of topology regarding regulatory connectivity are summarized in Table **3** and displayed in Fig. (**5**). The higher regulatory connectivity of a protein means more direct interactions with other proteins, such as c-Myc (85) and TGFB1 (63). The lower regulatory connectivity of a protein means fewer direct interactions with other proteins, such as Tob1 (4), KLF2 (2), REST (13), and Ski (18). The topology A is a network constructed for specimen-1 and B means network reconstructed for specimen-2 results also confirmed that only very few gene changes finally results in a significant change in topology values between two individual patients.

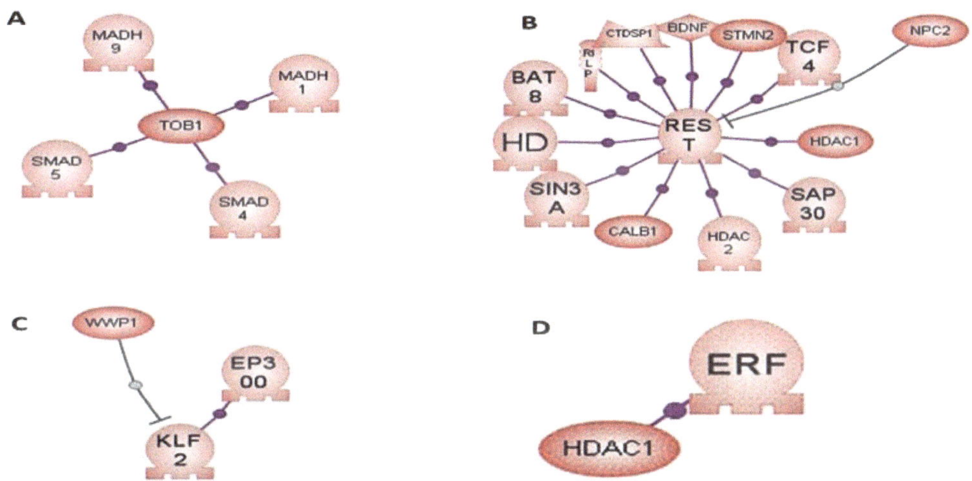

Fig. (5). Regulatory connectivity of four of eight seed proteins.

Table 3. Regulatory connectivity and betweenness centrality.

Nodes	Both Connectivity	Betweenness Centrality		
		(Both Specimens)	Specimen One	Specimen Two
Tob1	4	0.22	0.092	0.142
Ski	18	0.31	N/A	0.451
Sno	0	0	N/A	0
TGFB1	63	0.012	0.121	N/A
KLF2	2	0.092	0.098	0.098
ERF	1	0.35	N/A	0.512
REST	13	0.38	0.113	0.214
c-myc	85	0.012	0.142	0.112

Betweenness centrality (BC) is an important measurement for the downstream targeting hub. Here we used a formula to study BC, or a pair of nodes (s, t) as report [73], the shortest pathway through v point is denoted by $\sigma\,(s, t)$. Although regulatory connectivity is similar to shared proteins in both specimens as results are shown above, the values for BC are greatly different in some hubs such as c-Myc, ERF, REST, and Tob1 between specimen-1 and specimen-2 as shown in Table **3** and Fig. (**6**).

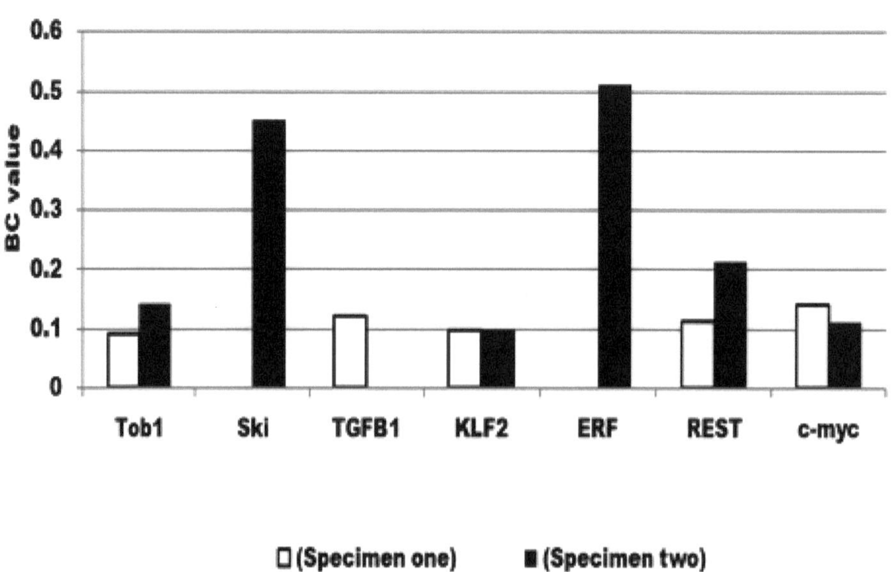

Fig. (6). Betweenness from Specimen 1 and Specimen 2.

Recently, therapeutic targeting such as drug targeting, small molecule targeting, Ab target, and RNA-interfering therapy has focused on GES based on topology analysis. Most publications focused on two parameters in topology, DC, and BC. Theoretically, both BC and DC all play an essential role in cell function, while DC is also likely to be toxic due to their system-wide influence; thus, we search GES with higher BC and low DC. A high BC value indicates a significant targeting node because it is a very important hub in the functional cell network, and low DC means very few branches without their system-wide influence to cause whole-cell functional toxicity. This study has a similar DC so that we discovered higher betweenness as key nodes. After GES was defined by topology analyses, the nodes were used to mine drugs, small molecule, and other molecular therapy agents. The resulting drug candidates were combined with GES and to predict therapeutic targeting. For example, we predicted that drugs like etoposide and taurine could inhibit quiescent CD8 cells in specimen-1 as Fig. (**7A**) and loratadine and taurine could directly inhibit quiescent CD8 cells in specimen-2 as Fig. (**7B**).

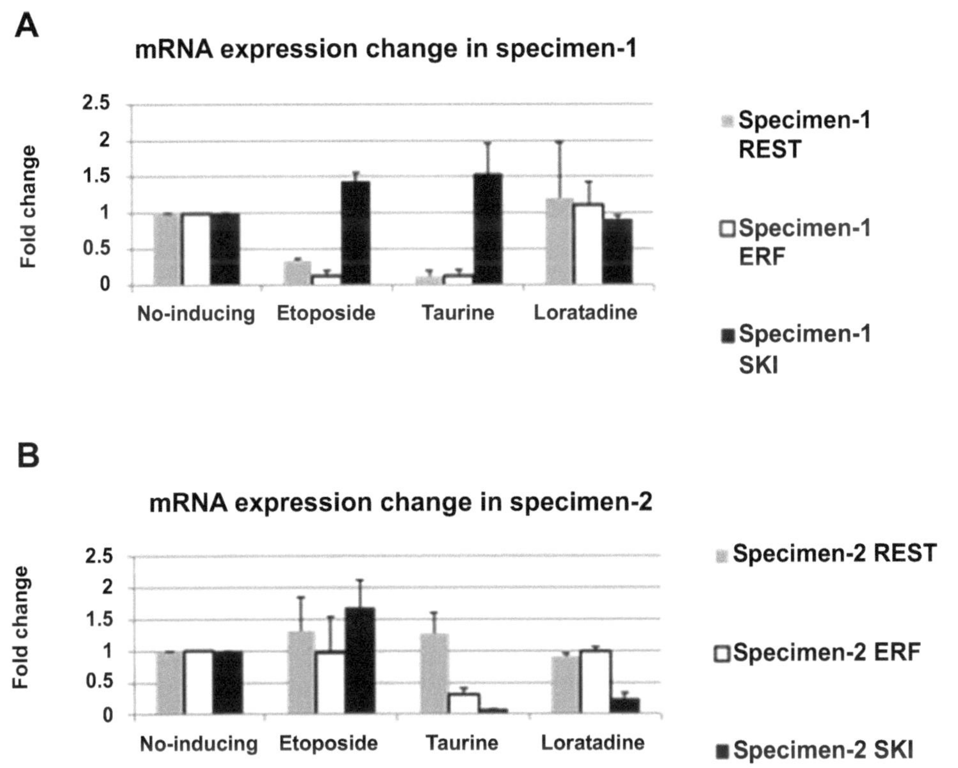

Fig. (7). Gene expression change after therapeutic targeting. **A** is gene expression after drug treatment for Specimen 1 and **B** is gene expression after drug treatment for Specimen-2.

According to previous evidence for TIL CD8+cells quiescent status, we studied two sets of compounds at culture day-4 with 72 hour's induction. After culturing at day-7, inhibition of targeted gene expression was confirmed that etoposide could, respectively, inhibit 65% and 87% REST and ERF gene expression but without SKI gene inhibition; taurine can inhibit 88% and 87% REST and ERF gene expression but without SKI gene inhibition while loratadine has not any obvious inhibition for REST, ERF and SKI in specimen-1. Taurine inhibited ERF, and SKI expression and loratadine only inhibit SKI in Specimen-2.

In order to study the TIL CD+8 cell killing tumor cells and study heterogeneous responses in an activated network, four genes (pre-TCR, TRAIL, Perforin, and

TNF receptor) were applied for the activated network which is high expression in activated CD8 cells. As compared to the quiescent CD8 cells from both specimens, we also constructed a network from four genes obtained from activated CD8+cells. In this analysis, the network contains four seed proteins, 81 neighbors, and a totally of 85 proteins in the whole network.

Following inhibiting and activating analysis of CD8+cells, cytotoxic T lymphocyte (CTL) assays were used to study cytotoxicity of TIL activity. Cytotoxic T lymphocyte (CTL) was measured for effector: target ratio by 1:50 using autogenously tumor cell as Fig. (**8A**). The results of killing activity showed $61\pm5.6\%$, $45\pm9\%$ and $21.2\pm3\%$ inhibited by etoposide, taurine and loratadine, respectively, in specimen-1 and $19.2\pm3.2\%$, $48\pm6\%$ and $45\pm4\%$, respectively, in specimen-2. The mechanism of heterogeneous responses of TIL was confirmed by a Western blot using an anti-granzyme-B antibody and anti-perforin antibody. Results of Q-rtPCR and Western blot demonstrated granzyme-B and perforin were highly expressed by etoposide and taurine to inhibit REST and ERF at specimen-1 while granzyme-B and perforin were highly expressed by inhibition of loratadine and taurine to SKI and ERF in specimen-2 as Fig. (**8B**) and Fig. (**8C**). As most inhibiting compounds, we also see that drugs interfere TIL growth curve to compare normal TIL cells as Fig. (**8D**).

In order to study heterogeneous responses, we used almost similar two patients' specimens with similar history and pathological results as our results above, a tiny change of key nodes can be magnified in network analysis. In order to overcome this kind of challenge, we applied for data generated from single-cell mRNA differential display and single-cell RNA-seq to analyze the network. We selected the seed proteins obtained from differentially expressed genes in single-cell level and analyzed networks based on these seed proteins and their neighbor proteins.

Up to now, genomics profiles have been successfully used in the analysis for clinical application [63]. New generation medicine such as "precision medicine" has encouraged physicians to develop an accurate genomics diagnosis with network construction to apply for the new fields. Here, we first used the data generated from "pure" genomic data to study a network. This aim is to study subtle individual immune response to further apply for personalized immunotherapy.

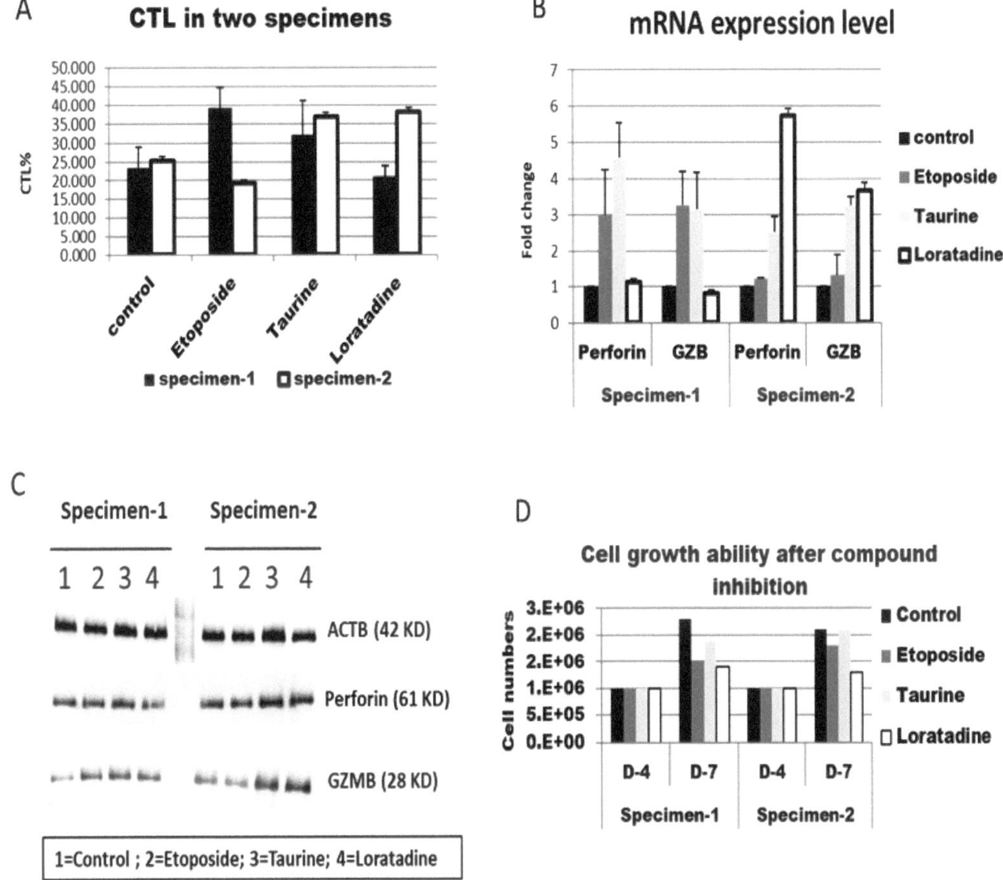

Fig. (8). Experimental confirmation. **A** is a diagram of CTL combination results of therapeutic targeting mining with GES mining from individual networks of Specimens 1 and 2. **B** is mRNA expression change after inducing quiescent pathway for Specimen 1-2. **C** is Western blot after inducing quiescent pathway for Specimen 1-2. **D** is cell growth after drug treatment GES change for Specimen 1 and 2.

In conclusion, network construction, with their analysis, including BC and DC, will play an important role in therapeutic targeting [64]. In these data from two specimens, we obtained some similar nodes (including four genes: c-Myc, Tob-1, ERF, and REST) from two specimens indicating a shared response in the quiescent network. After networking analysis to study the complexity of individual responses of CD8+cell quiescent, once one or more proteins are added into the network, such as TGFB1 increase from specimen-1, it could result in individual pathway shifts in a network. Although DC and BC all play an important role in therapeutic targets, here, a high BC value is defined as significant targeting nodes because they belong to very important hubs in functional cell network without more toxicity [65]. Following the results of system modeling, we defined REST and ERF as GES for therapeutic targets in specimen-1 and Ski, Tob1, and ERF in specimen-2. Drugs inhibiting GES further support our network analysis. As described above, etoposide and taurine could inhibit REST and ERF in specimen-1, and loratadine and taurine could directly inhibit Ski, Tob1, and ERF in specimen-2. Moreover, etoposide and taurine can significantly increase CTL in specimen-1, while taurine and loratadine increase CTL in specimen-2. Mechanism analysis of individual responses of TIL demonstrated granzyme-B and perforin were highly expressed by etoposide and taurine at specimen-1 while granzyme-B and perforin were highly expressed by inhibition of loratadine at specimen-2 as Fig. (9). Our results demonstrated that network analysis could be employed for personalized immunotherapy [66].

CLINICAL STUDY OF FUNCTIONAL T-CELL THERAPY

After two questions regarding quiescent TIL CD3+ and CD8+cell" with their genomic profiles and the heterogeneous response of TIL CD8+cells to response to tumor-cells were addressed, we study a clinical experiment with a primary hepatocellular cancer (51 years old, female) with size about 8 x 9 cm mass before treatment [67].

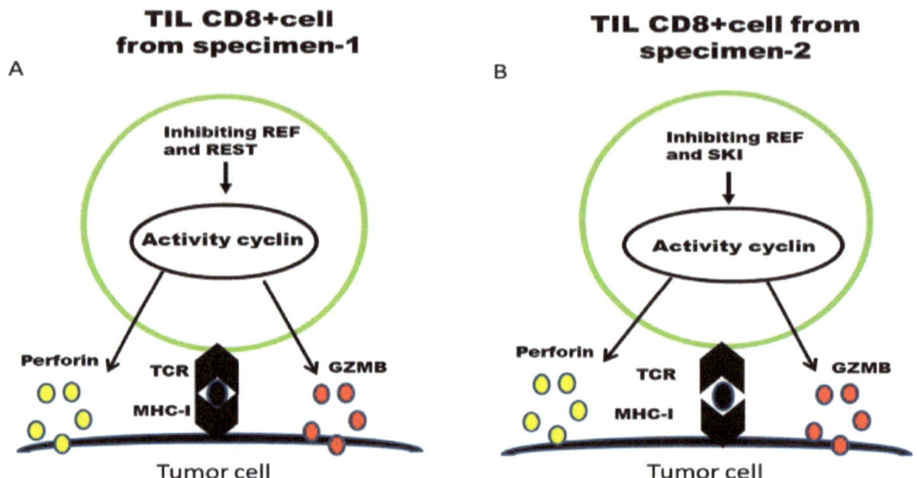

Fig. (9). Diagram of gene expression signature for TIL CD8+cells heterogeneous responses in specimens 1 and 2.

After we uncovered TIL CD8+cell genomics, mRNA expression was confirmed by quantitative real-time PCR; the differentially expressed genes were constructed for network construction; topology of genomic signatures used by Degree Centrality (DC) and Betweenness Centrality (BC) was established to study the communications between each pair of nodes; targeting biomarker was discovered from GES; experimental results achieved TIL cytotoxic activity to treat uncured liver cancer. Finally, we successfully reported as Fig. (**10**).

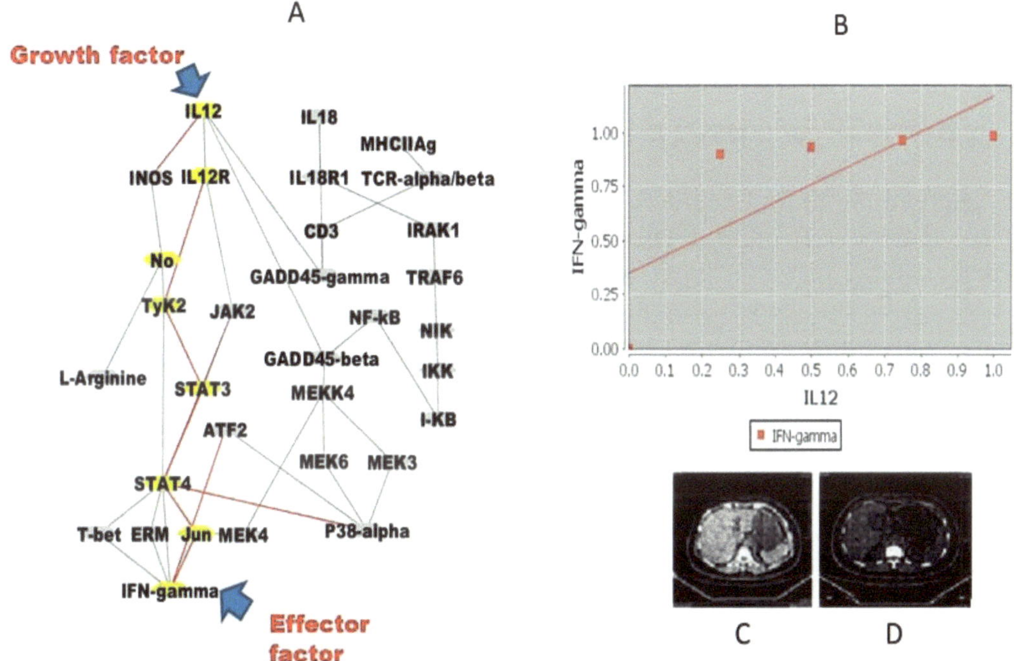

Fig. (10). Clinical experimental of functional cell immunotherapy.

Our clinical data have indicated a good response by the personalized functional T-cell immunotherapy [67]. Generally, the T-cells based on system modeling (or GWAS) has at least four advantages to compare genetically-modified adoptive immunotherapy: (a) induced T-cells are based on system biology rather than any genetic modification performance so that personalized immunotherapy can keep T-cells optimal proliferation during culture; (b) CD8+cell culture based on personalized genomic profiles with their network also can release some special substances (such as TNF-α and IFN-γ) or inhibiting some genes expression (such as inhibiting TGF-β) after the functional T-cell *in vivo* infusion; (c) functional inducing or inhibiting T-cells could be much safer than genetically-modified T-cell immunotherapy cells; (d) to treat the patient with a good efficacy as Fig. (**10C**) and Fig. (**10D**) . In the future, once new antibodies, antigens, cytokines, growth factors, and receptors are discovered such as antibody to anti-PD-1 and anti-cytotoxic T-lymphocyte antigen-4 (CTLA-4), individual T-cell genomic profiles related to the network linking the new compounds can be quickly applied to personalized immunotherapy for different patients.

A. specific growth factors can be used to culture TIL from the patient genomic biomarkers. Red color indicates inducing growth factors to produce a higher level of INF-gamma in culture TIL; B. IL12 can induce γ-IFN higher expression in the patient; C. A primary hepatocellular cancer (51 years old, female) with size about 8x9 cm mass before treatment; D. Tumor mass decreased to 6x7 cm with liquefaction after 5 months of personalized functional T-cell immunotherapy.

FUTURE OF FUNCTIONAL T-CELL THERAPY

Cell engineering of immune-cell therapy has the capacity to directly-act or release soluble factors to kill tumor cells. Functional cell therapy may have the ability to produce soluble factors *ex vivo*, resulting in inhibit or activate other immune cells of TME. Although genetically modified T-cell therapy has successfully involved in the treatment of several tumor diseases, which is related to viral or non-viral vector to genetic manipulation *in vitro,* these cells are required a strict regulation by Food and Drug Administration (FDA) to ensure the highest requirement of clinical safety. Functional cell engineering based on system modeling will give us a new consideration to clinical adoptive T-cell immunotherapy.

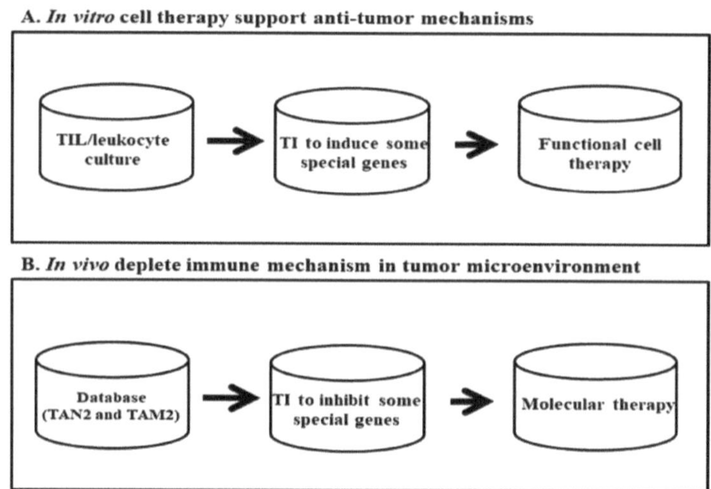

Fig. (11). Strategies of adoptive functional cell immunotherapy.

Clinically, functional cell therapy at least have four advantages [73]: (A) because of *ex vivo* bioprocessing without any genetic modification performance, the primary cell can keep very good proliferation rate and very good differentiation situation so that it can support enough cell number to treat patients; (B) because of e*x vivo* bioprocessing without any viral or non-viral vector genetic-modification performance, the functional primary cell can support much safer cells than genetically-modified cells to treat patients; (C) after *in vivo* infusion, the primary cell can support a special function as Fig. (**11**) and Fig. (**12**).

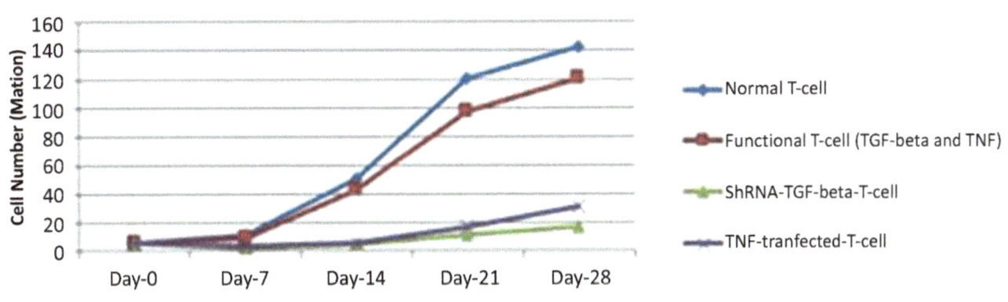

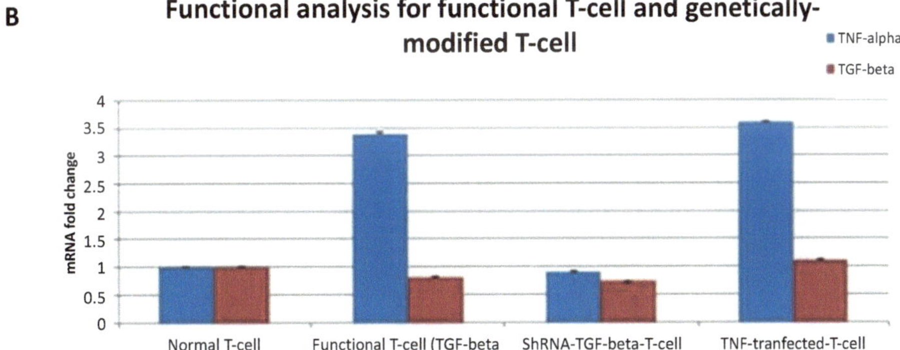

Fig. (12). Strategies of adoptive cell immunotherapy. Growth curve difference between shRNA-TGF-bet- -T-cell/Retroviral vector-TNF-alpha-T-cell and functional T-cell (**A**) and Gene expression fold change among genetically-modified-T-cell and Functional T-cell (**B**).

Once special functional TIL is inducing some specific genes (such as increasing TNF-α), it can play a special function to perform cell therapy for cancer patients. Moreover, because of depleting some genes (such as inhibiting TGF-β as Fig. (**12**)), it should more regress tumor disease by inhibiting TAM2 and TAN2 *in vivo* microenvironment mechanism; (D) several evidences have indicated that responses of CD8 cells MART-1 mutations for melanoma, NYESO-1 for metastatic synovial cell sarcomas, ERBB2IP mutation for bile duct cancer and CD-19 for chronic lymphocytic leukemia [68 - 72], if we used functional TIL proliferation, the functional TILs from tumor tissues can replace or partially replace genetically modified T-cell based on GWAS related immunologic reactivity against individual somatic mutations or abnormal expression. As Fig. (**13**) demonstrated, they have specific therapeutic targeting molecu-les/stimulating agents to perform individual "heterogeneous" immune responses for personalized T-cell immunotherapy.

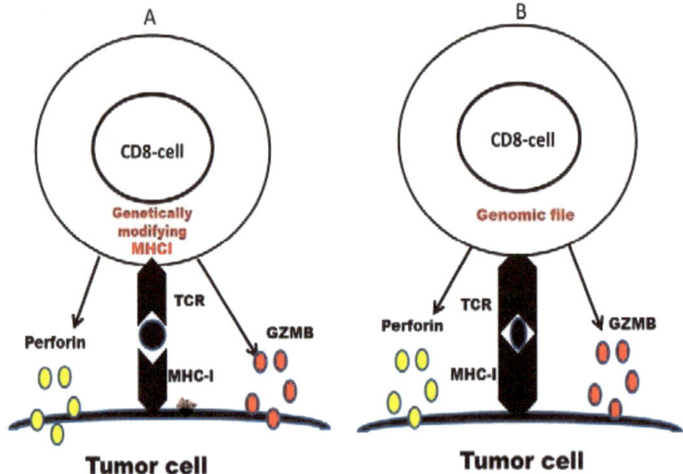

Fig. (13). Diagram of GWAS and GES. **A** is genetically modifying T-cell such as MART-1, NYESO-1 or ERBB2IP from GWAS (red color), and **B** is GES (red color) related to gene expression signature for heterogeneous responses by system modeling.

The new strategy and technique of T-cell culture based on genomic analysis and supported by system biology have excellent prospects for adoptive T-cell therapy because oncologists can safely and effectively utilize the new strategy for personalized immunotherapy shortly.

CONSENT FOR PUBLICATION

Not applicable.

CONFLICT OF INTEREST

The authors declare no financial interests.

ACKNOWLEDGEMENTS

We had set up single-cell methods to analyze genomic profiles, including CD3+, CD3+CD8+ from liver cancer during 1999-2007 when we worked in Case Western Reserve University. BL set up a single cell genomic technique to analyze the immune cells, GL set up bioinformatics analysis, and ZJ contributes topology study.

The mention of trade names or commercial products in this article is solely to provide specific information and does not imply recommendation.

REFERENCES

[1]   Berggren JR, Tanner CJ, Houmard JA. Primary cell cultures in the study of human muscle metabolism. Exerc Sport Sci Rev 2007; 35(2): 56-61.
[http://dx.doi.org/10.1249/JES.0b013e31803eae63] [PMID: 17417051]

[2]   Brevini TA, Antonini S, Cillo F, Crestan M, Gandolfi F. Porcine embryonic stem cells: Facts, challenges and hopes. Theriogenology 2007; 68 (Suppl. 1): S206-13.
[http://dx.doi.org/10.1016/j.theriogenology.2007.05.043] [PMID: 17582486]

[3]   Teng M, Geng Z, Huang L, Zhao X. Stem cell transplantation in cardiovascular disease: an update. J Int Med Res 2012; 40(3): 833-8.
[http://dx.doi.org/10.1177/147323001204000301] [PMID: 22906255]

[4]   Li Y, Tsai YT, Hsu CW, *et al.* Long-term safety and efficacy of human-induced pluripotent stem cell (iPS) grafts in a preclinical model of retinitis pigmentosa. Mol Med 2012; 18: 1312-9.
[http://dx.doi.org/10.2119/molmed.2012.00242] [PMID: 22895806]

[5]   Hughes CS, Radan L, Betts D, Postovit LM, Lajoie GA. Proteomic analysis of extracellular matrices used in stem cell culture. Proteomics 2011; 11(20): 3983-91.
[http://dx.doi.org/10.1002/pmic.201100030] [PMID: 21834137]

[6]   Kuettner H. Verimpfung an stelle der transplantation hochwertiger organe. Journal of the International Academy of Preventive Medicine 1977; 40: 74- 82.

[7]   Kuhnau WW. [Pituitary fresh cell implantation as endocrine stimulation]. Med Klin 1955; 50(28): 1187-9.
[PMID: 13244199]

[8]   Takata K, Kitamura Y. Molecular approaches to the treatment, prophylaxis, and diagnosis of Alzheimer's disease: tangle formation, amyloid-β, and microglia in Alzheimer's disease. J Pharmacol Sci 2012; 118(3): 331-7.
[http://dx.doi.org/10.1254/jphs.11R10FM] [PMID: 22382659]

[9]   Foreman PJ, Ward J. An evaluation of cell therapy in Down syndrome. Aust Paediatr J 1987; 23(3): 151-6.
[http://dx.doi.org/10.1111/j.1440-1754.1987.tb00234.x] [PMID: 2959248]

[10]   Howard Levy vs Dr Gabriel Cousens, No 333704, Superior Court for the State of Arizona in and for the County of Pima, Plaintiff's initial disclosure statement 1999. filed Oct 13.

[11]   Wislet-Gendebien S, Laudet E, Neirinckx V, Rogister B. Adult bone marrow: which stem cells for cellular therapy protocols in neurodegenerative disorders? J Biomed Biotechnol 2012; 2012601560
[http://dx.doi.org/10.1155/2012/601560] [PMID: 22319243]

[12]   Dausset J. [The HLA complex. 3. Implications in transplantation and transfusion]. Nouv Presse Med 1976; 5(22): 1413-6.
[PMID: 6945]

[13]   Larijani B, Esfahani EN, Amini P, *et al.* Stem cell therapy in treatment of different diseases. Acta Med Iran 2012; 50(2): 79-96.
[PMID: 22359076]

[14]   Dickerson JB. Provenge: revolutionary technology or ethical bust? Hum Vaccin 2011; 7(4): 477-80.
[http://dx.doi.org/10.4161/hv.7.4.14189] [PMID: 21451262]

[15]   Busca A. The use of monoclonal antibodies for the treatment of graft-*versus* -host disease following allogeneic stem cell transplantation. Expert Opin Biol Ther 2011; 11(6): 687-97.
[http://dx.doi.org/10.1517/14712598.2011.566852] [PMID: 21391897]

[16]   Barriga F, Wietstruck MA. Search for unrelated donor umbilical cord blood units for allogeneic stem cell transplantation: results in two time periods. Transplant Proc 2007; 39(3): 629-30.
[http://dx.doi.org/10.1016/j.transproceed.2006.12.025] [PMID: 17445562]

[17]   Zhdanov RI, Podobed OV, Vlassov VV. Cationic lipid-DNA complexes-lipoplexes-for gene transfer and therapy. Bioelectrochemistry 2002; 58(1): 53-64.
[http://dx.doi.org/10.1016/S1567-5394(02)00132-9] [PMID: 12401571]

[18]   Li B, Ding J, Larson A, Song S. Tumor tissue recycling--a new combination treatment for solid tumors: experimental and preliminary clinical research. *In Vivo* 1999; 13(5): 433-8.
[PMID: 10654199]

[19]   Stein JL, de la Torre-Ubieta L, Tian Y, *et al.* A quantitative framework to evaluate modeling of cortical development by neural stem cells. Neuron 2014; 83(1): 69-86.
[http://dx.doi.org/10.1016/j.neuron.2014.05.035] [PMID: 24991955]

[20]   Thiele I, Palsson BØ. A protocol for generating a high-quality genome-scale metabolic reconstruction. Nat Protoc 2010; 5(1): 93-121.
[http://dx.doi.org/10.1038/nprot.2009.203] [PMID: 20057383]

[21]   Shi M, Wu M, Pan P, Zhao R. Network-based sub-network signatures unveil the potential for acute myeloid leukemia therapy. Mol Biosyst 2014; 10(12): 3290-7.
[http://dx.doi.org/10.1039/C4MB00440J] [PMID: 25313005]

[22]   Lv S, Xu Y, Chen X, *et al.* Prioritizing cancer therapeutic small molecules by integrating multiple OMICS datasets. OMICS 2012; 16(10): 552-9.
[http://dx.doi.org/10.1089/omi.2012.0005] [PMID: 22917481]

[23]   Ratcliffe E, Thomas RJ, Williams DJ. Current understanding and challenges in bioprocessing of stem cell-based therapies for regenerative medicine. Br Med Bull 2011; 100: 137-55.
[http://dx.doi.org/10.1093/bmb/ldr037] [PMID: 21852279]

[24]   Brindley DA, Davie NL, Culme-Seymour EJ, Mason C, Smith DW, Rowley JA. Peak serum: implications of serum supply for cell therapy manufacturing. Regen Med 2012; 7(1): 7-13.
[http://dx.doi.org/10.2217/rme.11.112] [PMID: 22168489]

[25]   McCoy R, Hoare M, Ward S. Ultra scale-down studies of the effect of shear on cell quality; Processing of a human cell line for cancer vaccine therapy. Biotechnol Prog 2009; 25(5): 1448-58.
[http://dx.doi.org/10.1002/btpr.229] [PMID: 19634174]

[26]   Pahwa R, Jaggaiahgari S, Pahwa S, Inverardi L, Tzakis A, Ricordi C. Isolation and expansion of human natural T regulatory cells for cellular therapy. J Immunol Methods 2010; 363(1): 67-79.
[http://dx.doi.org/10.1016/j.jim.2010.10.006] [PMID: 20977911]

[27]   Takeuchi S. [A new look at the history of tumor immunotherapy--for its fruitful future through overcoming the widespread cynicism]. Hum Cell 1996; 9(1): 1-10.
[PMID: 9183623]

[28]   Rosenberg SA, Spiess P, Lafreniere R. A new approach to the adoptive immunotherapy of cancer with tumor-infiltrating lymphocytes. Science 1986; 233(4770): 1318-21.
[http://dx.doi.org/10.1126/science.3489291] [PMID: 3489291]

[29]   Ortegel JW, Staren ED, Faber LP, Warren WH, Braun DP. Modulation of tumor-infiltrating lymphocyte cytolytic activity against human non-small cell lung cancer. Lung Cancer 2002; 36(1): 17-25.
[http://dx.doi.org/10.1016/S0169-5002(01)00472-X] [PMID: 11891029]

[30]   Leong SP. Immunotherapy of malignant melanoma. Surg Clin North Am 1996; 76(6): 1355-81.
[http://dx.doi.org/10.1016/S0039-6109(05)70520-X] [PMID: 8977556]

[31]   Lippman SM, Spier CM, Miller TP, Slymen DJ, Rybski JA, Grogan TM. Tumor-infiltrating T-lymphocytes in B-cell diffuse large cell lymphoma related to disease course. Mod Pathol 1990; 3(3): 361-7.
[PMID: 2194216]

[32]   Li B, Tong SQ. Higher activity TIL Isolation and Analysis. Immunol J 1994; 10(1): 44-7.

[33]   Li BR, Tong SQ, Zhang XH, Lu J, Gu QL, Lu DY. A new experimental and clinical approach of combining usage of highly active tumor-infiltrating lymphocytes and highly sensitive antitumor drugs for the advanced malignant tumor. Chin Med J (Engl) 1994; 107(11): 803-7.
[PMID: 7867384]

[34]   Wang Z, Hu H, Zheng J, Li B.

[35]   Tao J, Zhang G, Ding J, Li B, Tong SQ. Experimental Study on Human Tumor Necrosis Factor α Genes Delivery *via* Receptor-mediated Endocytosis. Shanghai Second Medical University 2000; 1: 3-12.

[36]   Ding J, Qian G, Li B, *et al.* Primary research and application by TNF gene transducing into TIL. Zhongguo Zhongliu Shengwu Zhiliao Zazhi 1995; 2(1): 11-5.

[37]   Zhang W, Ding J, Qu Y, *et al.* Genomic expression analysis by single-cell mRNA differential display of quiescent CD8 T cells from tumour-infiltrating lymphocytes obtained from *in vivo* liver tumours. Immunology 2009; 127(1): 83-90.
[http://dx.doi.org/10.1111/j.1365-2567.2008.02926.x] [PMID: 18778280]

[38]   Owen MR, Sherratt JA. Pattern formation and spatiotemporal irregularity in a model for macrophage-tumour interactions. J Theor Biol 1997; 189(1): 63-80.
[http://dx.doi.org/10.1006/jtbi.1997.0494] [PMID: 9398504]

[39]   Caras I, Tucureanu C, Lerescu L, *et al.* Influence of tumor cell culture supernatants on macrophage functional polarization: *in vitro* models of macrophage-tumor environment interaction. Tumori 97(5): 54-647.
[http://dx.doi.org/10.1177/030089161109700518]

[40]   Wada N, Zaki MA, Hori Y, *et al.* Tumour-associated macrophages in diffuse large B-cell lymphoma: a study of the Osaka Lymphoma Study Group. Histopathology 2012; 60(2): 313-9.
[http://dx.doi.org/10.1111/j.1365-2559.2011.04096.x] [PMID: 22211289]

[41]   Beatty GL, Chiorean EG, Fishman MP, *et al.* CD40 agonists alter tumor stroma and show efficacy against pancreatic carcinoma in mice and humans. Science 2011; 331(6024): 1612-6.
[http://dx.doi.org/10.1126/science.1198443] [PMID: 21436454]

[42]   Coward J, Kulbe H, Chakravarty P, *et al.* Interleukin-6 as a therapeutic target in human ovarian cancer. Clin Cancer Res 2011; 17(18): 6083-96.
[http://dx.doi.org/10.1158/1078-0432.CCR-11-0945] [PMID: 21795409]

[43]   Wendt MK, Schiemann WP. Therapeutic targeting of the focal adhesion complex prevents oncogenic TGF-beta signaling and metastasis. Breast Cancer Res 2009; 11(5): R68.
[http://dx.doi.org/10.1186/bcr2360] [PMID: 19740433]

[44]   Cortez-Retamozo V, Etzrodt M, Newton A, *et al.* Origins of tumor-associated macrophages and neutrophils. Proc Natl Acad Sci USA 2012; 109(7): 2491-6.
[http://dx.doi.org/10.1073/pnas.1113744109] [PMID: 22308361]

[45]   Fridlender ZG, Albelda SM. Tumor-associated neutrophils: friend or foe? Carcinogenesis 2012; 33(5): 949-55.
[http://dx.doi.org/10.1093/carcin/bgs123] [PMID: 22425643]

[46]   Blanks MJ, Stehle JR Jr, Du W, *et al.* Novel innate cancer killing activity in humans. Cancer Cell Int 2011; 11: 26.
[http://dx.doi.org/10.1186/1475-2867-11-26] [PMID: 21813015]

[47]   Kilinc MO, Rowswell-Turner RB, Gu T, Virtuoso LP, Egilmez NK. Activated CD8+ T-effector/memory cells eliminate CD4+ CD25+ Foxp3+ T-suppressor cells from tumors *via* FasL mediated apoptosis. J Immunol 2009; 183(12): 7656-60.
[http://dx.doi.org/10.4049/jimmunol.0902625] [PMID: 19923444]

[48]   Xu Y, Hu H, Zheng J, Li B. Feasibility of whole RNA sequencing from single-cell mRNA

amplification. Genet Res Int 2013; 2013724124
[http://dx.doi.org/10.1155/2013/724124] [PMID: 24455282]

[49]   Li B, Liu G, Hu HL, Ding JQ, Zheng J, Tong A. Biomarkers Analysis for Heterogeneous Immune Responses of Quiescent CD8+cells -A Clue for Personalized Immunotherapy. Biom J 2015; 1: 1-11.

[50]   Haaland RE, Yu W, Rice AP. Identification of LKLF-regulated genes in quiescent CD4+ T lymphocytes. Mol Immunol 2005; 42(5): 627-41.
[http://dx.doi.org/10.1016/j.molimm.2004.09.012] [PMID: 15607822]

[51]   Tzachanis D, Li L, Lafuente EM, Berezovskaya A, Freeman GJ, Boussiotis VA. Twisted gastrulation (Tsg) is regulated by Tob and enhances TGF-beta signaling in activated T lymphocytes. Blood 2007; 109(7): 2944-52.
[http://dx.doi.org/10.1182/blood-2006-03-006510] [PMID: 17164348]

[52]   Chan WK, Rujkijyanont P, Neale G, *et al.* Multiplex and genome-wide analyses reveal distinctive properties of KIR+ and CD56+ T cells in human blood. J Immunol 2013; 191(4): 1625-36.
[http://dx.doi.org/10.4049/jimmunol.1300111] [PMID: 23858032]

[53]   Obara W, Ohsawa R, Kanehira M, *et al.* Cancer peptide vaccine therapy developed from oncoantigens identified through genome-wide expression profile analysis for bladder cancer. Jpn J Clin Oncol 2012; 42(7): 591-600.
[http://dx.doi.org/10.1093/jjco/hys069] [PMID: 22636067]

[54]   Li B, Chang T, Larson A, Ding J. Identification of mRNAs expressed in tumor-infiltrating lymphocytes by a strategy for rapid and high throughput screening. Gene 2000; 255(2): 273-9.
[http://dx.doi.org/10.1016/S0378-1119(00)00330-9] [PMID: 11024287]

[55]   Li B, Perabekam S, Liu G, Yin M, Song S, Larson A. Experimental and bioinformatics comparison of gene expression between T cells from TIL of liver cancer and T cells from UniGene. J Gastroenterol 2002; 37(4): 275-82.
[http://dx.doi.org/10.1007/s005350200035] [PMID: 11993511]

[56]   Daraselia N, Wang Y, Budoff A, *et al.* Molecular signature and pathway analysis of human primary squamous and adenocarcinoma lung cancers. Am J Cancer Res 2012; 2(1): 93-103.
[PMID: 22206048]

[57]   Lim D, Kim NK, Park HS, *et al.* Identification of candidate genes related to bovine marbling using protein-protein interaction networks. Int J Biol Sci 2011; 7(7): 992-1002.
[http://dx.doi.org/10.7150/ijbs.7.992] [PMID: 21912507]

[58]   Brandes U. A faster algorithm for betweenness centrality. J Math Sociol 2001; 25: 163-77.
[http://dx.doi.org/10.1080/0022250X.2001.9990249]

[59]   Bessarabova M, Ishkin A. JeBailey L, Nikolsky T. Knowledge-based analysis of proteomics data. BMC Bioinformatics 2012; 13: 13.
[http://dx.doi.org/10.1186/1471-2105-13-S16-S13]

[60]   Hulbert A, Jusue-Torres I, Stark A, *et al.* Early Detection of Lung Cancer Using DNA Promoter Hypermethylation in Plasma and Sputum. Clin Cancer Res 2017; 23(8): 1998-2005.
[http://dx.doi.org/10.1158/1078-0432.CCR-16-1371] [PMID: 27729459]

[61]   Perambakam S, Li B, Preisler H. Quantitation of interferon regulatory factor transcripts in patients with acute myeloid leukemia. Cancer Invest 2001; 19(4): 346-51.
[http://dx.doi.org/10.1081/CNV-100103129] [PMID: 11405174]

[62]   Wang JH, Tong SQ, Li B. Immunologic character of tumor infiltrating lymphocytes in ovarian carcinoma. Chin J Cancer Res 2000; 12(2): 99-104.
[http://dx.doi.org/10.1007/BF02983432]

[63]   Conesa A, Mortazavi A. The common ground of genomics and systems biology. BMC Syst Biol 2014; 8(2) (Suppl. 2): S1.
[http://dx.doi.org/10.1186/1752-0509-8-S2-S1] [PMID: 25033072]

[64]   Bonaz B. Inflammatory bowel diseases: a dysfunction of brain-gut interactions? Minerva Gastroenterol Dietol 2013; 59(3): 241-59.
[PMID: 23867945]

[65]   de Chassey B, Meyniel-Schicklin L, Aublin-Gex A, André P, Lotteau V. New horizons for antiviral drug discovery from virus-host protein interaction networks. Curr Opin Virol 2012; 2(5): 606-13.
[http://dx.doi.org/10.1016/j.coviro.2012.09.001] [PMID: 23025912]

[66]   Rosenberg SA, Restifo NP. Adoptive cell transfer as personalized immunotherapy for human cancer. Science 2015; 348(6230): 62-8.
[http://dx.doi.org/10.1126/science.aaa4967] [PMID: 25838374]

[67]   Li B. Breakthroughs of 2015-Personalized Immunotherapy Based on Individual GWAS and Biomarkers. Biom J 2015; 1: 1-2.

[68]   Powell MR, Sheehan DJ, Kleven DT. Altered Morphology and Immunohistochemical Characteristics in Metastatic Malignant Melanoma After Therapy With Vemurafenib. Am J Dermatopathol 2016; 38(9): e137-9.
[http://dx.doi.org/10.1097/DAD.0000000000000619] [PMID: 27541173]

[69]   Tran E, Turcotte S, Gros A, *et al.* Cancer immunotherapy based on mutation-specific CD4+ T cells in a patient with epithelial cancer. Science 2014; 344(6184): 641-5.
[http://dx.doi.org/10.1126/science.1251102] [PMID: 24812403]

[70]   Morgan RA, Dudley ME, Wunderlich JR, *et al.* Cancer regression in patients after transfer of genetically engineered lymphocytes. Science 2006; 314(5796): 126-9.
[http://dx.doi.org/10.1126/science.1129003] [PMID: 16946036]

[71]   Robbins PF, Morgan RA, Feldman SA, *et al.* Tumor regression in patients with metastatic synovial cell sarcoma and melanoma using genetically engineered lymphocytes reactive with NY-ESO-1. J Clin Oncol 2011; 29(7): 917-24.
[http://dx.doi.org/10.1200/JCO.2010.32.2537] [PMID: 21282551]

[72]   Kochenderfer JN, Wilson WH, Janik JE, *et al.* Eradication of B-lineage cells and regression of lymphoma in a patient treated with autologous T cells genetically engineered to recognize CD19. Blood 2010; 116(20): 4099-102.
[http://dx.doi.org/10.1182/blood-2010-04-281931] [PMID: 20668228]

[73]   Li B, Hu HL, Ding JQ, Yan D, Yang LM. Functional cell proliferation and differentiation by system modeling for cell therapy. International Journal of Latest Research in Science and Technology 2015; 2: 180-7.

CHAPTER 13

Biobank for Personalized Immunotherapy

Biaoru Li[1],*

Georgia Cancer Center and Department of Pediatrics, Medical College at GA, Augusta, GA 30912, USA

Abstract: A biobank is a resource for keeping blood and tissue samples, which is going to play an increasing role for personalized immunotherapy, called precision immunotherapy. Moreover, large profits from biobanks are their futures of patients' personalized immunotherapy. A new generation of immunotherapy often relies on a person's tissues/cells/molecules/data so that personalized immunotherapy starts to deposit the patient's specimens and clinical information with genomics data. If tumor patients can save their specimens such as tumor tissues or blood before treatment, furthermore, if patients can achieve some genomic data for future treatment, the specimens saved in biobanks and the genomics data observed from their tissues can contribute clinical physicians and clinical scientists to develop a new generation of treatment, for example, patients respond to immunotherapy predicted by individualized measurement and undergoing personalized T-cell immunotherapy. This chapter introduces biobank, one of the most up-to-date personalized immunotherapies, which enable conducting research and development (R&D) for professional collection of clinical specimens and clinical data. The chapter aims at describing the concept of biobank and future potential to treat patients. It also includes sample preservation protocols and data management as well as online service of samples and clinical data. Thus, some standard operating procedures apply for personalized immunotherapy of diagnostic and treatment procedures. Finally, ethics for sampling, clinical information, and genomics data are mentioned to support the biobank chapter.

Keywords: Biobank, Data-banking, Personalized immunotherapy, Precision medicine.

INTRODUCTION

T-cell adoptive immunotherapy and cytokine treatment of tumor diseases have come out several decades [1, 2]. For example, Steven Rosenberg had applied for lymphokine-activated killer cell (LAK) and tumor-infiltrating lymphocyte (TIL)

---

* **Corresponding author Biaoru Li**: Georgia Cancer Center and Department of Pediatrics, Medical College at GA, Augusta, GA 30912, USA; Tel: 440-317-1443; E-mail: bli@augusta.edu

to treat renal cancer and melanoma of patients during early 1980s [3, 4], and we had also used TIL to treat solid tumors for several hundred of tumor patients within the 1980s-the 1990s [5, 6]. Immunotherapy has developed so quickly that a few new methods have emerged during the 30 years [7, 8]. On the other hand, personalized medicine is also going to be quickly developed [9, 10]. Precision medicine is a new medical model that relied on individual characteristics of each patient rather than "one size fits all" treatment.

Since the 1980s, LAK, TIL, natural killer cells (NK cell), cytokine-induced killer cells (CIK), dendritic cells, and cytokine-induced killer cells (DC-CIK) have been increasingly developed as adoptive T-cell immunotherapy in translational medicine and different stages of clinical trials [11 - 16]. However, the cells only achieved 11-30% partial and complete responses (PR and CR) in clinics [17]. In order to increase immunotherapy effect, two subspecialties have developed during the last thirty years: (1) genetically engineering some particular substances, such as TNF-α, TGF-β, IL2, IL12, and IFN-γ, have mainly been introduced into T-cells [18 - 20]; (2) recently, genetically engineering some higher affinity substances between tumor cells and T-cell such as modified TCR (T-cell receptor) and chimeric antigen receptors T-cell (CAR-T cells) have been also successfully reported to treat B-cell leukemia/lymphomas as well as other tumor diseases [21 - 24].

When the human genome sequence was decoded in 2004 [25], scientists and physicians have primarily studied workflows from biobank and genomic profile/system modeling *in silico* to functional inducing T-cells *ex vivo* and genetically-engineering cell *in intro/ex vivo* related to the new techniques [26 - 28]. We have been studying the fields from tumor-tissue biobank such as T-cells' and primary tumor cells' isolation, storage, and culture into single T-cell/single tumor cell genomics and system biology for more than 30 years [29 - 31]. Fortunately, Rosenberg first reported the efficacy of T-cell personalized immunotherapy of different patients related to individual GWAS (genome-wide association study) in 2015 [32]. Now, personalized immunotherapy has been increasingly reported in the new generation of immunotherapy.

All in all, optimal immunotherapy requires excellent support of biobank so that personalized immunotherapy begins to save patient's specimens such as tumor tissue biobanking with their T-cells and tumor cells storage, including their molecules and genomics data. Once the system established, clinical scientists and medical doctors can readily use their biobanks for clinical administration of their tumor diseases at a hospital and undergoing immune therapy. Furthermore, the goal of this biorepository is to collect tumor tissue, blood, and data from patients undergoing immune-based therapy, so that they can use for correlative evaluations in optional protocols [33]. The specimens and data are linked to the patient, thus allowing for personalized immunotherapy. Furthermost, they provide continuous treatment such as those that evaluate the correlation of tumor biomarkers with patient variables to treat cancer, as well as those that identify interactions between biomarkers and immunotherapy [34].

Along with the R&D of new techniques in tumor tissue storage, T-cells/tumor cells storage, thawing, and cultures, the methodology significantly improves specimen biorepository to patient treatment and clinical care [35, 36]. If a patient can store his/her tumor and blood specimens, the vast choice of patient treatment can resolve the challenge of the patient himself with tumor disease, for example, patient specimens can be used by next-generation sequence (NGS) for personalized therapy once the patients have their tumor recurrence. Finally, the following knowledge explosion in this era, the possibility of applying for new treatment and new compounds should increasingly depend on the possibility of storage of tumor specimens.

BIOBANKS FOR PERSONALIZED IMMUNOTHERAPY

Concept of Biobanks

Because extensive diversity relied on purpose and role on biobanks, it is not easy to give an optimal concept for biobank [37]. Generally, biobanks are professional biorepositories of clinical samples regarding storing specimens at a harvested time, including clinical, epidemiological, and general source data. Also, processed samples are analyzed and optimally preserved for clinical patients with sharing to hospitals for the patients and clinical/scientific community for their clinical and translational researches [38]. An ideal biobank consists of the acquisition, delivery, preservation method under the regulation of Standard Operating Procedures (SOPs) to ensure correct performance of all components (such as specimens anonymization, patients' acquisition, delivery, preparation, analysis, proper storage conditions and specimens' sharing in hospitals under ethics). In short, the concept of the biobank is to set up an SOP tissue storing system for patients with a wide variety of data for the R&D requirements, translational medicine, and clinical application.

Concept of Biobank for Immunotherapy

1. T-cells of immunotherapy involve LAK, TIL, CIK, DC-CIK [39]. Moreover, these cells have significantly been developed into a new generation of immunotherapy, such as genetically engineering a type of the patient's own disease-fighting T-cells to killing own tumor cells so that the T-cells isolated from the patient's blood are altered by inserting a gene, which is reprogramed

to recognize and kill tumor cells as TCR-T-cells or CAR-T cells [40 - 42]. The altered cells are then reinfused into the patient's body in which the modified T-cells spread and further expand to identify and kill rapidly growing tumor cells *in vivo* [43]. T-cell biobank is one of the essential steps for the performance of personalized immunotherapy. The biorepository has three characteristics for application of T-cells personalized immunotherapy:

A. **Specificity**: T-cell immunotherapy produced from its immune system targets explicitly the own tumor cells in the body.

B. **Strength**: T-cell immunotherapy has a powerful killing function that systematically attacks its tumor cells in the body.

C. **Side-effect low**: the immunotherapy utilizes its immune system to kill its tumor cells, so that side effect is much lower for the patient treatment than those from heterogenous T-cell sources.

1. Personalized immunotherapy involves the tumor cells' biobanks, called tumor banks [44], aiming at exploring the biological features of tumor cells by harvesting and comparing healthy cells and the tumor cells. In general, four advantages are introduced by the tumor biobank for precision medicine (personalized immunotherapy and personalized therapy) [45]:

A. **Understanding the molecular basis of new feasible biomarkers for personalized therapy**: This purpose requires the isolation of molecule particles such as DNA, RNA, and proteins, which discuss below.

B. **Understanding T-cell sensitivity of killing tumor cell**: As described above, at present, adoptive T-cell immunotherapy such as LAK, TIL, CIK, DC-CIK, and modified T-cells as TCR T-cell and CAR-T cells have been increasingly applied for immunotherapy at different stages of clinical trials. However, a different type of T-cells is different responses to different patients and different tumor diseases. If a patient can store his/her tumor cells with the T-cells, cultured T-cells can use primary tumor cells to test CTL of these tumors by *ex vivo* sensitivity assay of T-cells for immunotherapy [46].

C. **Understanding drug sensitivity of tumor cells:** If a biobank has functional storing tumor cells from patients, the tumor cells' bank should be used to drug sensitivity assay (*in vitro/ex vivo*-chemosensitivity assay, CSA) [47] to decide on sensitive drug's selection of personalized chemotherapy to patient treatment. Our early researches indicated that results of combined TIL and sensitive drugs by using CSA were much better than those of only T-cell immunotherapy such as TIL treatment or those of only chemotherapy for patients from 1989-1999 [48].

D. **Understanding sensitive response to tumor cells for molecular targeting therapy**: If a biobank has proper storage of tumor cells from patients, the tumor cells from biobank can be used to screen molecular targeting Ab and small molecule for their therapy [49]. The screening assay can give doctors to select more sensitivity and more affordable molecular targeting compounds for these patients [50].

The biorepository for tumor cells from patients also has three characteristics in personalized therapy:

A. **Specificity**. The personalized therapy, including personalized immunotherapy, personalized chemotherapy, and personalized molecular therapy specifically target the own tumor cells in the body.

B. **Strength**. The personalized therapy, including personalized immunotherapy, personalized chemotherapy, and personalized molecular therapy, has a powerful killing function that systematically attacks own tumor cells in the body.

C. **Side-effect low**. The personalized therapy, including personalized immunotherapy, personalized chemotherapy, and personalized molecular therapy, kill only own tumor cells, so that side effect is very lower for the patient treatment.

1. Personalized therapy involves in tumor tissue, regulating cells, and regulating molecules from the tumor microenvironment (TME) [51]. TME researches aim at exploring the biological features by identifying molecules (protein and RNA), regulating cells, and tumor tissue matrix [52]. In general, the TME advantage from biobank includes identifying molecules and cell regulation for personalized targeting therapy.

A. **Identifying the molecular regulation of TME for personalized therapy**: the purpose will be discussed as our book mentioned below.

B. **Identifying the cellular regulation of TME for personalized therapy and personalized immunotherapy**: this purpose is to assay different genes' and proteins' expression at cell levels and matrix tissue level in TME [53]. If a biobank has a proper storage of tumor tissue from patients, the tumor tissue bank, including TME matrix, cells, and molecules, significantly improves the effects of personalized therapy of patient treatment.

C. **Identifying check-point inhibitors to regulating tumor cells growth and T-cell immunity** [54]: If a biobank has proper storage from patients, the TME from biobank is used to screen molecular targeting therapy of check-point inhibitors. The screening system can give patients to much support molecular targeting therapy.

In the future, except for tissue-based biobank for immunotherapy and personalized immunotherapy, an ideal biobank also requires the disease-based unit and population-based unit of biobanks for immunotherapy. The purpose of a disease-based unit of biobank is to determine specific exposure factors and tumorigenesis related to inhibitors for a development of tumor disease by a careful collection of specimens from a patient, often comprising various specimens harvesting by time-course and location from the same patient or various specimens achieved by time-course from similar diseases of different patients. For instance, we have studied the developmental model from myelodysplastic syndrome (MDS) to chronic myeloid leukemia (CML) and acute myeloid leukemia (AML) during the 1990s. Because we had an excellent biorepository to support the researches of development lineage of lymphoma-MDS-CML-AML, we could discover that IL4 and IL10 immunotherapy can increase the effect of amifostine for a particular period from MDS transferring into AML [55]. Population-based units consist of specimens, epidemiological information, and clinical data collected from volunteers or patients without specific standards to study some multiple factors (inclusion or exclusion criteria) [56]. The purpose mirrors the special status of one disease and thus comparable to the general population without the disease. We had selected several dozens of donors' specimens from healthy lung tissues and other positive and negative controls to compare a patient with advanced NSCLC (non-small cell lung cancer), for whom he selected for personalized therapy. Finally, we discovered therapeutic targeting drugs for the patient [57]. The results indicated that personalized therapy requires a population-based unit of biobanks. Now, GEO (gene expression omnibus) and SRA (Sequence Read Archive), ENCODE (Encyclopedia Of DNA Elements), and TCGA (The Cancer Genome Atlas) have stored a lot of these kinds of information [58 - 60]. If we can develop a population-based biorepository biobank itself, it contributes more information for immunotherapy and personalized immunotherapy.

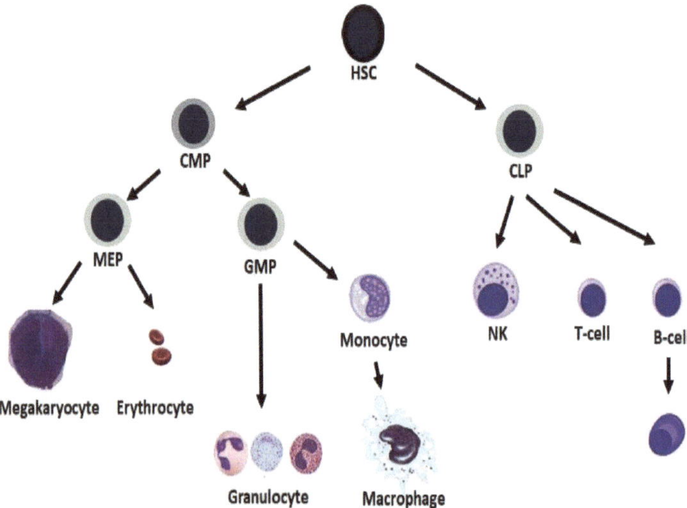

Fig. (1). Hematopoiesis. The formation of lymphopoiesis as B cells and T cells. After maturation, the lymphocytes enter the circulation and peripheral blood.

BIOBANK COMPONENTS

Basic Component of Biobanks

According to concept of biobanks as introduced above, biorepository provides all service or components for the R&D and clinical application with general features [61].

A. Collecting, shipping and storage of patient's materials such as tumor tissue and blood combined with general information, medical history, epidemiological data;

B. Performing Standard Operating Procedures (SOP);

C. Applying specimens' anonymization for the donor and patient privilege;

D. Dynamically developing the biorepository for a long-term service;

E. Monitoring and ongoing research project, R&D, translational medicine and current/future clinical application;

F. Monitoring ethical issues and legal prevention to the biobank.

Biobank Components of Immunotherapy

1. **Immune cells (such as T-cell biorepository) from the blood**. In the blood, immune cells include lymphocyte and macrophages as well as others, which come from bone marrow as Fig. (**1**). This process is called hematopoiesis. All lymphocytes originate from a common lymphoid progenitor (CLP) of stem cells; thus, differentiating into their distinct lymphocyte types. The formation of lymphopoiesis as B-cells mature from the gut-associated lymphoid tissue.
(GALT) in humans, while T-cells migrate to and mature in the thymus. After maturation, the lymphocytes enter the circulation and peripheral blood, which we can extract. The circulation lymphocytes include T-cells such as, CD3 (CD4 helper cell and CD8 cytotoxic cells), B-cell such as CD19 cells and NK cells (CD16/CD56) [62 - 64]. At present, T-cells of immunotherapy like LAK, CIK, DC-CIK are coming from the peripheral blood.
Moreover, these cells can be engineered as TCR-T-cells or CAR-T cells or expressing specific substances, so that much T-cell immunotherapy requires the peripheral blood to store to treat patients with tumor diseases [65, 66]. The activated T-cell or altered T-cells are reinfused back into the patient's body to kill tumor cells *in vivo*. Biorepository from peripheral blood contains almost all components for T-cells of immunotherapy as below;

   a. Cultured and activated T-cells such as LAK, CIK, DC-CIK, and engineered T-cells such as TCR-T-cells and CAR-T cells, which I have primarily presented as above.

   b. Although B-cells are poorly researched for human immunotherapy, B-cells have been confirmed to infiltrating into solid tumors [67]. Up to now, B-cells have been discovered not only producers of antibodies but also immune function as antigen-presenting cells (APC) [68]. The potential of B-cells of cell therapy is increasingly studied in animals [69]. For example, the CD40L/CD40 signaling pathway remains in B lymphocytes. The CD40-activated B cells functionally induce specific T-cell responses as APC [70]. Furthermore, CD40-activated B cell-based cancer immunotherapy can directly induce effective antitumor function. In the human, some early-stage clinical studies involving B-cell based cancer vaccines and B-cell-based immunotherapy are to study for safety and toxicity at phase-1 [71]. A phase-2, some results demonstrated that B-cell immunotherapy has an antitumor mechanism of T-cell responses [72]. In a pharmaceutical company, GMP performances are subject to set up the isolation and culture system for B-cell projects [73]. Therefore, we should consider lymphocyte biorepository, including B-cells for future translation medicine and clinical application such as CD40-activated B cells.

c. NK-cells from peripheral blood have mainly been studied for tumor disease and have been increasingly reported to administer tumor disease. The results of NK-cells administration have demonstrated a low side-effect for patients with tumor diseases [74]. CD16/56-cultured cells functionally play for antitumor effect because CD16/56-cultured cells may directly kill tumor cells without complex immunoregulation. In a pharmaceutical company, some GMP performances are to be used the NK cells isolation and culture system; thus, NK-cells should be considered under the biorepository of a future application for translation medicine and clinical administration.

d. Other T-cells such as NKT-cell and double negative T-cell (DN-T-cells). The potential of NKT-cells is not only NK function but also have some T-cell special receptors [75]. Moreover, DN T-cells are early T-cell biomarkers such as CD3 without CD4/CD8 [76]. Now both have been increasingly studied in the killing-tumor mechanism for cell therapy *in vivo* and *in vitro*. For example, some of the results of NKT-cells/DN T-cells demonstrated that both could effectively kill tumor cells in animal and human experiments [77]. In a pharmaceutical company, GMP performances have been set up the isolation and culture system for their cells so that we also should consider the T-cell biorepository, including those cells in future translation medicine and clinical care.

1. **Immune Cells (such as TIL Biorepository) using sources from tumor tissue for immunotherapy and personalized immunotherapy**
In tumor tissue, immune cells for immunotherapy and personalized immunotherapy include lymphocyte and macrophages. The T-cells are called TILs we had studied and applied for adoptive immunotherapy more than thirty years. In our early researches, we administered TIL combined with sensitive chemotherapy drugs tested by CSA for tumor cells from patients. Our results indicated 27% partial and complete responses for advanced tumor patients during the 1980s-1990s [78, 79]. Tumor-infiltrating B-lymphocyte, as discussed above, has been increasingly confirmed to act as potent antigen-presenting cells to tumor cells, although they are poorly investigated for immunotherapy. As discussed above, CD40-activated B-cells can specifically induce T-cell responses *in vitro* and *in vivo*. Now several early-stages of clinical studies were involved in B-cell based cancer vaccines. Also, the B-cells of TILs can lead to antitumor T-cell responses after different clinical trials [80]. All components for immunotherapy are illuminated as Fig. (**2**).
According to a few results of experimental and clinical researches, tumor-

infiltrating lymphocytes have two features: (I) specificity. The T-cell immunotherapy obtained by tumor tissues and induced from tumor cells can specifically target own tumor cells in the body; (II) Strength. T-cell immunotherapy is more than 100-fold ability to kill tumor cells to compare those from peripheral blood [81].

2. **Tumor cells and components of TME.** In tumor tissue, tumor cells, as described above, and tumor microenvironment (TME) around a tumor, are playing an essential role in personalized immunotherapy, personalized therapy, and personalized targeting therapy. In tumor tissue, TME consists of three components as Fig. (**3**):

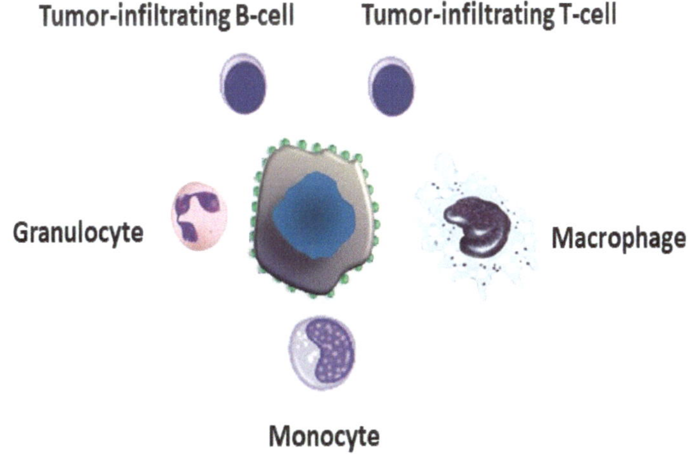

Fig. (2). Tumor-infiltrating lymphocyte and macrophage.
Tumor-infiltrating lymphocyte (T-cell and B-cell) for immunotherapy induced from tumor cells so that the lymphocyte specifically targets the own tumor cells in the body.

(I) Tissue called as extracellular matrix (ECM) with epithelium, basement and endothelium (Fig. **3A**) [82].

(II) Regulating cells including carcinoma-associated fibroblasts, myeloid-derived suppressor cells (MDSC), tumor-associated macrophages (TAM), tumor-infiltrating lymphocyte (TIL), neutrophils and so on Fig. (**3B**) [83].

(III) Signaling molecules which can influence tumor growth by releasing extracellular signals, promoting tumor angiogenesis, inducing immune tolerance and affecting the growth of tumor cells. Although TME is poorly researched for biobank establishment, TME will be developed once TME techniques are matured. For example, currently, pathologists can identify genes' and proteins' expression by immunocytochemistry techniques [84]; moreover, 10X genomics techniques can use different barcodes of identified cells to define genomics expression pattern [85]. Now we require to set up a optimal biorepository at a level of tumor tissues to keep complete TME, so that the biorepository can be utilized to future application in translational medicine and clinical care for personalized immunotherapy, personalized chemotherapy, and personalized targeting therapy.

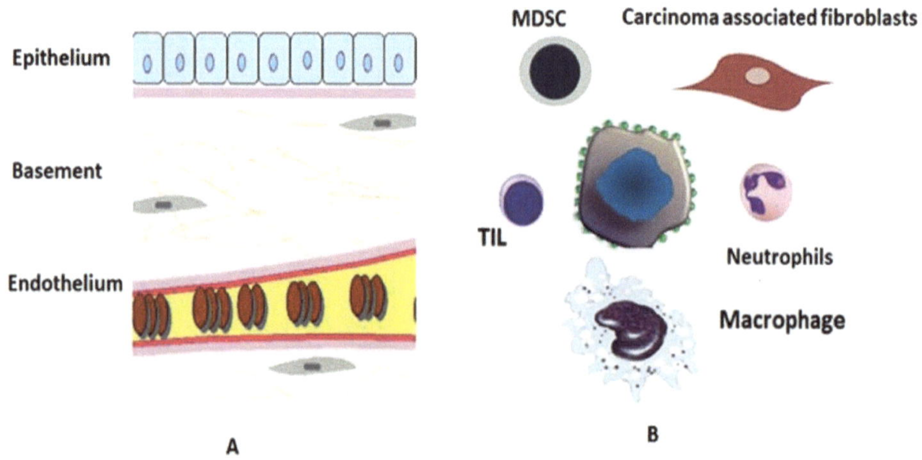

Fig. (3). Tumor cells and TME. Extracellular matrix (ECM) with epithelium, basement, and endothelium as Fig. (**3A**); Fig. (**3B**) demonstrates regulating cells including MDSC, tumor-associated macrophages, tumor-infiltrating lymphocyte and neutrophils with their signaling molecules by releasing extracellular signals for promoting tumor angiogenesis, inducing immune tolerance and affecting the growth and evolution of tumor cells.

BIOBANK PROTOCOLS FOR IMMUNOTHERAPY

1. Protocol Requirement for Personalized Immunotherapy

Personalized immunotherapy, as one of precision medicine, also has four functions as precision medicine of clinical application: prediction, prevention, prognostic estimation, and personalized therapy.

A. **Prediction:** the ability to conduct precise analysis of risk for tumor disease and then the effective prediction of immunotherapy. Although the traditional concept of immunotherapy is involved in T-cell infused into the body to play in immunotherapy, personalized immunotherapy has prediction function as same as precision medicine. For example, the patient was discovered genetic profiles with an SNP, which is sensitive to imatinib to treat so that medical doctors can use the imatinib to treat the patient [86]. Moreover, if a substantial differentiating T-cells are being kept in a biobank, they can be used by *in vitro/ex vivo*-immunotherapy sensitivity assay for different tumor diseases [87]. Now, biobanks play an essential role in discovering new predictive factors such as TME and tumor cells by which biobank data can be facilitated by correct prediction from those of tumor cells and TME.

B. **Prevention:** a biobank storing T-cells, B-cells, or whole blood also has the preventive function of tumor diseases. For example, as I mentioned above, CD40-activated B-cells seem to have effects as preventive vaccination [88]. Because CD40-activated B-cells can specifically induce T-cell responses, now several early-stage clinical studies involve in B-cell based cancer vaccines so that personalized immunotherapy contains the mechanism of tumor prevention.

C. **Prognostic estimation**: soon, it is possible to elevate the prognostic value if we set up genome data with T-cell/B-cell/tumor cell biorepository. The biobank finally leads to physicians to quick and accurate diagnosis and enable to estimate right treatment on time for patients with tumor diseases [89]. Several reports have indicated that biorepository of T-cells, B-cells, and tumor cells, as well as TME, can present a new plan for tumor diseases, treatment options, and response for these treatments.

D. **Personalized therapy**: If different SNPs and genomic expression from biorepository kept for patient biobank, they have importantly impacted on treatment efficacy. We have reported a dozen of cases by using genomic data to support T-cell personalized immunotherapy and personalized chemotherapy [90]. In 2015, Rosenberg also reported that GWAS data influence T-cell immunotherapy [91]. Recently next genomic sequences are more affordable so that the precision diagnosis can significantly increase the effectiveness of treatment. Biobanks are vital to storing patients' materials such as RNA, DNA, and proteins. Biobanks are going to develop a center for personalized immunotherapy, personalized chemotherapy, and personalized molecular targeting therapy.

2. Basic Protocols

According to a biobank concept and components, a biobank of personalized immunotherapy provides all SOP service as Fig. **(4)** (SOP-1) such as good biorepository, SOP performance, specimens' analysis, IT and database management, ethical document management as well as specimen application including R&D and long-term specimen management as the below:

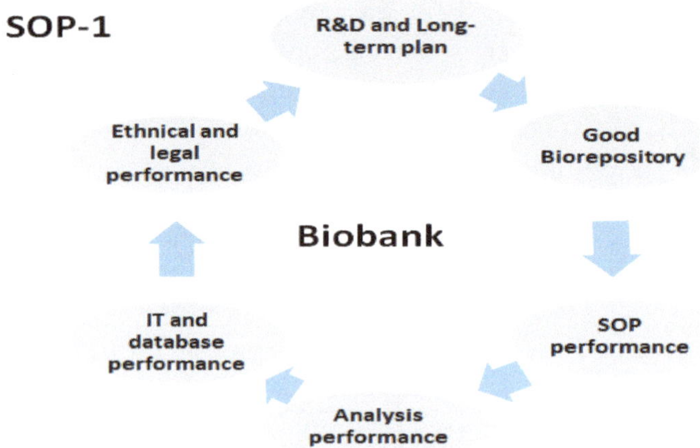

Fig. (4). Biobank performance.

A. **Biorepository**. Collecting, shipping and storage of clinical specimens such as tumor tissue and blood combined with general information, medical history, epidemiological data;

B. **Performing Standard Operating Procedures** (SOP) for all process in A;

C. **Biospecimens analysis** routinely;

D. **Biospecimens IT management** with the database under artificial intelligence; Performing ethnic and legal management;

E. **Cooperating patient's doctors** related application scientists to set R&D and translational medicine and clinical application plan.

3. Protocol for Biorepository of Immunotherapy

In general, according to **(I)** biobank concept of immunotherapy, three repositories of immunotherapy related cells and tissue are processed, such as immune cells (T-cells/B-cells), primary tumor cells and tumor microenvironment. According to **(II)** biobank components of immunotherapy, three components involved in the repositories, such as immune cells (T-cells and B-cells) from blood; immune cells from tumor tissue and tumor microenvironment including tumor cells and TME such as matrix tissues, regulating cells and regulating molecules within tumor tissues. According to **(III)** clinical application of precision medicine, four employments involved in the biorepository of personalized immunotherapy: prediction, prevention, prognostic, and personalized therapy. According to **(IV)** necessary process, biobanks consist of six items and performances, biorepository, SOP performance, routine analysis, IT/database management, ethical/legal performance, and R&D and long-term management.

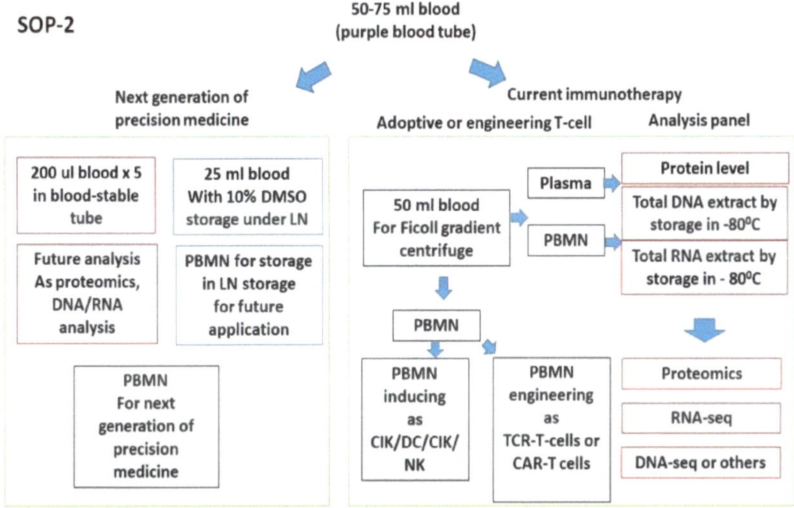

Fig. (5). illuminated as SOP-2 indicated all process from blood.

All in all, a suitable biobanking protocol of personalized immunotherapy agrees all over four prerequisites: "concepts," "components," "precision medicine," and "basic management of biorepository." Fortunately, we had set up TIL/tumor cell isolation and storage with the first clinical application of TIL immunotherapy and sensitive chemotherapy by CSA since 1989, we have an increasing experience to develop the protocol since the 1980s [92].

For example, no matter how early tumor tissues and immune cells/tumor cells were stored in our laboratory, we always kept patients' tumor tissues as FFPE, OCT and fresh frozen with their components. Now along with new techniques and knowledge in the era, our MD can use our patients' specimens for current precision medicine such as prediction, prevention, prognostic estimation, and personalized immunotherapy [93]. Because we early consider their biorepositories related to their future diagnoses and application, nowadays, our medical doctors can use our biorepository to develop their, at present, diagnosis and treatment. Here are concluded as below (SOP-2 and SOP-3).

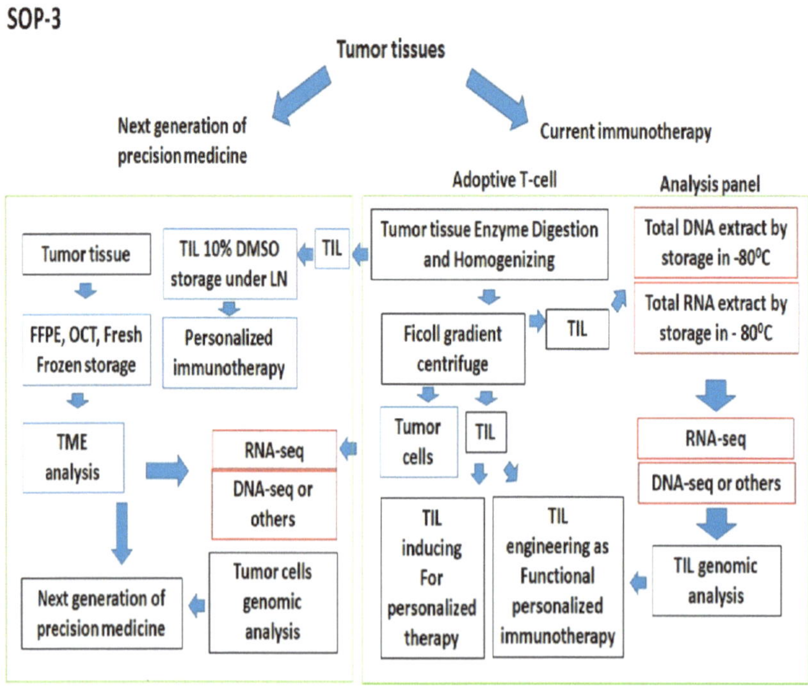

Fig. (6). Biorepository from Tumor Tissue (SOP-3).

BIOBANK ANALYSIS FOR IMMUNOTHERAPY

Because immunotherapy has some unique characteristics as our early publication in 1999 [94], analyses of biobanks of personalized immunotherapy much more focus on immune cells for treatment and tumor cells for diagnosis or assay. As I called the procedure as "tumor tissue re-cycle" during sampling procedures as Fig. (7) with five steps:

1. **Gating analysis** (Fig. 7A). Biobank starts general patient information with informed consent from the patient. Because patients' biobank begins to medical procedures, three parallel steps in clinical medical doctors, laboratory doctors such as pathologists and diagnostic lab, and biobank staff for the sharing system.

2. **Initial analysis of biobank** (Fig. 7B). Once patients' specimens are stored into biobank, initial analyses will begin, including (I) an analysis of proper specimens' collection such as blood clot or not and tumor tissue necrosis or not, tumor tissue *VS* healthy tissue; (II) blood or tissues within sterile manner and temperature condition; (III) aliquoting a smaller piece according to our protocol above to analysis; (IV) sharing of samples for hospital without thawing; (V)

completing survey data and record for further analysis. These multi-analyses require SOP workflow to keep reproducibility.

3. **First analysis of biobank.** The collected clinical samples, including blood and tumor tissue, requires proper preparation and preservation protocol. The first step of analysis is to perform a replicable and feasible aliquoting workflow with proper labeling, which should be compatible with the IT system to ensure correct storage for the first set of sample access. In personalized immunotherapy, molecules, including DNA, RNA, and protein and primary cells, including immune cells and primary tumor cells, require an aliquoting workflow as Fig. (**7C**). The purpose of analysis can study specimens of first storage for current personalized immunotherapy and future precision medicine.

4. **Following Analysis of Biobank**. Human tissue samples will lose quality during storage, although specimens are stored in liquid nitrogen situation. The essential step of following analytical samples' management is to perform an available, precise, and replicable aliquoting workflow. In personalized immunotherapy, molecules (including DNA, RNA, and protein) and primary cells (including immune cells and primary cells) require an aliquoted part as Fig. (**7D**). The purpose of analysis can study specimens' situation for ongoing personalized immunotherapy or precision medicine.

5. **R&D Analysis and Long-term Analysis**. Immunotherapy cells require a very strict analysis as Fig. (**7E**). Once patients' specimens are decided for R&D purpose and translational medicine such as CAR-T-cell immunotherapy, R&D analyses include (I) the cell viability from specimens' collection such as PBMN from blood or TIL or primary tumor cells from tumor tissue; (II) purity for each cells such as T-cells or primary tumor cells after purifying; (III) GMP assay such as HIV-1/HIV2, HBV, HCV from clinical specimens with their culture; (IV) Cell numbers from specimens' collection with their immune cells and primary tumor cells after purifying.

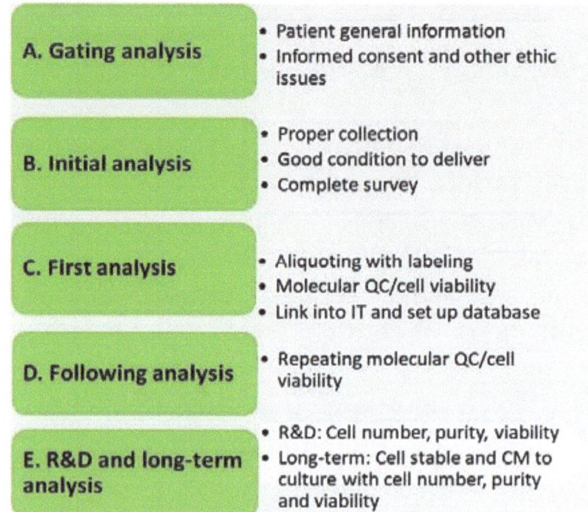

Fig. (7). Biobank analysis for immunotherapy.

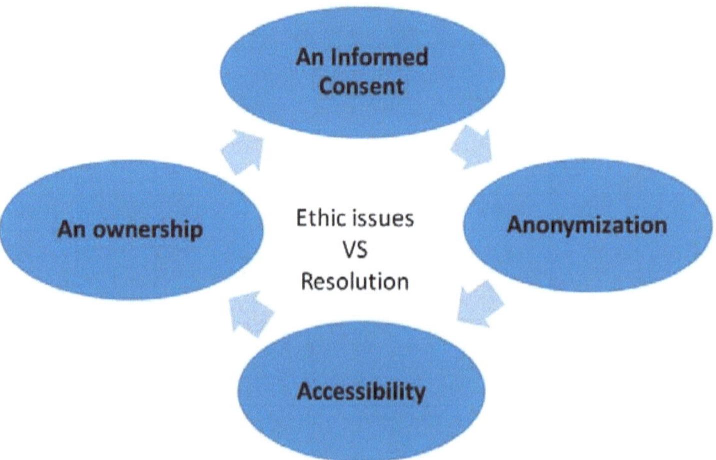

Fig. (8). Ethical issues and their resolution.

Long-term analyses of immunotherapy cells require much stricter than those of R&D as Fig. (**7E**). Once long-term storage are used to translational medicine such as T-cells of adoptive immunotherapy from patients' specimens, long-term analyses include as R&D analysis: (I) the cell viability from specimens' collection such as PBMN from blood or TIL or primary tumor cell from tumor tissue; (II) purity for each cells such as T-cells or primary tumor cells after purifying; (III) GMP analysis such as HIV-1/HIV2, HBV, HCV from clinical specimens with their cultures; (IV) cell numbers from specimens' collection with their immune cells and primary tumor cells after purifying; (V) stability for a storage for long-term service and clinical scientists service to perform a protocol from thaw cells until their culture medium.

ETHICAL ISSUES AND LEGAL RESOLUTION

Biobanks have several ethic issues as those of clinical pathology and clinical genetics so that their resolution, most of them, are performed as same as clinical pathology and clinical genetics, although several issues are different from those of pathology and clinical genetics [95]. Here, four ethical issues are involved in biobanks, called as four "A": **An Informed Consent, Anonymization, Accessibility, An ownership:**

1. **An Informed Consent with their Resolution**. Optimal agreements of informed consent documents are crucial in gating biobank. Proper informed consent can give clinical scientists and doctors enough to support to process biorepository and to utilize those by patients, researchers, and doctors for their projects. A biobank form of informed consent includes general consent as clinical pathology and clinical genetics. They also have a patient's extent permission to use their specimens for both present research and future applications without re-application from the patient [96]. At present, most of biobanks still need re-application of consent form if the configuration of biobanks alters their systems such as service and application beyond first informed consent. Fortunately, the development of an IT service can keep continuous and dynamic consent performance. This kind of service works as same as "Save Account" in a bank, which can be easy to access to keep a connection with the patients-doctors and to manage their biospecimens [97] dynamically. For example, doctors can report some discoveries from update information of biobank; patients can inform biobanks some progress for their diseases. IT-based informed-consent support-system give patients great benefits for health care or essential discovery while conducting clinical researches. As a publication, a recent study on the Australian biorepository showed that 94,4% of people responded that informed consent so that they can play an essential role in patients' health and treatment from biobank [98].
Two ethical issues are still not clear from biobanks: (I) about children specimens, biorepository obtained from children should require a parent or legal guardian consent. Tissues obtained from children and granted by parent consent and those used by maturation are not clear in ethic performance [99]; (II) about international biorepository, there is no international consensus on the informed consent because of differences among each legal system of each country [100].

2. **Anonymization for patient's privilege.** Anonymization is a critical concept for ethical issues in biorepository performance [101]. Especially, specimens' R&D performance and long-term storage of clinical diagnosis and treatment require full-anonymization with their identification procedures. For example, the USA and Europe provide professional and safe data management guidance [102]. In the biorepository for personalized immunotherapy, most of the performances follow the conventional clinical performance as same as pathology. Once patients' specimens are gating into a biobanking laboratory, data anonymization by coding is split into two workflow systems (coding system for biobanking performances and real information system from patients) [103]. Thus, specimen coding is done in an ordered performance by using a designed code for all specimens. Finally, identification data on patients combined with a coding symbol (code and barcode) with real patients' information are completed by decoding from both systems under the SOP. The anonymization secures researchers and clinical doctors either correctly perform their data or make avoid to contacting patients' information accidentally.

3. **Accessibility with that prevention**. After genomic data are involved in biobank with their application, such as NGS (next-generation sequence) data storage, patients and donors begin to concern their data and specimens in a biobank. Now the security of patient data and specimens has been increasingly questioned [104]. For example, researchers without ethic education use genomic sequence data, including their analyses to survey patient treatment so that their activities increase exposure possibility of patients' health status. Therefore, broad prevention steps are executed in each step of specimens' performance and analysis. Moreover, researcher units and clinical units use "Double-Blind", as medical data management, to access both genomics data and medical data so that biobank is very well prevented by this kind of accessibility [105].

4. **An ownership**. Ownership rights or their giving-up rights should be set up from the startup of a biobank because ownership plays an essential role in transferring specimens between foreign researchers/medical doctors (Material Transfer Agreement, MTA) [106] even if specimens are utilized after patients' death. Now clinical scientists should understand the issue of ownership. If clinical scientists and MDs want to use their specimens for R&D, translational medicine rather than patient rights himself, they must obey the ownership regulation including research goals such as biomarkers discovery and new drug discovery for new drug targets or a novel treatment except that the patient becomes participant for the results and benefits of the biorepository.

One ethical issue of ownership remains to argue in biobanks: For example, specimens from some countries such as those from China. Because medical doctors and patients' family in some countries want to decrease panic of the patient suffering from tumor disease, they rarely inform patients for their tumor diseases so that ownership of the specimen is not clear rather than that of this family member or doctors if biobanking receives a specimen from tumor patient.

Generally, biobanks from different countries face legal issues which should need to match their legal system so that they require to set up their solutions according to their legal systems [107].

DATABASE MANAGEMENT AND ONLINE SERVICE

The database is one of the crucial issues in biobanks so that a few of bioinformatics specialists serve in biobanks, who make biorepository fully support and correct analysis. Besides, strict accessibility, proper management, and anonymization require several IT engineers to perform hardware and software highly. Accordingly, international standards enable to share of harmonizing databases under structures of international organizations such as NCI, ISBER, and EC-JRC, which increases proper management by which the project can bring profits for the international corporation [108].

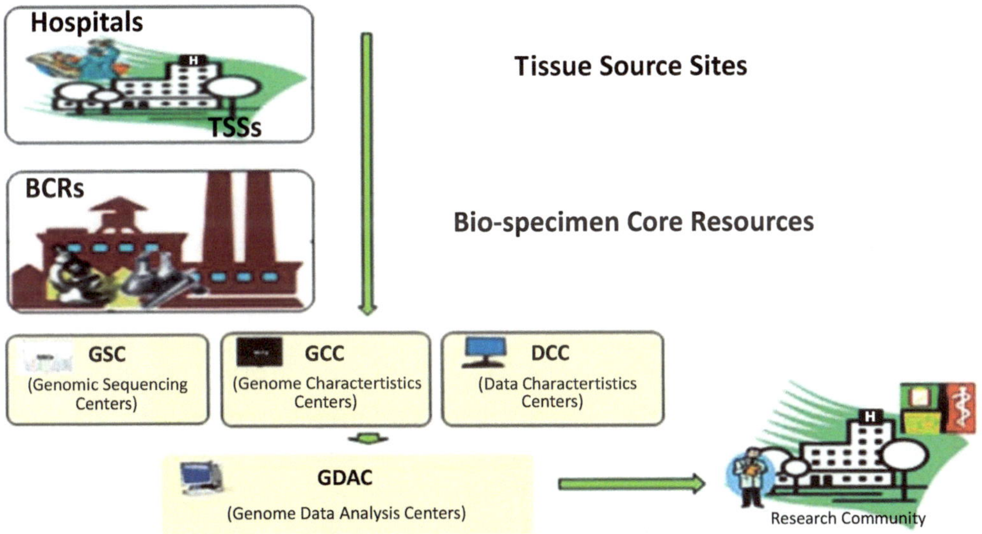

Fig. (9). TCGA system to support both biobank and database.

1. **Biobank Data.** Many database systems support biobank, while several biobanks require sound database systems. Here we introduce an excellent

system combining both mutual supports (biobank-database) called The Cancer Genome Atlas (TCGA). TCGA is the first feasible platform analyzing genetic mutations for cancer to improve to diagnose, treat, and prevent cancer launched by the National Cancer Institute and the National Human Genome Research Institute. During 2006-2009, three types of human cancers' integrated genomic data (glioblastoma multiforme, lung, and ovarian cancer) were stored and studied in TCGA [109]. After 2009, an additional 33 types of tumor integrated genomics were characterized by the platform [110]. Now their projects and techniques include gene expression profiling, copy number variation profiling, SNP genotyping, genome-wide DNA methylation profiling, microRNA profiling, and exon sequencing. The TCGA has a routine workflow from Tissue Source Sites (TSSs) working for clinical data collection, preliminary pathology data, and specimens' collection, to Biospecimen Core Resource (BCR) processing molecular analyte isolation and Quality Control (QC), eventually into genomic processing and analyzing [111]. To thoroughly study genomic data, four centers to generate data and analyze data for genomic processing: Genome Sequencing Centers (GSC), Genome Characterization Centers (GCC), Data Coordinating Center (DCC), and Genome Data Analysis Centers (GDAC). As Fig. (**9**). We can see a comprehensive biobank-database system as TCGA with TSS (Tissue Source Sites)-BCR (Biospecimen Core Resource)-QC-Analysis system (GSC/GCC/DCC/GDAC). Soon, we should believe that a database of personalized immunotherapy, as same as those of TCGA, plays a vital role in personalized immunotherapy for tumor diseases.

2. **Online Service of Biobanks.** As described above, broad scopes of data in biobanks include (I) basic facts such as demographics, ethnical, medical, environmental, genetic information collected from the patient, (II) medical information such as history, symptom, laboratory, imaging and pathological results and (III) biobank information such as specimens' storage. All biobanks require an excellent system supported by feasible and complex IT management and online service. Because of those complicated tasks, online services are essential to perform the data compatible with hospitals, biobank, and patients. Now software has served the system such as XTENS, which has a web portal, an internal database, and a data grid storage element [112]. Because the systems perform much sensitive information with legal prevention, researchers and clinicians need an available and permissible online with some tools under legal regulations sharing in their countries. Biobanks with IT systems and online services require understanding ethical issues prevented by their own country for the three steps of patients-doctors-biobank so that the biorepository can quickly support patients and doctors.

CONCLUSION

During the 1950s, some universities and hospitals began to store their surgical and pathological specimens in their facilities [113]. Because clinical scientists discovered many benefits for their storages of clinical specimens, biobanks are quickly developed in more and more hospitals, universities, and blood centers since the 1980s [114]. According to reports from different journals and organizations, there are 636 biobanks constructed in the USA in 2013 [115] and more than 300 biobanks in Europe before 2011 [116]. As described above, we began to consider storing tumor tissues since we set up TIL treatment and tumor-cells' CSA during the 1980s-1990s [5]. Along with developments of new techniques and matures of storage methods, such as re-thaw tumor cells to test drug sensitivity by CSA and TILs freshly frozen with their re-cultures to treat patients from fresh-frozen tumor tissues so that we start to design and re-utilizing tumor tissue projects [94]. Since 1995 we start formal storage protocols for patients' bone marrow and solid tumors guided by Dr. Preisler [117]. We also reported how to study tumor tissue "recycle work" as our publication in 1999 [94]. During half a century, research and development of specimens' biorepositories depend on the development of new techniques, such as new equipment of frozen techniques, new techniques of primary cell cultures and surging new techniques of molecular biology, genomics emerging (especially NGS) as well as TME. Now IT management and online service (such as artificial intelligence), and ethical issues with legal prevention, are also involved in a biorepository.

The development of biobanking techniques is so rapid that many medical centers have their own biobanks, let medical doctors select these emerging techniques to treat their tumor diseases at the hospital. However, we still face two questions in biobank system with those emerging techniques:

Establishing educational and training subjects of "**Biospecimen Science**" at degrees of Master or Ph.D./MD. Our generation of biobank scientists come from pathologists and clinical MD with the background of surgeons or pediatricians, obstetricians-gynecologists. Because every biobank scientist has its medical background of different experiences so that most of the biobanks are variable to storing performance and application. The experiences challenge their SOPs with their clinical researches and application. If we have standard education for biobank so that we can make avoid these kinds of problems. Now, genomics subjects emerge in the educational system of the university, such as genetic counselor (MS), bioinformatics (MS/Ph.D.) and genomics (MS/MA/Ph.D.). If a biospecimen science (MS/Ph.D./MD) is established, biospecimen can be unanimously used to avoid of the specimens' variables. Once biospecimens are considered as "Science" in the classroom, a new generation of medical scientists can study biobank categories such as biobank physiology, specimen collection, and influence factors to address the questions and resolve the challenges.

Establishing "**International Networks**". (I) Because biobanks involve several thousands of diseases to comparison such as positive controls and negative controls, (II) because different countries have different levels of biorepositories, if we set up an international network of biobank, the cooperation can increase the impact of the new generation of personalized therapy by international support. Unfortunately, although it is essential for patients to keep their specimens, biobanks from different countries face legal issues as previous-mentioned, for instance, "International Networks" should agree on legal systems of different countries. To resolve the questions, some clinical scientists begin to consider some new ways to help patients, doctors, and hospitals in "developing countries", such as the "World Health Organization" or "Ambassador of Society".

In short, personalized immunotherapy begins to deposit patients' tumor tissues or blood with their T-cells and tumor cells. Once the biorepositories set up, patients suffering from tumor diseases can readily use their biorepositories to treat their tumor diseases at the hospital and undergoing personalized immunotherapy. Moreover, the specimens and data will be linked to patients to provide continuous treatments once the patients have their tumor recurrences. Extensively and eventually, along with emerging techniques or new generation of drugs, their specimens can further support the possibility of applying for some new treatments and new compounds.

CONSENT FOR PUBLICATION

Not applicable.

CONFLICT OF INTEREST

The authors declare no financial interests.

ACKNOWLEDGEMENTS

Under the support of Dr. H. D. Preisler, we have set up different methods and models to set up a biobank and analyze genomic profiles such as CD3, CD4, and CD8 from immune and tumor diseases related personalized therapy. This clinical application was previously supported by National Cancer Institute IRG-91-0-2-09, USA (to BL).

The mention of trade names or commercial products in this article is solely to provide specific information and does not imply recommendation.

REFERENCES

[1]   Hamilton TC, Ozols RF, Longo DL. Biologic therapy for the treatment of malignant common epithelial tumors of the ovary. Cancer 1987; 60(8) (Suppl.): 2054-63.
[http://dx.doi.org/10.1002/1097-0142(19901015)60:8+<2054::AID-CNCR2820601518>3.0.CO;2-0]
[PMID: 2443236]

[2]   Khavari P. Cytotoxic cellular mediators of the immune response to neoplasia: a review. Yale J Biol Med 1987; 60(5): 409-19.
[PMID: 3321723]

[3]   Rosenberg SA, Spiess P, Lafreniere R. A new approach to the adoptive immunotherapy of cancer with tumor-infiltrating lymphocytes. Science 1986; 233(4770): 1318-21.
[http://dx.doi.org/10.1126/science.3489291] [PMID: 3489291]

[4]   Muul LM, Spiess PJ, Director EP, Rosenberg SA. Identification of specific cytolytic immune responses against autologous tumor in humans bearing malignant melanoma. J Immunol 1987; 138(3): 989-95.
[PMID: 3100623]

[5]   Li BR, Tong SQ, Zhang XH, Lu J, Gu QL, Lu DY. A new experimental and clinical approach of combining usage of highly active tumor-infiltrating lymphocytes and highly sensitive antitumor drugs for the advanced malignant tumor. Chin Med J (Engl) 1994; 107(11): 803-7.
[PMID: 7867384]

[6]   Li BR, Tong SQ, Hu BY, *et al.* [Study on the influence of enzymatic digestion upon tumor-infiltrating lymphocytes]. Shi Yan Sheng Wu Xue Bao 1994; 27(1): 103-7.
[PMID: 8042406]

[7]   Johnston MP, Khakoo SI. Immunotherapy for hepatocellular carcinoma: Current and future. World J Gastroenterol 2019; 25(24): 2977-89.
[http://dx.doi.org/10.3748/wjg.v25.i24.2977] [PMID: 31293335]

[8]   Marin-Acevedo JA, Chirila RM, Dronca RS. Immune Checkpoint Inhibitor Toxicities. Mayo Clin Proc 2019; 94(7): 1321-9.
[http://dx.doi.org/10.1016/j.mayocp.2019.03.012] [PMID: 31272574]

[9]   Saadeh C, Bright D, Rustem D. Precision Medicine in Oncology Pharmacy Practice. Acta Med Acad 2019; 48(1): 90-104.
[PMID: 31264437]

[10]   Kawazoe A, Shitara K. Next-generation sequencing and biomarkers for gastric cancer: what is the future? Ther Adv Med Oncol 2019; 111758835919848189
[http://dx.doi.org/10.1177/1758835919848189] [PMID: 31258627]

[11]   Swan D, Lynch K, Gurney M, O'Dwyer M. Current and emerging immunotherapeutic approaches to the treatment of multiple myeloma. Ther Adv Hematol 2019; 102040620719854171
[http://dx.doi.org/10.1177/2040620719854171] [PMID: 31244984]

[12]   Subklewe M, von Bergwelt-Baildon M, Humpe A. Chimeric Antigen Receptor T Cells: A Race to Revolutionize Cancer Therapy. Transfus Med Hemother 2019; 46(1): 15-24.
[http://dx.doi.org/10.1159/000496870] [PMID: 31244578]

[13]   Steffin DHM, Hsieh EM, Rouce RH. Gene Therapy: Current Applications and Future Possibilities. Adv Pediatr 2019; 66: 37-54.
[http://dx.doi.org/10.1016/j.yapd.2019.04.001] [PMID: 31230699]

[14]   Wang SS, Bandopadhayay P, Jenkins MR. Towards Immunotherapy for Pediatric Brain Tumors.

Trends Immunol 2019; 40(8): 748-61.
[http://dx.doi.org/10.1016/j.it.2019.05.009] [PMID: 31229353]

[15]   Lee YG, Chu H, Lu Y, *et al.* Regulation of CAR T cell-mediated cytokine release syndrome-like toxicity using low molecular weight adapters. Nat Commun 2019; 10(1): 2681.
[http://dx.doi.org/10.1038/s41467-019-10565-7] [PMID: 31213606]

[16]   Harrer DC, Schuler G, Dörrie J, Schaft N. CSPG4-Specific CAR T Cells for High-Risk Childhood B Cell Precursor Leukemia. Int J Mol Sci 2019; 20(11)E2764
[http://dx.doi.org/10.3390/ijms20112764] [PMID: 31195686]

[17]   Mardiana S, Solomon BJ, Darcy PK, Beavis PA. Supercharging adoptive T cell therapy to overcome solid tumor-induced immunosuppression. Sci Transl Med 2019; 11(495): 2293.
[http://dx.doi.org/10.1126/scitranslmed.aaw2293] [PMID: 31167925]

[18]   Balza E, Mortara L, Sassi F, *et al.* Targeted delivery of tumor necrosis factor-alpha to tumor vessels induces a therapeutic T cell-mediated immune response that protects the host against syngeneic tumors of different histologic origin. Clin Cancer Res 2006; 12(8): 2575-82.
[http://dx.doi.org/10.1158/1078-0432.CCR-05-2448] [PMID: 16638868]

[19]   Namba K, Kitaichi N, Nishida T, Taylor AW. Induction of regulatory T cells by the immunomodulating cytokines alpha-melanocyte-stimulating hormone and transforming growth factor-beta2. J Leukoc Biol 2002; 72(5): 946-52.
[PMID: 12429716]

[20]   Lussow AR, Fanget L, Gao L, Buelow R, Pouletty P. Targeting of activated T-cells with natural cytotoxic antibodies *via* an IL2-hapten conjugate prolongs graft survival. Transplant Proc 1996; 28(2): 571-2.
[PMID: 8623277]

[21]   Uttenthal BJ, Chua I, Morris EC, Stauss HJ. Challenges in T cell receptor gene therapy. J Gene Med 2012; 14(6): 386-99.
[http://dx.doi.org/10.1002/jgm.2637] [PMID: 22610778]

[22]   Baitsch L, Fuertes-Marraco SA, Legat A, Meyer C, Speiser DE. The three main stumbling blocks for anticancer T cells. Trends Immunol 2012; 33(7): 364-72.
[http://dx.doi.org/10.1016/j.it.2012.02.006] [PMID: 22445288]

[23]   Kotch C, Barrett D, Teachey DT. Tocilizumab for the treatment of chimeric antigen receptor T cell-induced cytokine release syndrome. Expert Rev Clin Immunol 2019; 15(8): 813-22.
[http://dx.doi.org/10.1080/1744666X.2019.1629904] [PMID: 31219357]

[24]   Osipov A, Murphy A, Zheng L. From immune checkpoints to vaccines: The past, present and future of cancer immunotherapy. Adv Cancer Res 2019; 143: 63-144.
[http://dx.doi.org/10.1016/bs.acr.2019.03.002] [PMID: 31202363]

[25]   Sella G, Barton NH. Thinking About the Evolution of Complex Traits in the Era of Genome-Wide Association Studies Annu Rev Genomics Hum Genet 2019.
[http://dx.doi.org/10.1146/annurev-genom-083115-022316]

[26]   Shay T, Kang J. Immunological Genome Project and systems immunology. Trends Immunol 2013; 34(12): 602-9. [27].
[http://dx.doi.org/10.1016/j.it.2013.03.004] [PMID: 23631936]

[27]   Haen SP, Rammensee HG. The repertoire of human tumor-associated epitopes--identification and selection of antigens and their application in clinical trials. Curr Opin Immunol 2013; 25(2): 277-83.
[http://dx.doi.org/10.1016/j.coi.2013.03.007] [PMID: 23619309]

[28]   Sadatomi D, Tanimura S, Ozaki K, Takeda K. Atypical protein phosphatases: emerging players in cellular signaling. Int J Mol Sci 2013; 14(3): 4596-612.
[http://dx.doi.org/10.3390/ijms14034596] [PMID: 23443160]

[29]   Li B, Perabekam S, Liu G, Yin M, Song S, Larson A. Experimental and bioinformatics comparison of

gene expression between T cells from TIL of liver cancer and T cells from UniGene. J Gastroenterol 2002; 37(4): 275-82.
[http://dx.doi.org/10.1007/s005350200035] [PMID: 11993511]

[30] Zhang W, Ding J, Qu Y, *et al.* Genomic expression analysis by single-cell mRNA differential display of quiescent CD8 T cells from tumour-infiltrating lymphocytes obtained from *in vivo* liver tumours. Immunology 2009; 127(1): 83-90.
[http://dx.doi.org/10.1111/j.1365-2567.2008.02926.x] [PMID: 18778280]

[31] Xu Y, Hu H, Zheng J, Li B. Feasibility of whole RNA sequencing from single-cell mRNA amplification. Genet Res Int 2013; 2013724124
[http://dx.doi.org/10.1155/2013/724124] [PMID: 24455282]

[32] Rosenberg SA, Restifo NP. Adoptive cell transfer as personalized immunotherapy for human cancer. Science 2015; 348(6230): 62-8.
[http://dx.doi.org/10.1126/science.aaa4967] [PMID: 25838374]

[33] Torikai H, Cooper LJ. Translational Implications for Off-the-shelf Immune Cells Expressing Chimeric Antigen Receptors. Mol Ther 2016; 24(7): 1178-86.
[http://dx.doi.org/10.1038/mt.2016.106] [PMID: 27203439]

[34] Han H, Wang S, Hu Y, *et al.* Monoclonal antibody 3H11 chimeric antigen receptors enhance T cell effector function and exhibit efficacy against gastric cancer. Oncol Lett 2018; 15(5): 6887-94.
[http://dx.doi.org/10.3892/ol.2018.8255] [PMID: 29849787]

[35] Roselli M, Formica V, Cereda V, *et al.* The association of clinical outcome and peripheral T-cell subsets in metastatic colorectal cancer patients receiving first-line FOLFIRI plus bevacizumab therapy. OncoImmunology 2016; 5(7)e1188243
[http://dx.doi.org/10.1080/2162402X.2016.1188243] [PMID: 27622042]

[36] Gu QL, Lin YQ, Yin HR, Li B. Preliminary study on cryopreservation of tumor infiltrating lymphocytes Journal of Immunology 1995; 04.

[37] Fransson MN, Rial-Sebbag E, Brochhausen M, Litton JE. Toward a common language for biobanking. Eur J Hum Genet 2015; 23(1): 22-8.
[http://dx.doi.org/10.1038/ejhg.2014.45] [PMID: 24713663]

[38] Bønnelykke K, Sleiman P, Nielsen K, *et al.* A genome-wide association study identifies CDHR3 as a susceptibility locus for early childhood asthma with severe exacerbations. Nat Genet 2014; 46(1): 51-5.
[http://dx.doi.org/10.1038/ng.2830] [PMID: 24241537]

[39] Jafferji MS, Yang JC. Adoptive T-Cell Therapy for Solid Malignancies. Surg Oncol Clin N Am 2019; 28(3): 465-79.
[http://dx.doi.org/10.1016/j.soc.2019.02.012] [PMID: 31079800]

[40] Mardiana S, Lai J, House IG, Beavis PA, Darcy PK. Switching on the green light for chimeric antigen receptor T-cell therapy. Clin Transl Immunology 2019; 8(5)e1046
[http://dx.doi.org/10.1002/cti2.1046] [PMID: 31073403]

[41] Magalhaes I, Carvalho-Queiroz C, Hartana CA, *et al.* Facing the future: challenges and opportunities in adoptive T cell therapy in cancer. Expert Opin Biol Ther 2019; 19(8): 811-27.
[http://dx.doi.org/10.1080/14712598.2019.1608179] [PMID: 30986360]

[42] Minutolo NG, Hollander EE, Powell DJ Jr. The Emergence of Universal Immune Receptor T Cell Therapy for Cancer. Front Oncol 2019; 9: 176.
[http://dx.doi.org/10.3389/fonc.2019.00176] [PMID: 30984613]

[43] Leung W, Heslop HE. Adoptive Immunotherapy with Antigen-Specific T Cells Expressing a Native TCR. Cancer Immunol Res 2019; 7(4): 528-33.
[http://dx.doi.org/10.1158/2326-6066.CIR-18-0888] [PMID: 30936089]

[44] Rush A, Matzke L, Cooper S, Gedye C, Byrne JA, Watson PH. Research Perspective on Utilizing and

Valuing Tumor Biobanks. Biopreserv Biobank 2019; 17(3): 219-29.
[http://dx.doi.org/10.1089/bio.2018.0099] [PMID: 30575428]

[45]   Doll S, Gnad F, Mann M. The Case for Proteomics and Phospho-Proteomics in Personalized Cancer Medicine. Proteomics Clin Appl 2019; 13(2)e1800113
[http://dx.doi.org/10.1002/prca.201800113] [PMID: 30790462]

[46]   Qian L, Zhang Y, Pan XY, Ji MC, Gong WJ, Tian F. IL-15, in synergy with RAE-1ε, stimulates TCR-independent proliferation and activation of CD8(+) T cells. Oncol Lett 2012; 3(2): 472-6.
[http://dx.doi.org/10.3892/ol.2011.495] [PMID: 22740934]

[47]   Kumi-Diaka J, Hassanhi M, Brown J, Merchant K, Garcia C, Jimenez W. CytoregR inhibits growth and proliferation of human adenocarcinoma cells *via* induction of apoptosis. J Carcinog 2006; 5: 1.
[http://dx.doi.org/10.1186/1477-3163-5-1] [PMID: 16401338]

[48]   Li B, Tong SQ, Zhang XH, Zhu YM, Gu QL. Research on TIL proliferation, phenotype and lethality of human malignant solid tumors. Modern Immunology 1994; p. 05.

[49]   Hirschhaeuser F, Walenta S, Mueller-Klieser W. Efficacy of catumaxomab in tumor spheroid killing is mediated by its trifunctional mode of action. Cancer Immunol Immunother 2010; 59(11): 1675-84.
[http://dx.doi.org/10.1007/s00262-010-0894-1] [PMID: 20652245]

[50]   Sylvan SE, Skribek H, Norin S, Muhari O, Österborg A, Szekely L. Sensitivity of chronic lymphocytic leukemia cells to small targeted therapeutic molecules: An *in vitro* comparative study. Exp Hematol 2016; 44(1): 38-49.e1.
[http://dx.doi.org/10.1016/j.exphem.2015.08.009] [PMID: 26325331]

[51]   Tandon I, Pal R, Pal JK, Sharma NK. Extrachromosomal circular DNAs: an extra piece of evidence to depict tumor heterogeneity. Future Sci OA 2019; 5(6)FSO390
[http://dx.doi.org/10.2144/fsoa-2019-0024] [PMID: 31285839]

[52]   52Toor SM, Sasidharan Nair V, Decock J, Elkord E. Immune checkpoints in the tumor microenvironment Semin Cancer Biol 2019; 1044-579X(19): 3-30123.

[53]   53Komi DEA, Redegeld FA. Role of Mast Cells in Shaping the Tumor Microenvironment Clin Rev Allergy Immunol 2019. 10.1007

[54]   Vigano S, Alatzoglou D, Irving M, *et al.* Targeting Adenosine in Cancer Immunotherapy to Enhance T-Cell Function. Front Immunol 2019; 10: 925.
[http://dx.doi.org/10.3389/fimmu.2019.00925] [PMID: 31244820]

[55]   Tao M, Li B, Nayini J, *et al.* *In vivo* effects of IL-4, IL-10, and amifostine on cytokine production in patients with acute myelogenous leukemia. Leuk Lymphoma 2001; 41(1-2): 161-8.
[http://dx.doi.org/10.3109/10428190109057966] [PMID: 11342369]

[56]   Sanderson E, Davey Smith G, Bowden J, Munafò MR. Mendelian randomisation analysis of the effect of educational attainment and cognitive ability on smoking behaviour. Nat Commun 2019; 10(1): 2949.
[http://dx.doi.org/10.1038/s41467-019-10679-y] [PMID: 31270314]

[57]   Li B, Senzer N, Rao DD, *et al.* Bioinformatics Approach to Individual Cancer Target Identification 11th Annual Meeting of the American Society of Gene Therapy.

[58]   Chou WC, Chen WT, Hsiung CN, *et al.* B-Myb Induces APOBEC3B Expression Leading to Somatic Mutation in Multiple Cancers. Sci Rep 2017; 7: 44089.
[http://dx.doi.org/10.1038/srep44089] [PMID: 28276478]

[59]   Oehl K, Kresoja-Rakic J, Opitz I, *et al.* Live-Cell Mesothelioma Biobank to Explore Mechanisms of Tumor Progression. Front Oncol 2018; 8: 40.
[http://dx.doi.org/10.3389/fonc.2018.00040] [PMID: 29527515]

[60]   Wang Z, Teng D, Li Y, Hu Z, Liu L, Zheng H. A six-gene-based prognostic signature for hepatocellular carcinoma overall survival prediction. Life Sci 2018; 203: 83-91.

[http://dx.doi.org/10.1016/j.lfs.2018.04.025] [PMID: 29678742]

[61]   K Andersson, F Bray, M Arbyn, *et al.* In etiological and clinical research–current and future The interface ofpopulation-based cancer registries and biobanks perspectives. Acta Oncol 49(8): 1227-34.

[62]   Maharaj D, Vianna P, DeCarvalho G, Pourkalbassi D, Hickey C, Gouvea J. Molecular remission using low-dose immunotherapy for relapsed refractory Philadelphia chromosome-positive precursor B-cell acute lymphoblastic leukemia post-allogeneic stem cell transplant. Future Sci OA 2019; 5(5)FSO380
[http://dx.doi.org/10.2144/fsoa-2019-0009] [PMID: 31245042]

[63]   Hsu FT, Chen TC, Chuang HY, Chang YF, Hwang JJ. Enhancement of adoptive T cell transfer with single low dose pretreatment of doxorubicin or paclitaxel in mice. Oncotarget 2015; 6(42): 44134-50.
[http://dx.doi.org/10.18632/oncotarget.6628] [PMID: 26683520]

[64]   Talkington A, Dantoin C, Durrett R. Ordinary Differential Equation Models for Adoptive Immunotherapy. Bull Math Biol 2018; 80(5): 1059-83.
[http://dx.doi.org/10.1007/s11538-017-0263-8] [PMID: 28382423]

[65]   Wilkins O, Keeler AM, Flotte TR. CAR T-Cell Therapy: Progress and Prospects. Hum Gene Ther Methods 2017; 28(2): 61-6.
[http://dx.doi.org/10.1089/hgtb.2016.153] [PMID: 28330372]

[66]   Pilunov AM, Kuchmiy AA, Sheetikov SA, *et al.* [Modification of Cytotoxic Lymphocytes with T Cell Receptor Specific for Minor Histocompatibility Antigen ACC-1Y]. Mol Biol (Mosk) 2019; 53(3): 456-66.
[PMID: 31184611]

[67]   Largeot A, Pagano G, Gonder S, Moussay E, Paggetti J. The B-side of Cancer Immunity: The Underrated Tune. Cells 2019; 8(5)E449
[http://dx.doi.org/10.3390/cells8050449] [PMID: 31086070]

[68]   Seledtsov VI, Goncharov AG, Seledtsova GV. Clinically feasible approaches to potentiating cancer cell-based immunotherapies. Hum Vaccin Immunother 2015; 11(4): 851-69.
[http://dx.doi.org/10.1080/21645515.2015.1009814] [PMID: 25933181]

[69]   Chen HW, Huang HI, Lee YP, *et al.* Linkage of CD40L to a self-tumor antigen enhances the antitumor immune responses of dendritic cell-based treatment. Cancer Immunol Immunother 2002; 51(6): 341-8.
[http://dx.doi.org/10.1007/s00262-002-0283-5] [PMID: 12111122]

[70]   Wennhold K, Shimabukuro-Vornhagen A, von Bergwelt-Baildon M. B Cell-Based Cancer Immunotherapy. Transfus Med Hemother 2019; 46(1): 36-46.
[http://dx.doi.org/10.1159/000496166] [PMID: 31244580]

[71]   Bekaii-Saab T, Wesolowski R, Ahn DH, *et al.* Phase I Immunotherapy Trial with Two Chimeric HER-2 B-Cell Peptide Vaccines Emulsified in Montanide ISA 720VG and Nor-MDP Adjuvant in Patients with Advanced Solid Tumors. Clin Cancer Res 2019; 25(12): 3495-507.
[http://dx.doi.org/10.1158/1078-0432.CCR-18-3997] [PMID: 30804020]

[72]   Grille S, Brugnini A, Nese M, *et al.* A B-cell lymphoma vaccine using a depot formulation of interleukin-2 induces potent antitumor immunity despite increased numbers of intratumoral regulatory T cells. Cancer Immunol Immunother 2010; 59(4): 519-27.
[http://dx.doi.org/10.1007/s00262-009-0768-6] [PMID: 19768458]

[73]   BenMohamed L, Gras-Masse H, Tartar A, *et al.* Lipopeptide immunization without adjuvant induces potent and long-lasting B, T helper, and cytotoxic T lymphocyte responses against a malaria liver stage antigen in mice and chimpanzees. Eur J Immunol 1997; 27(5): 1242-53.
[http://dx.doi.org/10.1002/eji.1830270528] [PMID: 9174617]

[74]   Lakhtin VM, Lakhtin MV, Mironov AY, Aleshkin VA, Afanasiev SS. [Lectin populations of NK cells against tumors coupled to viral infections (review of literature)]. Klin Lab Diagn 2019; 64(5): 314-20.
[http://dx.doi.org/10.18821/0869-2084-2019-64-5-314-320] [PMID: 31185156]

[75]   Bae EA, Seo H, Kim IK, Jeon I, Kang CY. Roles of NKT cells in cancer immunotherapy. Arch Pharm

Res 2019; 42(7): 543-8.
[http://dx.doi.org/10.1007/s12272-019-01139-8] [PMID: 30859410]

[76]   Prins RM, Incardona F, Lau R, *et al.* Characterization of defective CD4-CD8- T cells in murine tumors generated independent of antigen specificity. J Immunol 2004; 172(3): 1602-11.
[http://dx.doi.org/10.4049/jimmunol.172.3.1602] [PMID: 14734741]

[77]   Altomare E, Fallarini S, Biaggi G, Gattoni E, Botta M, Lombardi G. Increased frequency of circulating invariant natural killer T cells in malignant pleural mesothelioma patients. Cancer Biol Ther 2012; 13(9): 702-11.
[http://dx.doi.org/10.4161/cbt.20553] [PMID: 22684580]

[78]   Li B, Shen DH. Preliminary Study on the Resting Status of Tumor-infiltrating Lymphocytes. Chinese Microbiology and Immunology 1994; 14(6): 399-402.

[79]   Li B, Tong SQ, Hu BY, Zhu YM. Research on TIL proliferation, phenotype and lethality of human malignant solid tumors. Modern Immunology 1994; p. 05.

[80]   Affara NI, Ruffell B, Medler TR, *et al.* B cells regulate macrophage phenotype and response to chemotherapy in squamous carcinomas. Cancer Cell 2014; 25(6): 809-21.
[http://dx.doi.org/10.1016/j.ccr.2014.04.026] [PMID: 24909985]

[81]   Topalian SL, Muul LM, Solomon D, Rosenberg SA. Expansion of human tumor infiltrating lymphocytes for use in immunotherapy trials. J Immunol Methods 1987; 102(1): 127-41.
[http://dx.doi.org/10.1016/S0022-1759(87)80018-2] [PMID: 3305708]

[82]   Keane C, Tobin J, Gunawardana J, *et al.* The tumour microenvironment is immuno-tolerogenic and a principal determinant of patient outcome in EBV-positive diffuse large B-cell lymphoma. Eur J Haematol 2019; 103(3): 200-7.
[http://dx.doi.org/10.1111/ejh.13274] [PMID: 31211907]

[83]   Horiuchi H, Tamai N, Kamba S, Inomata H, Ohya TR, Sumiyama K. Real-time computer-aided diagnosis of diminutive rectosigmoid polyps using an auto-fluorescence imaging system and novel color intensity analysis software. Scand J Gastroenterol 2019; 54(6): 800-5.
[http://dx.doi.org/10.1080/00365521.2019.1627407] [PMID: 31195905]

[84]   Park D, Son K, Hwang Y, *et al.* High-Throughput Microfluidic 3D Cytotoxicity Assay for Cancer Immunotherapy (CACI-IMPACT Platform). Front Immunol 2019; 10: 1133.
[http://dx.doi.org/10.3389/fimmu.2019.01133] [PMID: 31191524]

[85]   Neal JT, Li X, Zhu J, *et al.* Organoid Modeling of the Tumor Immune Microenvironment. Cell 2018; 175(7): 1972-1988.e16.
[http://dx.doi.org/10.1016/j.cell.2018.11.021] [PMID: 30550791]

[86]   Hundal J, Kiwala S, Feng YY, *et al.* Accounting for proximal variants improves neoantigen prediction. Nat Genet 2019; 51(1): 175-9.
[http://dx.doi.org/10.1038/s41588-018-0283-9] [PMID: 30510237]

[87]   Ben Hassine I, Gharbi H, Soltani I, *et al.* hOCT1 gene expression predict for optimal response to Imatinib in Tunisian patients with chronic myeloid leukemia. Cancer Chemother Pharmacol 2017; 79(4): 737-45.
[http://dx.doi.org/10.1007/s00280-017-3266-0] [PMID: 28286932]

[88]   Wennhold K, Thelen M, Schlößer HA, *et al.* Using Antigen-Specific B Cells to Combine Antibody and T Cell-Based Cancer Immunotherapy. Cancer Immunol Res 2017; 5(9): 730-43.
[http://dx.doi.org/10.1158/2326-6066.CIR-16-0236] [PMID: 28778961]

[89]   Seminerio I, Descamps G, Dupont S, *et al.* Infiltration of FoxP3+ Regulatory T Cells is a Strong and Independent Prognostic Factor in Head and Neck Squamous Cell Carcinoma. Cancers (Basel) 2019; 11(2)E227
[http://dx.doi.org/10.3390/cancers11020227] [PMID: 30781400]

[90]   Li B, Liu G, Hu HL, Ding JQ, Zheng J, Tong A. A clue of persoanlized immunotherapy. Biom J 2015;

1: 3.

[91] Topalian SL, Wolchok JD, Chan TA, *et al.* Immunotherapy: The path to win the war on cancer? Cell 2015; 161(2): 185-6.
[http://dx.doi.org/10.1016/j.cell.2015.03.045] [PMID: 26042237]

[92] Li B. A strategy to identify genomic expression profiles at single-T-cell level and a small number of cells (review paper). J Biotechnol 2005; 71-82.

[93] Li B, Chang T, Larson A, Ding J. Identification of mRNAs expressed in tumor-infiltrating lymphocytes by a strategy for rapid and high throughput screening. Gene 2000; 255(2): 273-9.
[http://dx.doi.org/10.1016/S0378-1119(00)00330-9] [PMID: 11024287]

[94] Li B, Ding JQ, Larson A, Song SW. Tumor Tissue Recycling-A new combination therapy for solid tumor: experimental and Preliminarily clinical research. Anticancer 1999; 13(5): 1-6. [*IN VIVO*].

[95] Cadigan RJ, Lassiter D, Haldeman K, Conlon I, Reavely E, Henderson GE. Neglected ethical issues in biobank management: Results from a U.S. study. Life Sci Soc Policy 2013; 9(1): 1.
[http://dx.doi.org/10.1186/2195-7819-9-1] [PMID: 25401081]

[96] Steinsbekk KS, Kåre Myskja B, Solberg B. Broad consent *versus* dynamic consent in biobank research: is passive participation an ethical problem? Eur J Hum Genet 2013; 21(9): 897-902.
[http://dx.doi.org/10.1038/ejhg.2012.282] [PMID: 23299918]

[97] Fleming J, Critchley C, Otlowski M, Stewart C, Kerridge I. Attitudes of the general public towards the disclosure of individual research results and incidental findings from biobank genomic research in Australia. Intern Med J 2015; 45(12): 1274-9.
[http://dx.doi.org/10.1111/imj.12911] [PMID: 26390363]

[98] Colledge F, Persson K, Elger B, Shaw D. Sample and data sharing barriers in biobanking: consent, committees, and compromises. Ann Diagn Pathol 2014; 18(2): 78-81.
[http://dx.doi.org/10.1016/j.anndiagpath.2013.12.002] [PMID: 24485935]

[99] Tebbakha R. Biobank–Short Message Service for Linking Patients and Samples 2013.
[http://dx.doi.org/10.1089/tmj.2012.0231]

[100] Sariyar M, Schluender I, Smee C, Suhr S. Sharing and Reuse of Sensitive Data and Samples: Supporting Researchers in Identifying Ethical and Legal Requirements. Biopreserv Biobank 2015; 13(4): 263-70.
[http://dx.doi.org/10.1089/bio.2015.0014] [PMID: 26186169]

[101] Virani AH, Longstaff H. Ethical Considerations in Biobanks: How a Public Health Ethics Perspective Sheds New Light on Old Controversies. J Genet Couns 2014.
[PMID: 25348083]

[102] Pereira S, Gibbs RA, McGuire AL. Open access data sharing in genomic research. Genes (Basel) 2014; 5(3): 739-47.
[http://dx.doi.org/10.3390/genes5030739] [PMID: 25178093]

[103] Melas PA, Sjöholm LK, Forsner T, *et al.* Examining the public refusal to consent to DNA biobanking: empirical data from a Swedish population-based study. J Med Ethics 2010; 36(2): 93-8.
[http://dx.doi.org/10.1136/jme.2009.032367] [PMID: 20133403]

[104] Ravid R. Standard Operating Procedures, ethical and legal regulations in BTB (Brain/Tissue/Bio) banking: what is still missing? Cell Tissue Bank 2008; 9(2): 121-37.
[http://dx.doi.org/10.1007/s10561-007-9055-y] [PMID: 17985213]

[105] Artene SA, Ciurea ME, Purcaru SO, *et al.* Biobanking in a constantly developing medical world. ScientificWorldJournal 2013; 2013343275
[http://dx.doi.org/10.1155/2013/343275] [PMID: 24174912]

[106] Mahomed S, Behrens K, Slabbert M, Sanne I. Managing Human Tissue Transfer Across National Boundaries - An Approach from an Institution in South Africa. Developing World Bioeth 2016; 16(1):

29-35.
[http://dx.doi.org/10.1111/dewb.12080] [PMID: 25688848]

[107] Bartels P, Kotze A. Wildlife biomaterial banking in Africa for now and the future. J Environ Monit 2006; 8(8): 779-81.
[http://dx.doi.org/10.1039/b602809h] [PMID: 16896459]

[108] Gordy D, Tashjian RS, Lee H, Movassaghi M, Yong WH. Domestic and International Shipping of Biospecimens. Methods Mol Biol 2019; 1897: 433-43.
[http://dx.doi.org/10.1007/978-1-4939-8935-5_35] [PMID: 30539463]

[109] Tomczak K, Czerwińska P, Wiznerowicz M. The Cancer Genome Atlas (TCGA): an immeasurable source of knowledge. Contemp Oncol (Pozn) 2015; 19(1A): A68-77.
[http://dx.doi.org/10.5114/wo.2014.47136] [PMID: 25691825]

[110] Linehan WM, Ricketts CJ. The Cancer Genome Atlas of renal cell carcinoma: findings and clinical implications. 2019.

[111] Briz O, Perez-Silva L, Al-Abdulla R, *et al.* What "The Cancer Genome Atlas" database tells us about the role of ATP-binding cassette (ABC) proteins in chemoresistance to anticancer drugs. Expert Opin Drug Metab Toxicol 2019; 15(7): 577-93.
[http://dx.doi.org/10.1080/17425255.2019.1631285] [PMID: 31185182]

[112] Paskal W, Paskal AM, Dębski T, Gryziak M, Jaworowski J. Aspects of Modern Biobank Activity - Comprehensive Review. Pathol Oncol Res 2018; 24(4): 771-85.
[http://dx.doi.org/10.1007/s12253-018-0418-4] [PMID: 29728978]

[113] Otali D, Al Diffalha S, Grizzle WE. Biological, Medical, and Other Tissue Variables Affecting Biospecimen Utilization. Biopreserv Biobank 2019; 17(3): 258-63.
[http://dx.doi.org/10.1089/bio.2018.0094] [PMID: 31188629]

[114] Hartman V, Matzke L, Watson PH. Biospecimen Complexity and the Evolution of Biobanks. Biopreserv Biobank 2019; 17(3): 264-70.
[http://dx.doi.org/10.1089/bio.2018.0120] [PMID: 31188632]

[115] Linsen L, T'Joen V, Van Der Straeten C, *et al.* Biobank Quality Management in the BBMRI.be Network. Front Med (Lausanne) 2019; 6: 141.
[http://dx.doi.org/10.3389/fmed.2019.00141] [PMID: 31294024]

[116] Henderson GE, Cadigan RJ, Edwards TP, *et al.* Characterizing biobank organizations in the U.S.: results from a national survey. Genome Med 2013; 5(1): 3.
[http://dx.doi.org/10.1186/gm407] [PMID: 23351549]

[117] Devemy E, Li B, Tao M, *et al.* Poor prognosis acute myelogenous leukemia: 3--biological and molecular biological changes during remission induction therapy. Leuk Res 2001; 25(9): 783-91.
[http://dx.doi.org/10.1016/S0145-2126(01)00032-7] [PMID: 11489472]

SUBJECT INDEX